The WOMAN'S Encyclopedia of NATURAL HEALING

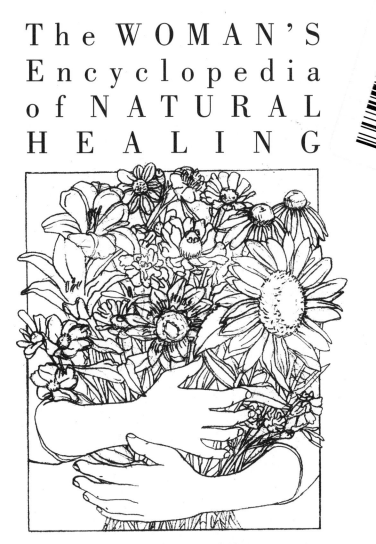

THE NEW HEALING TECHNIQUES
OF 100 LEADING
ALTERNATIVE PRACTITIONERS

DR. GARY NULL

INTRODUCTION BY VICKI HUFNAGEL, M.D.

SEVEN STORIES PRESS / New York, N.Y.

a c k n o w l e d g m e n t s

No book of this magnitude could be done without the collaborative efforts of outstanding transcribers, editors, and research assistants. I was fortunate to have all assisting on this project, namely, Loiz Zinn, Patrick Jennings, Vicki Riba Koestler, Vicki Hughes, Gabriole Van Bryce, Jeanne O'Neill, Miranda Ottewell, and Mikola De Roo. They all have my undying appreciation for their contributions.

This book is not intended to replace the services of a physician. Any application of the recommendations set forth in the following pages is at the reader's discretion. The reader should consult with his or her own physician concerning the recommendations made in this book.

Published by Seven Stories Press, New York, N.Y.

A Seven Stories Press First Edition

Library of Congress Cataloging-in-Publication Data

Null, Gary.
The women's encyclopedia of natural healing: the new healing techniques of 100 leading alternative practitioners / by Gary Null.
  p. cm.
  ISBN 1-888363-35-5
1. Women—Health and hygiene. 2. Women—Diseases—Homeopathic treatment. I. Title.
RX461.N85 1996
613'.042443—DC20   96-28291
                                                CIP

Book design by Cindy LaBreacht / Frontispiece by Tracy Kirshenbaum

Printed in the United States
10 9 8 7 6 5 4 3 2 1

contents

p r e f a c e

ALTHOUGH this is beginning to change, there has in the past been little research on women's health issues. And in many cases the research done on health issues affecting men and women equally has emphasized the men's side and understated differences pertaining to women. I've taken this unfair situation almost as an invitation, and it is one of the reasons I wanted to write an encyclopedic book that covered the major health areas affecting women, but from an alternative point of view. If doctors practicing Western medicine in the conventional way are going to ignore women's issues, let's see if the alternative medicine community can take up the slack. Let's see if we can help women keep themselves healthy by emphasizing good nutrition and all the individual alternative therapies that address the specific health concerns of women. There isn't another book out there that does this, so I wanted to fill the need and reach people.

I wanted my women's health book to be as up-to-date as possible, since so much is happening in this area in alternative health, so in the winter of 1995–96 I arranged interviews with over seventy-five alternative health practitioners whose work I respect, and who are treating patients successfully with tried and proven therapies your regular doctor may not even have heard about. At the same time I undertook a massive computer- and Internet-aided research project to exhaustively seek out every single article I could find, in both conventional and alternative medical journals, that pertained to alternative treatments of common health problems affecting women. Then I created summaries of every one of these articles in common language so that you don't have to have a medical degree to understand what the researchers have to tell you about alternative approaches to health problems you may be experiencing.

The combination of the hands-on clinical know-how of the alternative health practitioners whom I have interviewed for this book and the state-of-the-art scientific research that my associates and I collected and included at the back of each chapter give *The Woman's Encyclopedia of Natural Healing* its unique combination of essential information to help you find the most sensible solutions to your health concerns.

The natural healing tradition has always emphasized women's problems, since at many points in modern history, the natural healer was the only person women could go to have their problems taken seriously and taken care of. And natural healing techniques were often nearly exclusively a woman's domain. Just as doctors have traditionally been men, and midwifes and nurses traditionally women, women are still mostly excluded from the highest levels of the medical establishment—where the decisions are made as to which types of treatments to favor (typically those that rely on expensive drugs or even more expensive machines and procedures) and which to ignore (typically those involving substances that are not patent-protected, like vitamin C, or techniques that could be practiced by unlicensed, and hence uncontrollable, practitioners, including massage and herbal treatments).

We are at a moment in history when alternative approaches have, in theory, finally been accorded a newfound legitimacy in the eyes of the medical establishment. It is only right that now more and more people, and especially women, will turn to the long, strong, and wonderful natural healing tradition. International in scope, it spans many cultures and synthesizes ancient folkloric remedies together with cutting-edge technologies.

Some of you are longtime followers of natural healing ways; other readers are investigating alternative healing approaches here for the first time. To both groups, welcome.

introduction

Women as Healers

Early Stone Age man had one focus in life: survival. The complementary role of the healer fell to, and was embraced by, women. Women were naturally linked to healing in the first societies because of their ability to bleed monthly and give birth. These magical events, emanations from the female body, have naturally identified women as the primary source of healing power and knowledge among humankind.

Women once mixed earth with herbs, plants, minerals, and water to treat many illnesses and conditions. They were the first physicians and the first scientists. Out of the pain, trauma, and, often, death associated with childbirth, the mantle of healer fell to them out of necessity. Women, who saw death loom near so often during the birthing process, learned to work together to assist one another to prevent the tragedy of death from childbirth. Healing knowledge began to make a difference, increasing the odds of survival for all the human race.

Once a woman's maximum life span was twenty-five years. Family life was dedicated to lasting through to the next day. The concept of a future developed slowly. Fears — of famine, of natural disasters, of attack by predators, of accidents and mishaps — dominated our existence. Childbearing began at age fourteen and women bore sixteen children on average — of whom one might survive to adulthood, if the mother was strong, mindful, and fortunate.

Women need only look back on our past to be reminded of the harsh reality we have fought off one step at a time. The more informed and empowered we are, the more our bodies and our lives become our own. But today we are still working to have the right to control our reproductive rights and our sexual organs.

The Challenge

Gary Null has been a warrior working hard to educate the health care consumer. His gift is the ability to translate scientific data skillfully into language that everyone can understand. And he has examined important issues that others have either intentionally or unintentionally overlooked. Dr. Null is dedicated to empowering the consumer of health care. In this exciting book, he focuses on the needs of women.

Advances in medicine require enormous time and effort before they actually filter down to everyday clinical practice. My own work to bring to the public an awareness that hysterectomies are often performed unnecessarily began over sixteen years ago and has been a full-time effort for most of that time. Still, many men and women are unaware of the problem of unnecessary hysterectomies.

Traditional medicine rarely campaigns to change itself — however justified the change may be. In the case of hysterectomies, I have come to believe that public awareness of the facts of uterine function will not replace the standard myths in my lifetime. I am resigned to the opinion that it will take generations before it is accepted that the uterus has a function beyond holding a pregnancy.

The creation of *The Woman's Encyclopedia of Natural Healing* is an enormous step forward. In it Gary Null has given us an alternative woman's health care reference text, a text that by its very existence works to inform and change common practices.

The Alternative Path

Trained in traditional medicine, with gynecological surgery as my specialization, I have found change comes last to women's health care. In fact, the very existence of a specific field of expertise called "Women's Health Care" is still not accepted in traditional medicine.

While still in medical school I took a course given by Ida Rolf. She was teaching "rolfing," her personal form of deep tissue massage. I took this course for purely selfish reasons. I had undergone emergency gallbladder surgery and wanted to heal rapidly so I could get back to my classes. After the surgery I'd experienced pain and was unable to stand up straight. The effect of the rolfing class was dramatic. With each session I felt less pain. The experience of someone working on my body soothed me into a restful state. I was able to go back to my other classes in less than two weeks.

My surgeon was shocked at how fast I had healed. When I told him it was the rolfing, along with the vitamins I'd been taking, he laughed and insisted these things had nothing to do with my recovery. I did not tell him how the rolfing had also helped me deal with my anger. I had been misdiagnosed for two years by the Chairman of Internal Medicine at UCSF. My condition had been labeled psychosomatic and ignored until my gallbladder ruptured. The rolfing had helped me channel the rage I felt on account of my mistreatment into agressive positive motion. It was 1974 and this personal experience helped me choose to specialize in surgery instead of internal medicine.

The Healing Touch

In 1991 massage again became a central issue in my life. When I became pregnant I went to the head of Obstetrics at UCLA. Although this department at UCLA specialized in high-risk cases and I was by then well known both as an Ob/Gyn surgeon and an outspoken patient advocate, the doctor failed to diagnose my life-threatening condition. I had *placenta previa*, in which the placenta covers the birth canal. One morning I found myself hemorrhaging and nearly bled to death in a few minutes. To save my life, my obstetrician stated he had to sacrifice my pregnancy and he performed a crash Cesarean section. Had I been properly diagnosed none of this would have occurred. He took my fetal infant from my uterus at 26 weeks, 14 weeks premature.

I awoke in pain and was told I could not see my child because she was too ill and would not survive through the night, and that I was lucky this was the case since otherwise I would be taking home a vegetable instead of a healthy baby. The young resident who told this to me immediately after I had come out of surgery was breaking every rule of bedside manner and I told her so using every four-letter word I could think of. She stormed out and since no other support staff would venture anywhere near me, I pulled out my intravenous line and crawled on the floor until I found a wheelchair in the corridor. In severe pain, I wheeled myself to the neonatal intensive care unit to see my small fetal child, Demitra.

I won't detail the horror of that ward, the myriad tubes and intravenous lines, the constant transfusions, repeat chest x-rays, spinal taps and so forth, the infants in their plastic-sac containers, the terrified parents looking on, afraid even to touch their children for fear of harming them further. My own husband stood as if made of stone, staring at his child. I had to take his hand in mine for him to touch her.

The first thing I did was touch Demitra. The nurse raised her hand to stop me, and I glared at her. "She's not stable," she said. "I can see that," I answered. "Demitra may not survive the night," she added. I looked up as my hand reached for Demi: "Then it doesn't matter." My hand covered Demi's entire body. I talked to Demitra, telling her she was strong and would survive.

Every day thereafter I held, stroked, massaged, and spoke to Demitra. Back in the 1970s I would have been thrown out of the neonatal unit for touching my baby. I would have been told I was endangering my child's life. The scientific literature now supports the touching of premature infants as being beneficial. The infant apprehends through touch and sound that it is not simply a piece of cybermachinery attached to other machines through lines and tubes. A sense of belonging to life is transmitted through human contact. Demitra today is a strong, normal warrior-child with an IQ over 170, who dominates her kindergarten class, and is always protecting other children.

Data shows improved outcomes for premature infants born to touch and massage. Even so, traditional medicine has not fully embraced this work. The change in attitude in favor of touch therapies is still ongoing and change, as always, doesn't come easily. My work in Female Reconstructive Surgery resulted in the first surgical program using massage as part of the recovery protocol in the nation. That was in 1985. And today more than a decade later the change is still ongoing.

The Path Forward

Change in medicine takes far longer than in the pure sciences. Because medicine is tied to a huge economic structure, effecting change is a glacial process. Dr. Gary Null is part of the wave that is pushing medicine to deal with patients' needs. His work here in giving us *The Woman's Encyclopedia of Natural Healing* is fundamental. It will help provoke necessary changes in women's health care delivery.

Women want to have basic information about their bodies. Women know how important it can be to share our personal experiences. And many women have experienced misdiagnosis, victimization, and other traumas that are commonplace in traditional medical practice. And so we find ourselves seeking new options and alternative treatments.

Dr. Null has drawn on his expertise and skills in clinical research and applied them here in this encyclopedia to create a vast resource text that encompasses new concepts and therapies that have a clinical basis. The form of this book allows the reader to experience, through dialogue, the practitioners who are creating and providing these new innovative therapies.

Here the reader can hear the voice of the clinician to learn what motivated them in their work and what are the theoretical bases for the treatments. The text gives the reader easy access to the Who, Where, Why, and What of women's alternative medicine.

In my practice I see women every day who are on an odyssey seeking alternatives in care. Most of my patients have seen at least five physicians for second opinions before they find me. Before this text by Dr. Null there was no resource devoted to the work of the practitioners who are working to create alternatives for women. Women have spent countless hours searching the medical literature, attending lectures, and asking everywhere for help. Before now there has been no reference text to help them in their quest for answers and help.

The Woman's Encyclopedia of Natural Healing allows a woman rapid access to the clinical and scientific grounding that will enable her to formulate her own program of alternative care and treatment. It also looks at health in a comprehensive manner, including environmental impact, nutrition, nutritional supplements, and exercise. Each chapter concludes with a listing of supportive published medical literature and brief synopses of relevant articles. You can select the ones you feel are most informative, and get direct access to them through your computer on the world wide web and on Medline. Many people are unaware of the many medical libraries that exist. Medical libraries are located in teaching university medical centers, local hospitals, and at a variety of medical associations (i.e. your local county medical association). The librarians at these centers can teach you how to use the Index Medicus to look up topics and find the materials you need.

Enjoy this wonderful book as a tool for self empowerment. And from all of us practitioners, Gary, thanks for making our research a lot easier.

Vicki Hufnagel, M.D.
Medical Director, Center for Female Reconstructive Surgery
Founding Member, The Berkeley Women's Health Collective
Contributor, *Our Bodies, Ourselves* (First Edition)
Author of *No More Hysterectomies*
Los Angeles, October 1996

1. AGING

In our society, and in this century in particular, ageism has singled out women harshly. Sexual attractiveness is deemed to be the exclusive province of the young, but even more so for women than for men. Recent years have brought some new understanding of the causes of aging; in particular, several theories have led to new therapies offering women opportunities not only to improve their health but to slow down some of the aging processes. Some of the more prevalent current scientific hypotheses on why we age follow . . .

Causes

FREE RADICAL DAMAGE. It is well accepted that aging and degenerative diseases are the result of cellular damage brought on by free radicals, molecules that have become unstable after losing one of their orbiting electrons. These molecules' unpaired electrons make them highly reactive, and in an attempt to restore balance, a free radical will steal electrons from other molecules, causing damage and destruction.

Free radicals are produced through normal metabolism in the body, but increase with exposure to animal fat, alcohol, cigarettes, and other toxic chemicals. Dr. Christopher Calapai, a complementary medicine physician and M.D. practicing in New York City, gives an example of how this damage can occur: "Free radicals generated by cigarette smoke are huge in number. They steal healthy electrons from the lining of the lungs, thereby oxidizing lung tissue. When lung tissue is oxidized, cells break down and die. As hundreds of thousands of cells become oxidized and damaged, whole tissues and organs become affected throughout the body. Aging and disease are magnified."

LOW THYROID FUNCTION. Low thyroid functioning can prompt diseases associated with aging. According to distinguished scientific researcher Dr. Ray Peat, from Eugene, Oregon, in the early 1900s doctors were better informed about the importance of correcting this condition than they are today: "Most of the basic research on the thyroid was done before World War II. Pharmaceutical companies came in after the war with what they thought was the latest word in understanding the thyroid. It turns out they were wrong. Until 1940, it was accepted that 40 percent of Americans benefited from taking thyroid supplements. After faulty tests were established, it was believed that only 5 percent of Americans needed or benefited from thyroid supplements. In the 1930s indications of hypothyroidism included such things as too much cholesterol in the blood, insomnia, emphysema, arthritis, and failure of the immune system. Many conditions now considered mysterious diseases were recognized as traits of low thyroid. Very often these conditions would simply disappear when thyroid supplements were given.

"When the thyroid is low we have to rely on emergency systems—such as the production of adrenaline and cortisone—to adapt to stress. Cortisone and adrenaline are now recognized as factors that cause damage, setting degenerative diseases in motion and causing damage to the lining of blood vessels and brain cells, but very often people don't realize that it is thyroid that keeps us from relying excessively on these stress hormones."

BIOLOGICAL CLOCK. Dr. Lance Morris, a naturopathic physician from Tucson, Arizona, relates two other theories that attempt to explain the aging process. One of these holds that the body has a cellular biological clock that is set to self-destruct after a certain amount of time: "Interestingly, over the years, there has been a tendency to slowly increase the upside numbers. At this time, there is a feeling that the top limit is pushing 140 years. Individuals have actually lived to that age, and even longer."

SHRINKING THYMUS GLAND. Yet another theory, as Dr. Morris explains, relates aging to the thymus gland. "When we are born, this gland covers our entire chest. It's huge. As we grow up, it diminishes in size, a process known as thymic involution. One of the theories of aging is that if we could stop thymic shrinking we could stop the aging process altogether."

Symptoms

A wide variety of gradual bodily changes may be associated with aging. Often the aging process can lead to an increased susceptibility toward weight gain and fatigue. But this is not necessarily the case. There is no physiological reason why most people should grow obese or weary as they grow older: these are societal norms that have little to do with nature. It can be just as natural, for example, for people to eat and sleep a little less as they grow older to balance out any slowing down of metabolic processes, thus maintaining stable weight and energy levels.

Typical signs of aging also include changes in skin, hair, nails, and connective tissue. Decreases in memory, concentration, and sharpness may also accompany aging. Again, this need not necessarily be the case.

Often as women age, as is also true of men, they may suffer from elevated blood sugar, cholesterol, and triglycerides, and other chemical imbalances. Greater incidences of degenerative diseases such as cancer, heart disease, thyroid dysfunction, musculoskeletal problems, and gastrointestinal disorders also typically accompany the aging process in both women and men.

Clinical Experience

TESTS

Aging well means being healthy and balanced from within. To check that all systems are running optimally, Dr. Calapai recommends a full spectrum of tests, with special attention to the following areas: "The adrenal glands produce our anti-aging hormones. With age, some people start producing less. This can be from free radical damage, excessive stress, injuries, and all sorts of reasons. As a result we see changes in memory, concentration, skin, hair, hormonal fluctuations, and energy levels. We start to see problems with immune response and increases in blood sugar, cholesterol, and abdominal deposition of body fat. So we need to look at adrenal function.

"Certainly, tests should look at vitamin and mineral levels to check our digestive and absorptive abilities. Looking at the basic blood chemistry tells us how well we are absorbing protein. We need to look at the fat-soluble vitamins and cholesterol, triglyceride, and the ratio of good HDL cholesterol to bad LDL cholesterol, which can provide information about our fat absorption. I also recommend looking at enzymes of the pancreas to assess function, and a comprehensive stool analysis to see whether or not there are too many undigested particles in the stool. If parasites are present, this can decrease our absorptive ability. These are some of the main tests we need to perform to get a thorough picture of the individual."

YOUR DIET AND OTHER NUTRITION-BASED APPROACHES

An antiaging diet for women of all ages should consist of high-quality organic foods, emphasizing complex carbohydrates such as beans and whole grains, fruits, and vegetables. Girls and adolescents may need more of certain nutrients, as they are still growing. And individual women in specific age groups may have specific nutrient requirements that can be addressed through supplements. But a basic healthy diet will vastly improve the quality of life and reduce the aging process in women of all ages.

Antiaging diets contain few if any animal-based proteins, and fats are minimized. This high-fiber diet helps prevent common afflictions associated with aging, such as constipation, hemorrhoids, pressure in the intestines, ulcers, high blood pressure, colorectal cancer, and overall body toxemia. One of the principles of longevity is eating to the point of being not quite full. Especially as she gets older, a woman can eat small servings more frequently. Freezing unused portions can allow her to cook less often and still eat home cooking.

At least eight 8-ounce glasses of water should be drunk daily. Many senior citizens drink too little, and their brains dehydrate and shrink as a result. Water is necessary for the electrical charges in the body to do their work properly. Additionally, fresh juices, which are high in enzymes, should be a regular part of the diet: two to three 6-ounce glasses of fresh, organic mixed vegetable juice per day, with 1-2 mg of buffered Vitamin C added to each glass, or up to bowel tolerance.

FASTING AND OTHER DETOXIFICATION THERAPIES. The more toxic we are, the faster we age. Cosmetic changes such as face lifts or hair dye may temporarily make women appear younger, but they do not make a real difference. To keep youthful and healthy, women must address what is happening inside. "Everyone needs detoxification," says Susan Lombardi, founder and president of We Care Health Center in Palm Springs, California, and author of *Ten Easy Steps for Complete Wellness.* "I am vegetarian, and I take care of myself. Do I still need detoxification? Yes, because the air that we breathe is polluted, the water that we drink is full of chlorine, the clothing we wear is made of artificial fabrics and chemicals, the lotions and shampoos that we use all contain chemicals. Once these chemicals are inside us, we never fully eliminate them unless we go through a detoxification procedure." Lombardi recommends rejuvenating the system from the inside out by fasting on fresh raw vegetable juices once a week, along with these other simple yet effective detoxification therapies:

JUICE FASTING. Juice fasting gives the digestive system a rest and speeds up the growth of new cells, which promotes healing. (If you have any medical problems, do not fast without medical approval and supervision.)

On a juice fast, a person abstains from solid foods and drinks juice, water, and herbal teas throughout the day. "We should be drinking every half hour to an hour," advises Lombardi. "If we go for long periods of time without drinking anything, then a little glass of juice will not be able to sustain us. But if we are constantly drinking, the day will go by very smoothly."

Lombardi recommends a combination of the following:

Carrot juice. High in the antioxidant beta carotene, and full of wonderful enzymes.
Celery juice. High in sodium—not the artificial type poured from the salt shaker, which is bad for you, but the good, natural kind that promotes tissue flexibility.
Beet juice. Beets nourish the liver, one of the most important organs of the body, with hundreds of different functions. If your liver is functioning well, most likely everything else in your body will be too.
Cabbage juice. High in vitamin C.

Mix the juice from each vegetable in equal proportion, and drink this combination throughout the day. A little cayenne, which increases circulation, sending blood to every corner of the body to promote healing, can be added for flavor. Lemon juice in water and different herbal teas—some good ones are parsley and dandelion tea for the liver and kidneys, and pau d'arco for blood purification—can be added for variety. "Any herbal tea free of caffeine will be good," Lombardi says. "Since you need to drink on an hourly basis, you don't want to drink the same thing over and over."

DETOX DRINK. An excellent formula for colon cleansing is a drink made from ground flax seeds, psyllium seeds, and bentonite, which is a liquid clay. "Clay absorbs toxins," says Lombardi. "The seeds expand in the water and become like a brush. They brush the interior tubing, our pipe system. When the pipe system is completely clean, foods are absorbed through our digestive system."

ANTIOXIDANTS. Dr. Morris calls aging a catch-22. "Oxygen is the great substance that sustains and gives life, but unfortunately it is also the substance that destroys us through oxidation." For this reason, antioxidants are essential. Here are the most important:

Vitamin E. 400–800 IU per day, taken at the largest meal. Best in its natural form (as a mixed tocopherol or d-alpha tocopherol). Avoid synthetic vitamin E (dl-alpha).

Beta carotene. 25,000 IU per meal. Helps slow down aging and lessens cancer risk. Nontoxic, since the body must convert beta carotenes into vitamin A and will not convert more than it can use.

Vitamin A. 1,000–3,000 IU per meal. Blood tests will determine whether or not a person is getting too much vitamin A, which can be toxic.

Selenium. 100 mcg per meal. One of the causes of premature aging and even death, particularly in professional athletes, is cardiomyopathy, an enlargement of the heart. This is usually associated with selenium deficiency. Adequate amounts of this critical nutrient are needed to help the body produce the antioxidant enzyme glutathione peroxidase, which is on the front line of aging defense.

Zinc. 30–90 mg daily. Zinc feeds over 100 enzyme systems in the brain, as well as various systems throughout the body. It is essential in the formation of stomach acid; without sufficient zinc, malabsorption syndrome occurs. Most older people are zinc deficient.

Vitamin C. 3,000–5,000 mg daily. In disease-fighting and antiaging protocols, higher doses are given.

Bioflavonoids. A minimum of 50 mg, three times daily, of grapeseed extract, a bioflavonoid that has the highest known antioxidant properties of any nutrient.

Superoxide dismutase. This important antienzyme nutrient is produced by the body. Not effective when taken orally, unless enteric-coated.

MORE SUPER SUPPLEMENTS

Sea algae. High in trace elements, antioxidant cofactors, flavonoids, and carotenoid.

Coenzyme Q10. Every cell in the body needs this coenzyme to create energy and build stamina.

NADH. Also known as coenzyme 1, NADH is a naturally occurring substance in the body that supplies energy to the cells, allowing them to live longer.

Thymus extract. Pure oral thymus extract enhances immune function and helps reverse the aging process.

Tyrosine. Strengthens the thyroid and adrenal glands, protecting against stress.

ENZYME THERAPY. Nina Anderson, author of *Over Fifty, Looking Thirty: The Secrets of Staying Young,* attributes slow aging to sufficient enzyme levels: "Many scientists say that people get old before their time due to enzyme exhaustion. Some people are old at forty because of the lack of enzymes, while others are young at eighty because of an abundance. Above all else, I would advise anybody who is trying to avoid looking and feeling older as they get older to take supplemental enzymes."

She goes on to explain what enzymes do that are so important: "Enzymes are molecule catalysts found everywhere in your body. In fact, there are over 1,300 different ones. They make everything happen. In my book I use this analogy: minerals are building blocks of your body. They are the nose, eyes, ears, bones, all the things that hold you together. Something has to build this. Enzymes are the construction workers that facilitate everything in the body going together."

Anderson recommends eating more raw foods, mineral supplements, and digestive plant enzymes to increase enzyme levels: "The mineral supplements to take should be crystalloid form with electrolytes. The crystalloid form goes right into the cell walls. This fortifies your body.

"Plant enzymes assist in the digestion of food right on through the intestinal tract. You want to help the digestive process for the whole length of the digestive tract. With supplemental enzymes, you won't have an upset stomach anymore or feel bloated and exhausted after a big meal. The skin will start to improve too. The skin manifests everything that happens inside. If your inner organs start to degenerate, if they are not functioning properly, this kind of stress shows up on your face. The first thing people do when they start getting older is look in the mirror and go, 'Oh my God, I've got wrinkles.' They spend millions trying to get rid of them. But what they have to realize is that wrinkles start from inside. You have to work on the inside to get the outside to reflect that good health.

"Without the proper enzymes, none of the other good things you do matters. For example, fat-soluble vitamins A, D, E, and K require fat for absorption. That fat has to be broken down by an enzyme, lipase. If lipase is not present in sufficient quantities, that fat will not be broken down. If the fat isn't broken down, the vitamins will not be released. Therefore, you can spend a fortune on vitamin pills, and if you don't have the proper enzymes to release those vitamins into your system, they are just going to be flushed out."

Enzymes can be used externally as well as internally for youthful effects: "There are amazing enzyme treatments for the skin. Papaya enzymes are wonderful. Or you can mix a plant enzyme powder and put it on as a mask. Not only does it take the lines out of your face, but it fills them in and builds up collagen. It can also get rid of age spots and shrink moles. When you use enzymes as a mud pack when you come in from the sun, it fights free radicals that otherwise might foster melanoma."

HERBS. Herbs are an important part of any antiaging nutritional protocol, and can be taken as capsules, powders, teas or tinctures.

Fo-ti. Rejuvenates the endocrine system and is an excellent digestive tonic.

Ginkgo biloba. The ginkgo tree has survived for hundreds of thousands of years due to its powerful immune system. An extract of the leaf of the tree improves circulation to the microcapillaries of the brain and heart so that needed nutrients and oxygen can get to all the tissues.

Ginseng is the best-known longevity herb. For centuries, the Chinese have revered ginseng for its rejuvenating effects. Research has shown that ginseng can stop free radical damage associated with aging. It helps people focus better when under stress, and increases overall energy levels.

Gota kola. Elephants, who browse on gota kola, are known to have excellent memories and to be long-lived. Gota kola is useful for increasing vitality and endurance, and may lower blood pressure.

Hawthorn berries support circulation and cardiac function.

Milk thistle protects liver function. The liver releases toxins from the body, promoting health and youthfulness.

Wild yam supports adrenal gland production of DHEA, a building block for the development of estrogen, progesterone, testosterone, and cortisols that decrease with age. As an adaptogen, wild yam balances the body's hormonal functions. It has also been shown to ameliorate numerous chronic conditions, including heart disease, cancer, arthritis, and autoimmune diseases. DHEA is extremely safe, with no known side effects.

EXERCISE AND OTHER PHYSICAL TECHNIQUES

When we exercise, we detoxify as we sweat through our skin and exhale from our lungs. Some good exercises include jogging or daily brisk walks, yoga stretches, and jumping on a mini-trampoline, which exercises every cell of the body. Exercise slows down the aging process because it stimulates detoxification.

Chiropractor Dr. Mitch Proffman says that traditional cultures have appreciated the connection between physical fitness and longevity, making athletic activities a part of women's ritual ceremonies: "In traditional Navajo society women would run three times daily as a formal part of the four-day rites of passage after the onset of menstruation. The first run was at dawn, and each subsequent run would be for a longer distance. It was believed that the total distance a woman could run would determine her longevity."

He goes on to state that recent research supports the connection between exercise and a longer life: "The *Journal of the American Medical Association* has reported that exercise increases people's life spans. Women walking forty to fifty minutes, three to four times per week, live longer. The same article claims that exercise decreases the chance of dying from all known diseases. This can be attributed to the fact that most major diseases, such as cancer, diabetes, and heart disease, are stress-related, and exercise reduces stress.

"Another important function of exercising is that people's mental abilities improve. In a recent study at the University of Illinois, Dr. William Greenboro, Ph.D., studied four different groups of rats. One group led a sedentary life. Another group played aimlessly on wood and plastic in their cages. A third group was on a special motorized wheel, and a fourth group walked through intricate mazes and ropes. The finding was that all rats who exercised in any manner had more capillaries in their brains and better brain function. This suggests that exercise fuels the brain with more oxygen and increases natural growth factors, in humans as well as in rats."

Dr. Joseph Pizzorno, N.D., president of John Bastyr College of Naturopathic Medicine in Seattle, Washington, says that strengthening exercises are the best defense against the dangers women face of increased frailty as they age: "It turns out that the majority of the debility of old age is simply due to people not using their muscles. The full strength of what one had at twenty and thirty is almost completely returned with weight strengthening exercises. There are a lot of different weight training programs out there. I have been doing some research. The one I find most effective, and am now using personally, is something called Super Slow. Weights are used in a very, very controlled, very, very intense way to get maximum effects from the exercise. I am quite impressed with what I have seen."

Stress release. "In my personal opinion, the single most important factor influencing aging and disease is stress," says Dr. Morris. "We need to control emotional anxieties and tensions, and learn how to not let life get to us. It is important to learn to let go and enjoy life." Methods Dr. Morris suggests to overcome stress include deep breathing exercises, tai chi, yoga, meditation, *qi gong*, mantras, massage, Reiki, and biofeedback. "These are things that I recommend that all of us do in the pursuit of health, longevity and wellness."

Since exercise increases oxygenation, it also has the potential of fostering free radical damage. To prevent undesirable effects, women may want to combine exercise with sufficient amounts of antioxidants, in the diet and/or as dietary supplements. *(See "Antioxidants," above.)*

BREATHING EXERCISES. Breathing exercises combined with physical activity increase the action of lymphatic cleansing. Detoxification expert Susan Lombardi explains, "For lymphatic cleansing, you want to synchronize your breathing with the movement of your legs and arms. When you are walking or jumping on the trampoline, inhale four times, and exhale four times. Move your arms and legs each time you take a little breath. Inhale through your nose and exhale through your nose or mouth.

"This breathing technique was learned from the Taromaro Indians, who live in the northern part of Mexico. They are famous for their fantastic health. They have no need of hospitals or homes for the elderly. They have no disease, no police force, no jails, and no mental institutions."

Skin brushing. Using a natural brush all over dry skin removes dead cells and leaves pores open, so that more toxins can be expelled. Lombardi explains why this is so important: "We are supposed to eliminate two pounds of toxins through the pores of the skin. Due to pollution, smog, the creams we use, the clothes we wear, and so forth, our pores are more closed than open. Always brush toward the heart.

SAUNAS. This is a good follow-up to dry skin brushing because it pushes toxins out through the skin. The main thing to remember with saunas is to be prudent. You want to perspire but not remain there for too long a time. Nor do you want too much heat. "Follow the directions," says Lombardi. "And wear a cooling drape on your head. You don't want to heat up the brain area."

There are multiple benefits from detoxification, explains Lombardi: "You will look and feel better. Your skin will be clear and you will not have constipation. Your nails will improve as well as your heart and digestive system. It will clear your mind, and improve concentration. Nothing will de-stress your body like a sauna."

In addition, here are two detoxification therapies that require the assistance of health practitioners, and two others that you can do on your own.

OTHER DETOXIFICATION THERAPIES

CHELATION THERAPY. Martin Dayton, M.D., from Florida, board certified in family medicine, chelation therapy, and clinical nutrition, says that chelation therapy has multiple benefits, and long life is one of them: "Dramatic increases in life span are found with chelation. While there are no longevity studies per se, this conclusion is implied indirectly by studies which show a lessening of killer degenerative diseases. In fact, chelation favorably impacts all four major causes of death in the United States. In 1990 there were approximately 700,000 deaths associated with heart disease, 500,000 due to cancer, 144,000 from cerebral vascular disease, and 86,000 as a result of chronic obstructive lung disease."

During the chelation process many beneficial changes occur at the cellular level. A manmade amino acid, called EDTA, is administered to the patient via intravenous drip. Once in the bloodstream, EDTA attaches itself to heavy metals such as lead, cadmium, and mercury and holds onto these toxic substances until they exit the body through the urine. Dr. Dayton explains why removal of these substances is vital to good health: "The toxic material prevents normal function and repair. For example, lead prevents normal enzymatic processes so that the body cannot function properly and repair itself. This leads to premature aging and the premature development of disease. Removal of toxic material through chelation keeps the body functioning optimally."

Dr. Dayton notes that even excess iron, which is necessary for life, accelerates free radical production and causes harm: "Periodic purging of iron from the body via menstrual bleeding is thought to protect women from hardening of the arteries. However, this protection is lost at menopause with the cessation of menstruation. At this time, arterial clogging accelerates. Chelation removes this excess iron."

Since the modern person is overwhelmed by pollutants, Dr. Dayton recommends chelation therapy for anyone over thirty. "Lead is found everywhere, in the air we breathe, the water we drink, the food supply. It is even found at the North Pole. Lead and other toxic pollutants are hard to avoid in today's world. As a matter of fact, the concentration of lead found in the human skeleton now is several hundred times greater than that found in our preindustrial revolution ancestors. In one study, where lead was thought to be involved, eighteen years following chelation therapy a tenfold decrease in cancer death rate was found for those who had the treatment versus those who had nothing."

Aside from its overall benefits, chelation therapy specifically helps aging individuals by improving brain function. Dr. Dayton cites the following evidence: "Research shows that circulation improves greatly in the brain and to the brain. One study of fifteen patients who had twenty infusions of chelation therapy found that fourteen out of fifteen demonstrated significant cerebral blood flow. Some showed dramatic improvement in cognitive abilities.

"In another study, thirty patients with carotid blockages were given thirty chelation treatments over a ten-month period. The carotid artery extends from the chest through the neck to the brain. It is the brain's main source of blood flow. Blockage decreased between 20 and 40 percent.

"Unclogging carotid blockage is vitally important because the American College of Physicians states that patients with an obstruction of 70 percent or greater are at a high risk for stroke. They even recommend chelation therapy as a preferred treatment. I take that to heart and use chelation therapy on these individuals. People who have carotid artery disease improve as their arteries open up. I see this happen over and over again."

COLON CLEANSING. Colon cleansing is an ancient and time-honored health practice for rejuvenating the system, used in Egypt over 4,000 years ago. Later, Hippocrates taught these procedures in his health care system. The large intestine, or colon, is healed, rebuilt, and finally restored to its natural size, normal shape, and correct function.

Colon therapist Anita Lotson explains the procedure and some of its physical and psychological benefits: "There are several stages of therapy. The first segment involves cleansing, a thorough washing of the large intestine. The colon is irrigated by a technique whereby water is gently infused into the large bowel, flowing in and out at steady intervals. Through this method, water is allowed to travel the entire length of the colon, all the way around to the cecum area. The walls of the colon are washed and old encrustation and fecal material are loosened, dislodged, and swept away. This toxic waste material has often been attached to the bowel walls for many, many years. It is laden with millions of bacterium, which set up the perfect environment for disease to take route and entrench itself in the system, wreaking havoc. As this body pollution is eliminated, many conditions—from severe skin disorders to breathing difficulties, depression, chronic fatigue, nervousness, severe constipation, and arthritis—are reduced in severity, providing great relief, especially when augmented with dietary changes and other treatment modalities.

"The next phases are the healing, rebuilding, and finally restoration of a healthy colon, functioning at maximum efficiency for the final absorption of nutrients, and the total and timely elimination of all remaining waste materials. During the healing phase, we begin to infuse materials into the bowel that will cool inflamed areas and strengthen weak sections of the colon wall. Flaxseed tea, white oak bark, and slippery elm bark all soothe, lubricate, and introduce powerful healing agents directly into the large intestine. These herbal teas may be taken orally as well. Simple dietary changes have been made by now, such as the addition of water. This simple measure spells the difference between success and failure in alleviating many bowel conditions. I ask all my clients to double their intake of water.

"I love to see people's change in attitude from the time they come in to the time that they leave. Sometimes people are very irritable when their bowels are backed up. They're often depressed, and sometimes nasty. By the time they leave, you can see a smile and a bounce in their step. It's a different person altogether."

MAGNETIC HEALING. Susan Bucci is a holistically trained nurse who has spearheaded the development of magnetic healing products. "Magnets oxygenate tissues and allow cell walls to absorb more oxygen," she explains. "They promote mental acuity and normalize pH balance by increasing alkalinity. Restorative sleep is enhanced. Therapeutically, they stop pain, fight infection, and reduce inflammation and fluid retention. Over time, fatty and calcium deposits dissolve and the circulatory system opens up. Put that all together and you've got healing from A to Z. Take that a step further: if you achieve optimal well-being, you can actually live a long, productive life."

In addition to promoting overall well-being, magnets can eliminate many specific signs and symptoms of old age. Nurse Bucci reports these antiaging benefits from her own use of magnetic healing techniques: "My energy level has increased. I used to have chronic fatigue in the worst way, but now that's gone. My immune system is functioning much better, so my susceptibility to viruses and colds has decreased dramatically. Allergies are basically gone, and there are no more killer sinus headaches. My circulation has improved so that I withstand weather a whole lot easier. Wounds heal quickly, and my spider veins have disappeared. Also, I was headed for an early menopause, but now my menstrual cycle is very much on track, very regular.

"Hair, skin, and nails have definitely improved. My hair grows faster, and has a much better quality to it. Within two weeks of using magnets on a daily basis, I was able to see new, thick, dark, hair growing. My grays started falling out and disappearing. I was going to color my hair about four years ago and I still haven't touched it with an ounce of anything. My skin definitely looks and feels younger. And my nails grow so well that if I break one, it doesn't upset me. I know that it will grow right back."

How is it that magnets can do so much? Simply stated, magnets perform a wide range of benefits because we are magnetic beings who derive energy from the earth's magnetic field. Bucci explains, "One reason we get sick is that the earth has lost a good deal of its magnetism which leaves the body in an unbalanced state. Additionally, we are bombarded by unhealthy energies." Magnets create overall benefit by restoring internal harmony.

It is important to realize that any old magnet will not do. The negative pole restores health and good energy to the system, while exposure to the positive pole is detrimental. This has been repeatedly proven in studies where a variety of creatures, from earthworms, mice, and chickens to larger animals, live twice as long as untested control groups when exposed to negative field magnets, and half as long when exposed to positive fields. Susan recommends unipolar magnets, marked by the Davis and Rawls system with an *N* or the word *negative* and a green label. "That's the healthy side, and that's the one we face toward the body." Negative field ions support biological systems, which help the body to heal itself. "The body is an amazing machine with a remarkable capacity to cure itself," Susan says. "Give it a boost in the right direction and it does the rest on its own. The negative field is completely safe and risk-free."

Susan finds that magnets work best when worn on a daily basis. During the day she wears a magnet over her heart to improve circulation and oxygenation. "It keeps the heart open and flowing and sends all that wonderful oxygen throughout my body," she says. At night, she takes the magnet off and sleeps with her head on a magnetic mattress pad. This is because the most important benefit while sleeping is increased melatonin production from the brain's pineal gland. "People are running out to buy melatonin, but guess what? We can encourage our own melatonin production.

"People ask me how long magnets should be worn. Generally speaking, the longer you wear them, the more healing takes place. You can wear them all night and during the day. Generally, the body will tell you when it has had enough. It also will tell you when a condition has healed, although you should check with a physician just to make sure." Magnets, and more information, can obtained from Susan Bucci's company, Imaginetics, at (800) 285-3430.

LIVE CELL THERAPY. This is the use of living embryonic cells to regenerate tissues. Dr. Lance Morris notes, "Research is being performed on Alzheimer's patients to regenerate brain cell tissue. This is very exciting work. There is also work being done using thymus gland tissue to reverse the aging process. Thymus glands that you get in the health food store are useful in supporting immune function and in helping with the aging process. That's a simple thing that you can do on your own and it's very safe to do." Live cell therapy enhances immune response by increasing stem cells, cells that can differentiate into a wide variety of immune and blood cells throughout the body.

Brain Aging

One of the most disturbing symptoms of aging in women is diminished brain function, which can cause everything from forgetfulness and loss of concentration to Alzheimer's and other serious diseases. Fortunately, modern research reveals that much can be done to keep the brain in top form your entire life. Here, two experts in antiaging discuss new advances in the field.

Dr. Eric Braverman, founder and director of Princeton Associates for Total Health (PATH), in

Princeton, New Jersey, says that brain aging affects people differently and brain health is a preventative process. "Even when you feel halfway decent in your fifties, sixties, and seventies, parts of your body may be breaking down," he cautions.

The part of the brain affected determines which symptoms manifest themselves. "Individuals age in all different shapes and forms, just as a face can have wrinkles on the brow or wrinkles under the eye," Braverman says. "The area of the brain that slows down can affect such things as general memory, concentration, or logic." Dr. Braverman believes that each person must be individually tested to determine weak areas of brain function and to devise a program that addresses specific needs. For overall general improvement, he endorses these important therapies.

AMINO ACIDS AND OTHER BRAIN NUTRIENTS. Amino acids build up in particular areas of the brain that need help. The dopamine system responds to the essential amino acids tyrosine and phenylalanine. Melatonin helps sleep and slows down aging by supporting the pineal gland. Choline builds memory, while gabba, available as gabbapentin, helps anxiety disorders. Choline, phosphatytyl serine, ginkgo, tryptophan, tyrosine, and phenylalanine all boost brain voltage.

CHELATION THERAPY. As described earlier *(see "Other Detoxification Techniques," above)*, chelation therapy pulls out aluminum and other heavy metals from the bloodstream, resulting in improved memory. It can also reverse or prevent other destructive conditions associated with the aging process, such as arthritis, hardening of the arteries, cataracts, and strokes.

ELECTROSTIMULATION. Amino acids and neurotransmitter precursors are more effective when accompanied by electrostimulation of the brain. A TENS unit, worn on the forehead and left wrist, helps drive these substances along a good pathway. A cranioelectrical stimulation (CES) device also helps electrical fields, and additionally enhances the entire neurotransmitter system.

EXERCISE. Research shows that the whole neurotransmitter system of the brain can be improved through exercise. *(See "Exercise and Other Physical Techniques," above.)*

MEDITATION. Meditation connects the body and mind electrically, creating harmony between the brain and other body systems.

NATURAL HORMONES. Women must get three hormones from natural sources to slow down the aging process: progesterone, testosterone, and estrogen. Without natural estrogen, the hair thins, the vagina dries, the nails break, the bones rot, and the brain weakens. Estrogen improves the absorption of nutrients into the brain, especially improving dopamine levels. Progesterone protects from the side effects of estrogen. Additionally, it is calming to the brain and improves sleep. Testosterone enhances the sex drive, builds stronger bones, and gives greater physical strength.

PHYSICAL TOUCH. Neurotransmitters are adversely altered when people are in isolation, when they don't have love in their life.

NUTRITION AND SUPPLEMENTS. Another leading researcher in the field of antiaging, Dr. Ross Pelton of San Diego, author of *Mind, Food, and Smart Pills*, agrees that our brains do not have to deteriorate as we age: "It is simply poor nutrition and abuse that allows this condition to develop. Virtually everyone can enhance their memory, learning capabilities, and intelligence." Dr. Pelton helps his women patients optimize brain functioning with two goals in mind: to slow down or stop the brain aging process, and to optimize the function that we have.

First and foremost, Dr. Pelton recommends building total body health with a healthy diet. An organic vegetarian diet supplies the body with more protective nutrients and healthful fiber, and at the same time decreases toxins. Additionally, Pelton believes that every woman should take a high potency multivitamin/mineral supplement and extra antioxidants with each meal: "We are no longer looking at the Recommended Daily Allowance (RDA) as the level of nutrients appropriate for people. I say RDA stands for Really Dumb Allowance. It's more like the minimum wage, the minimal amount you can get by on. If we want to get into lifestyles of antiaging and life extension, we need to consider not only healthy diets but a program of optimal nutritional supplementation. Antioxidants are among the most important protectors against the aging process in general and against brain aging in particular. They will stop the onset of senility, Alzheimer's disease, and other brain injuries."

Then Dr. Pelton utilizes special nutrients to enhance the brain:

Flaxseed oil. This major brain nutrient is the greatest source of the essential fatty acid omega-3 (eicosapentaenoic acid, or EPA). Omega-3 gets converted into another fatty acid, which nourishes the fat cells in the brain. One tablespoon of flaxseed oil is needed daily. It should be refrigerated, not cooked, and taken with the largest meal of the day.

Hydergine increases oxygen to brain cells, and makes a person less susceptible to free radical damage and aging. Dr. Pelton says this is one of the most important substances for preventing brain aging due to its oxygenating capabilities. Hydergine is available in the United States, although as a prescription drug;

Lucidril and Piracetam, which have similar properties (*see below*), must be ordered from overseas. Although classified as drugs by the FDA, Hydergine, Lucidril, and Piracetam do not have any side effects, according to Dr. Pelton—only positive effects on memory and the prevention of brain aging. Overseas mail order sources sell Hydergine in 4.5 mg tablets, while in the United States it is only available in 1 mg tablets. The higher dosage, taken twice a day, is highly effective in helping people with early signs of memory loss.

Piracetam. This prescription drug is not available in the United States; however, it is available in over eighty-five other countries worldwide, where it is appreciated for its remarkable qualities and its complete lack of toxicity. Like Hydergine, Piracetam is powerful for preventing brain cell destruction caused by a lack of oxygen. Piracetam also can increase the flow of electrical information between the left and right hemispheres of the brain, a process known as superconnecting. It has proven effective in treating the learning disorder dyslexia. When used in conjunction with high-potency lecithin, Piracetam is highly effective in helping some Alzheimer's patients improve cognition, memory, and recall.

Lucidril, as its name suggests, makes you more lucid. This exciting drug can actually reverse brain aging. Dr. Pelton explains: "The primary yardstick in brain aging is the buildup of lipofusion, the result of free radical damage over the years. This buildup is really cellular garbage that collects and coalesces inside the cells into a black, tarlike mass. In elderly people you can see this in the skin as liver spots or age pigment. It is theorized that when 60 to 70 percent of the brain cell is clogged, it breaks down and stops working. That's when the symptoms of senility kick in very quickly.

Lucidril actually dissolves and flushes out these garbage deposits from brain cells and restores the brain cell to a much younger state." Lucidril has been shown to extend the life of laboratory animals and to enhance intelligence, learning, and recall.

Depranil. This drug has been shown in animal studies to prevent the destruction of a specific group of neurons in the nigra striata, the area of the brain that goes bad when people develop Parkinson's disease. Moreover, it helps enhance intelligence and cognition when 5 mg are taken, once daily.

Melatonin is the one substance from the armamentarium of alternative medicine to get free play in the mainstream media recently; you've probably already heard a lot about melatonin. This is a brain hormone produced by the pineal gland, and it diminishes with age. Three mg once daily taken at bedtime can help normalize sleep cycles.

DMAE is a naturally occurring but little-known B vitamin that enhances memory, boosts natural energy, and improves sleep. Additionally, it helps learning problems in children that have short attention spans. DMAE is safe, but if too much is taken, it can produce mild headaches, insomnia, and muscle tension.

Unless otherwise noted, these important brain enhancers can be purchased in health food stores.

Patient Stories

Reiki is a type of massage therapy or body work in which pressure point techniques are used in order to move energy through the body, thus achieving balance and harmony.

REIKI THERAPIST NILSA VERGARA ON HER CLIENTS' EXPERIENCES

My first example is a fifty-nine-year-old woman who came to our healing circle feeling old and tired. She suffered from aches and severe pain in her neck and knee from car accidents. She was also going through job changes, and was estranged from her adult son.

Each week she received a fifteen-minute session, and she quickly began feeling better. She released a lot of emotional toxins via crying and verbal expression of what she was feeling. She decided to take a Reiki class so that she could give herself daily treatments.

Within a month, her changes were quite dramatic. She had a tremendous increase in energy and vigor. She told me she now feels like she is twenty-eight. With the Reiki, she now has very little pain. She feels emotional and vital. Her attitude has changed. She feels self-fulfilled and in control of her life. Her relationship with her son has greatly improved. To quote her, "I feel like my whole life is as it should be."

My next client is a sixty-five-year-old woman. When she first came to see us, she was depressed. She had been in therapy for years, but nothing seemed to lift the depression. She felt tired all the time and would catch colds easily. Emotionally, she felt like a victim, and others treated her as one.

After her first fifteen-minute session she felt immediately better. She knew that something powerful was happening. She returned and eventually studied Reiki. Today, she reports feeling much healthier. She has more energy and an optimistic outlook. She no longer feels like a victim, and if anyone tries to put her in that role, she is no longer afraid to set limits. In addition, she is much more able to tolerate the cold weather, which indicates that her body has improved its oxygen intake.

One of my students has an eighty-three-year-old mom who fell and broke her hip bone as well as the bone in her wrist and arm. She decided to give her mother Reiki regularly, and her mother responded quite well. She began feeling stronger and stronger. Within four weeks she was out of her cast, walking with just the aid of a cane, not a walker. This is pretty remarkable for an eighty-three-year-old, because a broken hip does not always lead to a good outcome. So, as you can see, Reiki really enhances the body's ability to recuperate.

Another client is a fifty-three-year-old woman who had some serious memory problems. Her thinking was scattered; emotionally, she was fearful and guilt-ridden; and she was estranged from her adult children.

I recommended Reiki to her to see if we could work through some of these emotional blockages and change these negative patterns. She took a Reiki class, and within six months, her memory improved tremendously. She was much more focused in her thinking, and her job performance improved greatly. She became more insightful, much less fearful. Now she can speak with her adult children and set limits, and she no longer feels anxious and guilt-ridden. In addition to using Reiki, she uses herbal teas for detoxification, drinks vegetable juices, fasts, and gets colonics.

Hot News

DHEA, a precursor to the hormones estrogen and testosterone, may be one factor that determines natural life span, since its production decreases with advancing age, reaching a low at maximum recorded age; a natural DHEA supplement is found in the wild yam. Also shown to decrease in the body with age are melatonin, a free radical scavenger, and the antioxidant coenzyme glutathione, both of which can be supplemented to good effect in the elderly. Other plant supplements such as *Ginkgo biloba* and American ginseng provide antiaging benefits and aid in preventing cerebral disorders.

Perhaps surprisingly, restriction of food in general has been shown to slow the aging process in animals, suggesting that caloric intake should be lessened with increasing age. More specifically, excess sucrose in the diet may accelerate aging, inducing hyperglycemia and hyperinsulinemia.

Studies suggest that mental deterioration in Alzheimer's patients can be slowed by supplementation of iron, vitamins B6 and B12, coenzyme Q10, and acetyl-L-carnitine. Irreversible brain damage may be preventable through the use of desferrioxamine, which binds aluminum, thus decreasing its level in the brain; huperzine-A is another promising treatment. *(See below.)*

NUTRITION

Fruits and vegetables are the primary source of vitamins C and E and the carotenoids, which protect us from the oxidant byproducts of normal metabolism. But only 9 percent of Americans eat the recommended five servings of fruits and vegetables a day.

B. N. Ames et al., "Oxidants, Antioxidants, and the Degenerative Diseases of Aging," *Proceedings of the National Academy of Sciences* 90 (Sept. 1993): 7915–22.

The lower the intake of fruits and vegetables, the higher the risk of cancer—of almost every type.

"Vitamin C, Cancer and Aging," *Age* 16 (1993): 55–58.

The elderly are at greater risk than the general population for low intake of vitamins B6, C, E, zinc, beta carotene, and iron. Supplementation was shown to produce improved immune response.

S. N. Meydani, "Vitamin/Mineral Supplementation, the Aging Immune Response and Risk of Infection," *Nutrition Reviews* 51, no. 4 (April 1993): 106–15.

A study of 32 subjects over age 60 shows that vitamin E enhances immune function in healthy aged subjects.

N. Simin et al., "Vitamin E Supplementation Enhances Cell-Mediated Immunity in Healthy Elderly Subjects," *American Journal of Clinical Nutrition* 52 (1990): 557–63.

Serum cholesterol was shown to be lower with increased consumption of vitamin E.

E. Cheraskin, "Chronologic Versus Biologic Age," *Journal of Advancement in Medicine* 7, no. 1 (spring 1994): 31–41.

When older individuals receive 800 IU of vitamin E per day, the effect of exercise-induced oxidative stress is reduced.

M. Meydani et al., "Vitamin E Requirement in Relation to Dietary Fish Oil and Oxidative Stress in Elderly," in I. Emerit and B. Chance, *Free Radicals and Aging* (Basel, Switzerland: Birkhauser Verlag, 1992): 411–418.

Vitamin E supplementation improved the antioxidant status of elderly individuals.

S. N. Meydani, "Dietary Modulation of Immune Response in the Aged," *Age* 14 (1991): 108–15.

Vitamin C is important in collagen formation and hormone and neurotransmitter synthesis, and as an antioxidant it's a free radical scavenger. Low levels of vitamin C, and low carotene, increase the risk of age-related eye diseases such as cataracts.

"Vitamin C, Cancer and Aging," *Age* 16 (1993): 55–58.

A study of three U. S. Healthcare practices showed that the ingestion of under 100 mg of ascorbic acid daily was associated with the greatest number of nonspecific symptoms. On the other hand, those who ingested 200 mg of C or more per day had the fewest symptoms, at all ages. Subjects age 50 or over who consumed the most C were clinically similar to subjects age 40 consuming the least C.

E. Cheraskin, "Chronologic Versus Biologic Age," *Journal of Advancement in Medicine* 7, no. 1 (spring 1994): 31–41.

Benefits were seen in a study of 143 elderly subjects given a vitamin injection of 1 mg B12, 1 mg folate, and 5 mg of B6 eight times over three weeks. The study suggests that vitamin deficiency is common in the aged, even if they have "normal" vitamin levels.

H. J. Narath et al., "Effects of Vitamin B12, Folate and Vitamin B6 Supplements in Elderly People with Normal Serum Vitamin Concentrations," *Lancet* 346 (July 8, 1995): 85–89.

Glutathione improves immune function, stabilizes red blood cells, and provides protection against external toxins and free radicals. In a study of 33 people aged 60 and over, those with chronic conditions (e.g., heart disease, arthritis, and diabetes) had lower levels of glutathione.

R. H. Fletcher and S. W. Fletcher, "Glutathione and Aging: Ideas and Evidence," *Lancet* 344 (November 19, 1994): 1379–80.

A study of people aged 60 or over showed that higher self-rated levels of health, lower cholesterol, lower body mass index, and lower blood pressure were all linked to higher levels of glutathione. In combination, glutathione, age, and level of suppressed anger accounted for 39 percent of the variance in an index of morbidity. By itself, glutathione accounted for 24 percent of the variance.

M. Julius, "Glutathione and Morbidity in a Community-Based Sample of Elderly," *Journal of Clinical Epidemiology* 47, no. 9 (1994): 1021–26.

Glutathione levels were 17 percent lower in subjects aged 60 to 79 compared to subjects aged 20 to 39.

C. A. Long et al., "Low Blood Glutathione Levels in Healthy Ageing Adults," *Journal of Laboratory and Clinical Science* 120, no. 5 (November 1992): 720–25.

When rats were placed on a diet containing 66 percent sucrose, their mean and maximal life spans were significantly shorter than those of animals on a corn starch or energy-restricted sucrose diet. The implication is that diets high in sucrose may age us by inducing hyperglycemia and hyperinsulinemia.

R. B. McDonald, "Influence of Dietary Sucrose on Biological Aging," *American Journal of Clinical Nutrition* 62 (Suppl.) (1995): 284S–93S.

High HDL cholesterol and the ratio of HDL to cholesterol are linked with longevity. Total carbohydrate and refined carbohydrate consumption are inversely related to HDL cholesterol. Endurance training enhances HDL cholesterol.

M. Nikkila and J. Heikkinen, "High Density Lipoprotein Cholesterol and Longevity," *Age and Aging* 19 (1990): 119–124.

DHEA is one of the few compounds that decreases gradually with advancing age and reaches a low at maximum recorded age. This suggests that DHEA is one factor responsible for setting the "clock" that determines life span. A study of 138 elderly subjects (over 85) and 64 controls (ages 20 to 40) shows DHEA levels four times higher in young controls than in the oldest.

E. G. Birkenhager-Gillesse et al., "Dehydroepiandrosterone Sulfate (DHEA) in the Oldest Old, Aged 85 and Over," *New York Academy of Sciences* (1994): 543–52.

DHEA was given at 50 mg to 13 men and 17 women (from 40 to 70). In only 2 weeks, DHEA sulfate serum levels were restored to those found in young adults. Treatment resulted in a remarkable increase in physical and psychological well-being for the majority.

A. Morales, "Effects of Replacement Dose of Dehydroepiandrosterone in Men and Women of Advancing Age," *Journal of Clinical Endocrinology and Metabolism* 78 (1994): 1360–67.

MELATONIN

Melatonin is an efficient endogenous free radical scavenger. Aged humans and animals are melatonin-deficient. Sensitivity to oxidative stress increases with age.

B. Poeggeler et al., "Melatonin, Hydroxyl Radical-Mediated Oxidative Damage, and Aging: A Hypothesis," *Journal of Pineal Research* 14 (1993): 151–68.

EXERCISE

Physical activity can reverse cardiac, pulmonary, musculoskeletal, and metabolic-endocrine changes associated with age and disease.

D. T. Lowenthal et al., "Effects of Exercise on Age and Disease," *South. Med. Journal* 87, no. 5 (May 1994): S5–12.

FOOD RESTRICTION

Rat, mouse, and hamster studies indicate that food restriction slows the aging process and extends the animals' maximum life span. While food restriction can delay immune system development, it can also preserve immune system function in rodents of advanced age. Food restriction reduces the ability to cope with cold, but the ability to cope with many other stresses increases.

E. J. Masoro, "Retardation of the Aging Process by Food Restriction: An Experimental Tool," *American Journal of Clinical Nutrition* 55 (1992): 1250S–52S.

HERBS/PLANT EXTRACTS

Ginkgo biloba extract is effective in all types of dementia, even cognitive disorders secondary to depression (because of its beneficial effect on mood).

D. M. Warburton, "Psycho-pharmacologie clinique de L'extrait de *Ginkgo biloba*," [Clinical Psychopharmacology of *Ginkgo Biloba* Extract], *Presse Med* 15, no. 31 (Sept. 25, 1986): 1595–1604.

Ginkgo biloba is prescribed for psychiatric and behavioral disorders, and for vascular and nervous system problems. Numerous clinical trials justify these prescriptions.

M. Allard, "Traitement des troubles du vieillissement par extrait de *Ginkgo biloba*: De la pharmacologie à la clinique" [Treatment of the Disorders of Aging with *Ginkgo Biloba* Extract: From Pharmacology to Clinical Medicine], *Presse Med* 15, no. 31 (Sept. 25, 1986): 1540–45.

The use of *Ginkgo biloba* for cerebral disorders due to aging was tested in a study of 166 patients and proven effective. After 3 months the difference between the *Ginkgo biloba* group and the control group became significant, and it increased over the following months.

J. Taillandier et al., "Traitement des troubles du vieillissement cerebral par l'extrait de *Ginkgo biloba*: Étude longitudinale multicentrique à double insu face au placebo," *Presse Med* 15, no. 31 (Sept. 25, 1986): 1583–87.

Animal research showing that aged garlic extract improves memory acquisition suggests that the extract may be useful for humans.

T. Moriguchi et al., "Prolongation of Life Span and Improved Learning in the Senescence Accelerated Mouse Produced by Aged Garlic Extract," *Biol. Pharm. Bull.* 17, no. 12 (December 1994): 1589–94.

A study of 71 subjects over 60 years of age showed that treatment with American ginseng prolonged functional age. Effectiveness for the treated group was about 90 percent.

J. Cui and K. J. Chen, "American Ginseng Compound Liquor on Retarding Aging Process," *Chung Hsi I Chief Ho Tsa Chih* 11, no. 8 (August 1991): 451, 457–60.

A study on humans shows treatment with the oriental herbal preparation huanshao dan has an antiaging effect.

X. Du et al., "Effect on Anti-aging and Treating Yang Deficiency of Kidney with Huanshao dan Capsules. A Clinical Report of 309 Cases," *Chung Kuo Chung Hsi I Chieh Ho Tsa Chih* 12, no. 1 (January 1992): 4-5, 20–22.

OZONE THERAPY

Ozone therapy given over a 4-month period improved the ocular condition of a majority of a study group.

E. Riva Sanseverino et al., "Effects of Oxygen-Ozone Therapy on Age-Related Degenerative Retinal Maculopathy," *Panminerva Med* 32, no. 2 (April–June 1990): 77–84.

TRANSCENDENTAL MEDITATION

A study of residents in 73 retirement homes (average age 81) showed that transcendental meditation improved blood pressure (systolic blood pressure was reduced, on average, from 140 to 128), vision, cognitive function (thinking/memory), hormone levels of DHEA, and longevity. After 3 years, all members of the TM group were still alive, while the death rate of the 478 retirement home residents not involved in the study was 62.5 percent.

"Can Transcendental Meditation Make You Live Longer and Prosper?" *New Scientist* (April 28, 1990): 40.

ALZHEIMER'S DISEASE

Low levels of vitamin B12 are characteristic of Alzheimer's patients.

T. Ikeda et al., "Vitamin B12 Levels in Serum and Cerebrospinal Fluid of People with Alzheimer's Disease," *ACTA Psychiatr. Scand.* 86 (1992): 301–5.

B12 levels were shown to be correlated with performance on the Mini-Mental State Examination.

A. J. Levitt et al., "Folate, Vitamin B12 and Cognitive Impairment in Patients with Alzheimer's Disease," *ACTA Psychiatr. Scand.* 86 (1992): 301–5.

Twenty patients with long-term sporadic Alzheimer's were given supplements of iron, vitamin B6, and coenzyme Q10. The results after a year: significant improvement in performance on mental and functional tests. Coenzyme Q10 may reduce free radicals produced by iron; B6 is important in neurotransmitter synthesis.

M. Imagawa, "Iron, B6 and Coenzyme Q10 in Alzheimer's," *Nutrition Report* 12, no. 10 (October 1994): 75; M. Imagawa, "Therapy with a Combination of Iron, Vitamin B6, and Coenzyme Q10 in the Long Term for Sporadic Alzheimer's Disease," *Neurobiology* A15 (1994): S101.

Zinc deficiency is linked to Alzheimer's; supplementation with zinc early in the disease may help.

"Zinc Deficiency Tied to Neurofibrillary Tangles in Alzheimer's," *Family Practice News* 20, no. 20 (October 15–31, 1990): 7.

A study of postmortem brain tissue from 11 Alzheimer's patients and 6 controls linked Alzheimer's to deficiencies in zinc and cesium, and to reduced selenium, which may decrease antioxidant activity.

F. M. Corrigan et al., "Reduction of Zinc and Selenium in Brain Alzheimer's Disease," *Trace Elements in Medicine* 8, no. 1 (1991): 1–5.

Oil of evening primrose, zinc sulfate, and sodium selenite, given daily, reduced saturated fatty acids in the plasma of phospholipids; there may be a defect in incorporation of fatty acids in the membranes of Alzheimer's patients.

F. M. Corrigan et al., "Dietary Supplementation with Zinc Sulfate, Sodium Selenite and Fatty Acids in Early Dementia of Alzheimer's Type II: Effects on Lipids," *Journal of Nutritional Medicine* 2 (1991): 265–71.

Alzheimer's is linked to essential fatty acid deficiency, as well as to aluminum buildup. Our Western diet tends to be high in saturated fatty acids and low in essential fatty acids. Dietary recommendations include more essential fatty acids.

P. E. Newman, "Could Diet Be One of the Causal Factors of Alzheimer's Disease?" *Medical Hypotheses* 39 (1992): 123–26.

Reduced levels of vitamins A and E, and of beta carotene, may promote nervous system degeneration and dementia. A study of 38 patients showed that both those with Alzheimer's and those with multi-infarct dementia had low levels of E and beta carotene; A was significantly reduced only in patients with Alzheimer's.

C. Zaman et al., "Plasma Concentrations of Vitamins A and E and Carotenoids in Alzheimer's Disease," *Age and Aging* 21 (1992): 91–94.

Vitamin E prevents some types of cell deaths, including such deaths caused by glutamate and cysteine starvation. E reduces glutamate toxicity, and this vitamin may play a role in slowing Alzheimer's and reversing some of the damage already caused by the disease.

C. Behl et al., "Vitamin E Protects Nerve Cells from Amyloid B Protein Toxicity," *Biochemistry and Biophysical Research Communications* 186, no. 2 (July 31, 1992): 944–50.

Treatment with acetyl-L-carnitine slowed deterioration in Mini-Mental Status and Alzheimer's Disease Assessment Scales, and normalized high-energy phosphate levels in a study of 5 probable Alzheimer's patients and 21 controls.

J. W. Pettegrew et al., "Clinical and Neurochemical Effects of Acetyl-L-Carnitine in Alzheimer's Disease," *Neurobiology of Aging* 16, no. 1 (1995): 1–4.

L-carnitine was shown to slow deterioration in 13 out of 14 measures of Alzheimer's disease, in a study of 130 patients.

A. Spagnoli et al., "Long-Term Acetyl-L-Carnitine Treatment in Alzheimer's Disease," *Neurology* 41 (November 1991): 1726–32.

Brain autopsies showed a 25 to 40 percent reduction in carnitine acetyltransferase activity in Alzheimer's patients, as opposed to controls. This finding provides a rationale for acetyl-L-carnitine treatment of these patients.

R. N. Kalaria and S. I. Harik, "Carnitine Acetyltransferase in the Human Brain and Its Microvessels Is Decreased in Alzheimer's Disease," *Annals of Neurology* 32, no. 4 (October 1992): 583–86.

Acetyl-L-carnitine, given at a dosage of 2 g/day for 1 year, slowed the progression of Alzheimer's disease in a placebo-controlled study.

"Acetyl-L-carnitine and Alzheimer's Disease," *Nutrition Reviews* 50, no. 5 (1992): 142–44.

Therapy with L-deprenyl was shown to be effective for treatment of memory disorder in dementia and Alzheimer's patients in a 6-month study.

G. Fianli et al., "L-Deprenyl Therapy Improves Verbal Memory in Amnesic Alzheimer's Patients," *Clinical Neuropharmacology* 14, no. 6 (1991): 523–36.

In a study of 40 patients, 20 were treated with 80 mg of *Ginkgo biloba* extract for 3 months rather than with a placebo. After 1 month of this double-blind study, the treated patients showed significant improvement in memory and attention, psychopathology, psychomotor performance, functional dynamics, and neurophysiology.

B. Hofferberth, "The Efficacy of Egb 761 in Patients with Senile Dementia of the Alzheimer Type: A Double-Blind, Placebo-Controlled Study on Different Levels of Investigation," *Human Psychopharmacology* 9 (1994): 215–22.

Ginkgo biloba extract increases cholinergic transmission in aged animals and addresses major elements involved in Alzheimer's disease.

M. Allard, "Treatment of Old Age Disorders with *Ginkgo biloba* Extract: From Pharmacology to Clinic," in E. W. Fungold, ed., *Rokan (Ginkgo Biloba)–Recent Results in Pharmacology and Clinic* (New York: Springer-Verlag, 1988): 201–11.

A study of 54 patients with mild impairment of everyday function showed that *Ginkgo biloba* extract improved accuracy and speed in tests of cognitive efficiency.

K. Wesnes et al., "A Double Blind Placebo-Controlled Trial of *Ginkgo biloba* Extract in the Treatment of Idiopathic Cognitive Impairment in the Elderly," *Human Psychopharmacology* 2 (1987): 159–69.

A study of 60 patients with mild to moderate primary degenerative dementia showed that treatment with *Ginkgo biloba* extract over 4–12 weeks improved the patients' clinical condition and their performance on psychometric tests. Short-term memory and vigilance also benefited.

W. U. Weitbrecht and W. Jansen, "Primary Degenerative Dementia: Therapy with *Ginkgo biloba* Extract," *Fortschr. Medicine* 104 (1986): 199–202.

The herbal formulation Mentat improves memory and cognition in patients who are aged or chronically ill.

S. K. Bhattacharya et al., "Effect of Mentat, an Herbal Formulation, on Experimental Models of Alzheimer's Disease and Central Cholinergic Markers in Rats," *Fitoterapia* 67, no. 3 (1995): 216–22.

Ten Alzheimer's patients with sleep disturbances were given bright light exposure for 2 hours per day between 7 and 9 p.m. for 1 week. For 8 out of these 10, their sleep-wakefulness patterns improved.

A. Satlin et al., "Bright Light Treatment of Behavioral and Sleep Disturbances in Patients with Alzheimer's Disease," *American Journal of Psychiatry* 149, no. 8 (August 1992): 1028–32.

Magnetic field applications produce effects of melatonin secretion and circadian organization similar to those of exposure to light. Circadian rhythms are severely disrupted in Alzheimer's patients; animal studies show that application of magnetic fields suppresses melatonin secretion and may synchronize circadian rhythms in humans.

R. Sandyk et al., "Age-Related Disruption of Circadian Rhythms: Possible Relationship to Memory Impairment and Implications for Therapy with Magnetic Fields," *International Journal of Neuroscience* 59 (1991): 259–62.

Animal, biochemical, and epidemiological studies show that aluminum plays a serious role in the progression of Alzheimer's disease.

D. R. Crapper McLachlan et al., "Would Decreased Aluminum Ingestion Reduce the Incidence of Alzheimer's Disease?" *Canadian Medical Association Journal* 145, no. 7 (1991): 793–803.

Reducing the level of aluminum in the brains of Alzheimer's patients slows mental deterioration by nearly 50 percent. Desferrioxamine, an aluminum binder, prevents irreversible brain damage. A study of 48 patients showed that after 2 years, the group treated with desferrioxamine were still able to live at home (with caretakers), while those who were untreated continued to deteriorate (some had to be admitted to nursing homes and several died).

"Effect of Aluminum on Brain Cells," *Press Digest* 22 (June 3, 1991): 3.

Epidemiological evaluation of 2,300 patients with Alzheimer's compared to 2,200 controls showed that the risk of this disease increases with increasing aluminum concentrations in the water supply.

L. Neri and D. Hewitt, "Aluminum, Alzheimer's Disease and Drinking Water," *Lancet* 338 (August 10, 1991): 390.

Smoking is linked to the risk of Alzheimer's, and to the age of onset. Smoking may damage the lining of the nose, providing an inroad for the causative agents of Alzheimer's.

R. C. A. Pearson et al., "Nicotine Intake in Alzheimer's Disease," *British Medical Journal* (August 10, 1991): 361.

Thirty minutes of transcutaneous electrical nerve stimulation (called short-term TENS), received daily, may improve memory and affective behavior in Alzheimer's patients. Alzheimer's sufferers given this treatment experienced improvement in some aspects of verbal and visual short-term and long-term memory, in mood, and in alertness.

E. J. Scherder et al., "Effects of Short-Term Transcutaneous Electrical Nerve Stimulation on Memory and Affective Behaviour in Patients with Probable Alzheimer's Disease," *Behavioural Brain Research* 67, no. 2 (1995): 211–19.

Huperzine-A is a promising agent for treatment of Alzheimer's; it enhances memory and cognition.

X. C. Tang et al., "Comparison of the Effects of Natural and Synthetic Huperzine-A on Rat Brain Cholinergic Function in Vitro and in Vivo," *Journal of Ethnopharmacology* 44 (1994): 147–55.

In a study of 101 patients with age-associated memory impairment and Alzheimer's, the effects of huperzine-A were compared to the effects of the drug Piracetam. For patients treated with huperzine-A, the improvement rate for memory was 73 percent, while for patients treated with Piracetam, the rate was 32 percent. In another study of 111 patients, huperzine-A and Piracetam yielded similar memory improvement rates.

Z. Wang et al., "A Double Blind Control Study of Huperzine-A and Piracetam in Patients with Age-Associated Memory Impairment and Alzheimer's Disease," *Neuropsychopharmacology* 10, no. 35 (May 1994): 763S.

2. ANEMIA

Anemia is a health condition characterized by red blood cells deficient in hemoglobin, the iron-containing portion of the blood. Hemoglobin enables the blood to transport oxygen from the lungs throughout the body, and to carry away carbon dioxide; the listlessness, pallor, and shortness of breath in the anemic reflect a lack of oxygen and buildup of carbon dioxide in the tissues.

Causes

Dr. Dahlia Abraham, a complementary physician from New York City, describes three major classifications of anemia, each of which is associated with a specific cause:

"The first cause of anemia is excessive blood loss. Chronic blood loss can occur in association with menstruation, or because of conditions such as hemorrhoids or a slow, bleeding, peptic ulcer.

"The second cause of anemia is excessive red blood cell destruction. Normally, old and abnormal red blood cells are removed from circulation. If the rate of destruction exceeds that of manufacture of new cells, then anemia can result. A number of factors can cause excessive red blood cell destruction, such as defective hemoglobin synthesis, injury, or trauma within the arteries.

"The third and most common type of anemia is caused by nutritional deficiencies in iron, vitamin B12, and folic acid. Of these, iron deficiency is most frequently seen. People require extra iron during growth spurts in infancy and adolescence. Pregnancy and lactation are other times when women need iron supplementation. During childbearing years, many women experience anemia caused by an iron deficiency.

"Supplementation may not solve the problem because many people have difficulty absorbing iron. They lack enough hydrochloric acid, the stomach acid that helps the body assimilate iron. This is common among the elderly, who generally produce less hydrochloric acid. Another cause of decreased iron absorption is chronic diarrhea.

"Vitamin B12 deficiency is most often due to a defect in absorption. B12 must be liberated from food via hydrochloric acid and bound to a substance called intrinsic factor, which is also secreted in the stomach. In order for B12 to be absorbed then, an individual must secrete enough hydrochloric acid and enough intrinsic factor. Women with this type of anemia may need to take supplements of B12, hydrochloric acid, and intrinsic factor.

"Folic acid deficiency may also cause anemia. Folic acid becomes totally depleted in alcoholics. It is also commonly deficient among pregnant women because the fetus demands so much of it. Folic acid is vital for cell production in the growing fetus, and prevents birth defects, such as neural tube imperfections. This is why prenatal vitamins must contain this nutrient. In addition, a number of pharmaceutical drugs, such as anticancer drugs and oral contraceptives, can drain the body of folic acid. Women taking either of these should be supplementing their diet with folic acid, especially since this nutrient is difficult to get in foods."

Dr. Pat Gorman, an acupuncturist and educator in New York City, explains anemia and other blood disorders in women from an Asian perspective: "In women, blood has an actual cycle that rises and falls every month. There is a building phase that occurs for about a week after your period. Then there is a peak phase where the blood reaches its richest moment; that's the moment you ovulate. This is followed by a storage phase. (If you are pregnant, the blood is stored.) A week before your period, you go through a cleansing phase where your organs release toxins into the blood. That's the week before your period when you can go through a PMS hell if the toxins are not being properly released. Next is the purging of the actual period."

Using this philosophy as her framework, Dr. Gorman holds that women become anemic when they are out of touch with their monthly cycles. In our fast-paced society, one of the major reasons for this condition is that women fail to rest at the appropriate times: "Women work all the time. They show no vulnerability, and just keep on going no matter what. There is no respect for the actual rhythm of the cycle. I believe that we need to bring back the menstrual hut. When you are bleeding, you need to stop working for a day or two. I know I am saying things that sound impossible, but if you have anemia—and 60 to 70 percent of the women that I see do—you need to face the fact and work with it."

She adds that another major reason why women become anemic is that they incorrectly approach pregnancy: "There is a law called the one-month, one-year law. After a pregnancy is terminated, whether in abortion, miscarriage or birth, one month of absolute rest is needed. Women say, 'That's not possible. I just gave birth but I have other children. I have to take care of things.' The Chinese say this is a straight road to a severe anemic problem.

"The one-year aspect of this is the avoidance of pregnancy for at least another year. Women who try to conceive, and who miscarry, often frantically begin again. They need to build up the blood for an entire year's cycle before trying to conceive again. It is very difficult for me to help anxious patients relax and understand that this is the way to overcome anemia and to have a really healthy baby."

Additionally, Dr. Gorman warns that birth control pills are unhealthy because they disturb the integrity of the blood's cycle. They fool the body into believing that it is continually pregnant by locking blood into its storage phase. By eliminating the cycle of building, peaking, storing, cleansing and purging, oral contraceptives create many problems.

Symptoms

General symptoms of anemia are weakness and a tendency to tire easily. When there is a B12 deficiency, the symptoms may include paleness; the tendency to tire easily; shortness of breath; sore, red, swollen tongue; diarrhea; heart palpitations; and nervous disturbances.

Clinical Experience

DIAGNOSIS

According to Dr. Abraham, the treatment of anemia is dependent on proper clinical evaluation by a physician. Too often, physicians assume anemia is from an iron deficiency, but this is just one possible reason. "It is absolutely imperative that a comprehensive laboratory analysis of the blood be performed," she says. "Do not be satisfied when your physician offers a simple diagnosis of anemia," she warns. "Insist that your doctor investigate the underlying causes."

While Dr. Gorman agrees that clinical studies help confirm a diagnosis, she adds that Asian physicians are trained to accurately detect anemia and other blood disorders through observation: "In Chinese medicine, you examine the body. Look at your tongue. Is it pale? Look at your lips. Are they pale? See if the mucous membranes under the eyes are pale. These signs indicate whether or not you are anemic."

YOUR DIET

Green, leafy vegetables are high in iron and folic acid. It is best to purchase organic vegetables, as pesticides interfere with absorption. Eating vegetables raw or lightly cooked preserves their folic acid content. Soy or shoyu sauce, miso, and tempeh are rich sources of vitamin B12.

Proteins should be eaten every day, preferably vegetarian proteins, such as from grains and legumes, like rice and beans, or oatmeal with soy milk. When animal protein is eaten, it should be from fish. Caffeine and alcohol are detrimental to healthy blood, and should be eliminated.

SUPPLEMENTS. According to Dr. Abraham, iron, B12, and folic acid should be prescribed as needed. Additionally, hydrochloric acid and intrinsic factor are often required to aid in the absorption of these nutrients.

Patient Story

YOLANDA

I was born in Nicaragua, Central America, and I used to be a very healthy person. But in June 1993, I went to the emergency room. My hemoglobin was down to 2.8; the normal count for a woman is between 12 and 14. There I was with aplastic anemia, meaning that my bone marrow was not making any blood cells: no red cells, no white cells, no platelets. I almost had no blood.

The doctor said that my sickness was idiopathic, meaning that they didn't know what caused it. They said that one possible cause was the use of an antibiotic. But the only one that I took in my life was fifteen years earlier. Another possible cause was exposure to chemicals or pesticides. A lot of towns in Nicaragua are surrounded by cotton plantations where cotton growers use a lot of pesticides to spray their crops.

In July 1993, I was referred to a bone marrow transplant unit and was put on a medication, a kind of chemotherapy. After one month of treatment, the medication failed to work. Then the doctors wanted to do a bone marrow transplant. I have seven siblings so I had donors, and one of them was a perfect match. But I had my reservations. A bone marrow transplant is very costly. Also, you get bone marrow that is working, but due to the chemotherapy or radiation, your liver, kidneys, pancreas and so forth, pay a terrible toll.

Prior to my sickness, I was following a macrobiotic diet. I was starting to use Oriental and alternative medicine, and I knew of the power of the body to heal itself. I decided to keep on my macrobiotic diet, and was able to, more or less, clean myself of the chemotherapy. During this time I did not even get a cold. I didn't sneeze through all my sickness.

I was clean, but my blood counts were still very low. I needed a transfusion every ten days. On one hand, the transfusions were very helpful, and I was grateful to be able to get them. But through transfusions I was also receiving a lot of genetic and other information completely foreign to my body. I could not control what the person who donated that blood was eating. So I was trying to clean my body of toxins and I decided to look for help.

I went to a naturopath who helped me a lot. Then I read an article on Ayurveda. That article said that Ayurveda is very specific, even with the use of grains and vegetables. There are grains and vegetables that are not appropriate for your body type. In early February 1994, I went to an Ayurvedic doctor. He gave me a very gentle treatment consisting of diet, aromatherapy, massage, and meditation. After three weeks of following that treatment, my blood count went up for the first time.

I keep up with this treatment still. My last checkup at the hospital showed normal white cells. Red cells were a little bit low. They were 3.83, and the normal count is four. But they are increasing day by day.

My energy level is excellent. I went back to work three months ago, and am now leading a completely normal life. I am very grateful to Ayurveda.

Hot News

Anemia may be due to folic acid deficiency, which is common in alcoholics and pregnant women. Antacids, calcium, and zinc interfere with iron absorption and should be taken separately; however, ascorbic acid and vitamin A both reduce anemia when taken together with iron.

Caution must be taken with iron supplementation; an excess has been linked to cancer and to liver, heart, and pancreas damage. *(See below.)*

IN GENERAL

Anemia may be due to iron deficiency (the most common cause), to B12 deficiency (usually due to an absorption problem rather than a dietary lack), or to folic acid deficiency, which can be a problem because the body does not store large amounts of this nutrient. Folic acid deficiency is common in alcoholics, pregnant women, and patients with chronic diarrhea or other malabsorptive states.

M. T. Murray and J. E. Pizzorno, *An Encyclopedia of Natural Medicine* (Rocklin, Calif.: Prima Publishing, 1991): 136–42.

NUTRITION

Antacids, calcium, and zinc interfere with iron absorption and should be taken separately.

J. F. Balch and P. A. Balch, *Prescriptions for Nutritional Healing* (Garden City Park, N.Y.: Avery, 1990): 91–92.

Iron-related indices of anemia normalized as a result of treatment with ferric ammonium citrate (the equivalent of 6 mg iron) in addition to vitamin C given over 9 weeks.

M. Taniguchi et al., "Improvement in Iron Deficiency Anemia through Therapy with Ferric Ammonium Citrate and Vitamin C and the Effects of Aerobic Exercise," *Journal Nutr. Sci. Vitaminol* 37, no. 2 (April 1991): 161–71.

Fifty or 100 mg of ascorbic acid daily raised hemoglobin and hematocrit levels and erythrocyte counts in healthy young women after 8 weeks.

O. A. Ajayi and U. R. Nnaji, "Effect of Ascorbic Acid Supplementation on Haematological Response and Ascorbic Acid Status of Young Female Adults," *Annals Nutr. Metab.* 34 (1990): 32–36.

Vitamin A plus iron markedly reduced anemia in pregnant women; 97 percent of a group treated with both A and iron became nonanemic. The effectiveness of the treatment is seen as one-third attributable to A and two-thirds attributable to the iron supplementation.

D. Suharno et al., "Supplementation with Vitamin A and Iron for Nutritional Anemia in Pregnant Women in West Java, Indonesia," *Lancet* 342 (November 27, 1993): 1325–28.

It's important that your iron supplementation be supervised by a doctor. Excess iron has been linked to cancer and to damage of the liver, heart, and pancreas, as well as to lymphocyte activity.

J. F. Balch and P. A. Balch, *Prescriptions for Nutritional Healing* (Garden City Park, N.Y.: Avery, 1990): 91–92.

Only 3 percent of pregnant women given iron supplements were anemic at delivery, compared to 30 percent of a group given placebos. The iron status of the babies at birth and 2 months after delivery correlated with their mothers' iron status, particularly during the 7th month of pregnancy.

C. De Benanze et al., "Prevention de l'anemie Ferriprive Au Cours de la Grossesse par une Supplementation Martiale Precoce: un Essai Controle," [Prevention of Iron-Deficiency Anemia in Pregnancy Using Early Iron Supplementation: A Controlled Trial], *Rev. Epidemiol. Sante Publique* 37 (1989): 109–18.

Iron and folate supplemenation reduced anemia in pregnant women from a level of 50 percent to below 6 percent in a particular community.

G. Izak et al., *Scandinavian Journal of Haematology* 11 (1973): 236.

Ten iron-deficiency anemic patients were treated for 3–6 weeks with iron and B12 supplements. Results: Red cell indices normalized.

P. Gram-Hansen et al., "Glycosylated Hemoglobin (HbAlc) in Iron and Vitamin B12 Deficiency," *Journal of Internal Medicine* 227 (1990): 33–136.

3. BIRTH CONTROL

In the United States of the 1990s, no subject is more volatile or more politicized than that of birth control. My goal in this chapter is not to add to any side of the debate but merely to make sure that the information already available to some in the alternative health community is available to all.

No currently available form of birth control is 100 percent effective and risk free, and no single form of birth control is right for everyone. A woman's fertility is always a highly personal matter, so the more you are able to feel in sync with your menstrual cycle and fertility, the better able you will be to make the right decisions for you and your partner about birth control.

Fertility Awareness

Fertility awareness, also called natural family planning, the Billings method (named after John and Evelyn Billings, two Australian researchers who helped popularize it), or mucous observation, among other names, is a much underrated but extremely effective method of pregnancy prevention. This is *not* the old rhythm method promoted by the Catholic church in the past, which was notoriously ineffective; each woman has her own "rhythm" that may change from time to time and may not fit into any established pattern.

Actually, fertility awareness might more accurately be characterized not as a method of birth control but as a way of life. That is, if you have a more accurate understanding of the dynamic physiological changes that occur during your menstrual cycles, you will be more aware of exactly when you are likely to get pregnant and can then take preventive measures or, if you are trying to become pregnant, enhance your chances.

Recently, researchers at Princeton University reanalyzed a mountain of data that had been collected by the World Health Organization (WHO) on couples who used fertility awareness, and found that this method was 97 percent effective in preventing pregnancy for those who understood its principles and used it as their sole method of contraception. This research impressively puts to rest the widely held myth that fertility awareness isn't very effective.

Two myths that prevent many people from using fertility awareness as their main method of birth control are that it is difficult to learn, and that women have to take their temperature every day and laboriously chart their menstrual cycles for the rest of their lives. This is definitely not the case. You can learn the basic principles of fertility awareness over a few months, and by knowing what to look for, you can learn to *intuitively* identify your fertile period with a high degree of accuracy without having to deal with charts and thermometers on a daily basis.

Essentially, there are a number of specific bodily changes that signal the onset of a woman's fertile time. These include changes in cervical mucus, body temperature, and sexual desire, and an ovulatory pain called "*mittleschmertz*" (middle pain).

Getting pregnant requires three factors: sperm, alkaline fertile mucus to nurture and transport the sperm, and a ripe egg in one of the egg (fallopian) tubes. The menstrual cycle is counted as beginning on the first day of menstrual bleeding, and the average cycle is twenty-seven to thirty days (although cycles as short as twenty-one days, or as long as three to nine months, are common). A viscous, "stretchy" mucous secretion, manufactured in the glands of the cervical canal, begins to ooze from the cervical opening about day 10 of the average cycle and increases daily, peaking at day 14 to 16. Using a plastic speculum, you can actually see the clear mucus, which looks a lot like egg white, oozing from the cervical opening.

As production increases, the stretchy mucus seeps from the vagina and makes a sort of crusty secretion on your underpants or can be picked up by toilet paper.

At the same time that fertile mucus is beginning to develop, a ripe egg pops through the side of one of your ovaries and begins its trip of three to five days down the egg tube. In the days approaching ovulation, your temperature rises gradually, and in most women it makes a sharp drop on the day of actual ovulation. If fertile mucus is present and you have unprotected intercourse, the sperm slip easily through the liquid highway of mucus into the cervical canal, where they are kept alive for several days to regroup, as it were, and swim up through the uterus in search of an unfertilized egg.

The idea in using fertility awareness for contraception is to avoid having any sperm in the vagina when fertile mucus might be present. By carefully looking for the signs of ovulation (fertile mucus, a drop in temperature, *mittleschmertz*, and other signs), you can identify pretty specifically when that time is. The first part of the cycle (including menstruation) is considered the "unsafe" time because fertile mucus can appear early, or at low levels—but *any* fertile mucus presents the *possibility* of pregnancy. Couples who use fertility awareness as a form of birth control avoid having penis-in-vagina sex at this time, but may enjoy other forms of sexual activity. Others use a barrier method of contraception until they are sure that ovulation has occurred. After ovulation, however, another egg will not appear, so this is considered the "safe" time. After that time, according to researchers, it is perfectly safe to have vaginal intercourse without worrying about getting pregnant.

You can quite effectively learn the tenets of fertility awareness from a number of excellent books, but many women and their partners find taking a workshop of several sessions the easiest and best way to learn it. There are now a wide array of fertility detection devices that can be fun to use and are quite accurate. To find the nearest fertility awareness instructor, contact the Ovulation Method Teacher's Association, Box 14511, Portland, OR 97214. Many Catholic hospitals also teach this method.

Resources for Fertility Awareness

Barbara Feldman, Director, Fertility Awareness Center and Birth Control the Natural Way, P.O. Box 2606, New York, N.Y. 10009; (212) 475-4490

Fertility Awareness Network, P.O. Box 1190, New York, N.Y. 10009. Send $4.00 and SASE for an eight-page introductory packet.

Barbara Kass-Annese, Los Angeles Regional Family Planning Council (LARFPC), 3600 Wilshire Boulevard, #600, Los Angeles, Calif. 90010; (213) 386-5614.

Diocesan Development Program for Natural Family Planning, 3211 Fourth Street, N.E., Washington, D.C. 20017; (202) 541-3240.

National Family Planning Center of Washington, D.C., 8514 Bradmore Drive, Bethesda, Md. 20817; (301) 897-9323.

The Condom

Condoms, latex rubber sheaths that unroll to cover the penis, are highly effective—from 90 to 98 percent—in preventing pregnancy and provide the best protection from sexually transmissible diseases (STDs). The effectiveness of condoms can be raised to nearly 100 percent by combining them with the cervical cap, diaphragm, Vaginal Contraceptive Film (VCF), or fertility awareness. Many people—both men and women—are reluctant to use condoms because direct skin-to-skin contact feels better. However, that thin rubber membrane may be all that stands between you and pregnancy or a variety of annoying or serious diseases. If you think of the entire body as being available for sexual stimulation, maybe covering up 1 percent of it isn't all that bad. Some people also worry that condoms cut down on sexual sensations and make it more difficult for a man to achieve orgasm. From a woman's perspective, many men ejaculate too readily anyway, so to somewhat delay the man's orgasm may be an advantage.

Condoms are often thought of as a "male-controlled" method, but actually, effective use of condoms requires the interest and willingness of both partners. Today, both men and women buy condoms and keep them in their backpacks or at the bedside for ready use. Because of low cost and wide availability, condoms are the most commonly used barrier method in the world. Condoms come in a variety of styles, different sizes, and with various aesthetic embellishments, with or without lubricants and/or spermicide.

In order to be effective, condoms must be used correctly. They should be unrolled along the shaft of the penis with a little space left at the tip to collect the ejaculate. Condoms may be lubricated or can be used with a variety of water-based lubricants (read the label), but they should *not* be used with petroleum-based lubricants such as Vaseline. When the penis is withdrawn after ejaculation, you or your partner should carefully hold the condom in place to insure that no sperm are spilled into the vagina. For pregnancy protection, condoms should be used for all vaginal insertions. (For STD protection, you may want to use them in other types of sex play as well, such as anal insertions.)

Because of rumors about a high breakage rate, many people believe that condoms are not all that effective. To counter these fears, the FDA has instituted more rigorous standards of testing, so breakage is minimal. Condoms that are old, or have been exposed to heat, may break more often. If you are worried about breakage, use two condoms at a time. Also, try to buy them in small quantities and at places where turnover is high, such as large discount drug stores. If a break occurs and you are aware of it, insert spermicidal cream or jelly into the vagina as soon as possible.

If you have a variety of sexual partners and vaginal or anal intercourse is a part of your sexual play, you should consider using condoms for each and every sexual session.

The Cervical Cap

According to women's health and sexuality advocate Rebecca Chalker, "The existence of the cervical cap is one of the best-kept secrets of the twentieth century." Here is an approach to birth control that is as safe and effective as the diaphragm but that offers a good measure of spontaneity and the convenience of the pill. In Europe there are a handful of cervical cap designs, but in the United States only one, the Prentif cavity-rim cervical cap made by Lamberts Ltd. of London, has been approved by the FDA for general use. The Prentif cervical cap has the appearance of a large thimble made of soft latex rubber. As described by Chalker in her book, *The Complete Cervical Cap Guide*, "a dollop of spermicide is placed in the dome, the cap rim is folded in half, tipped into the opening of the vagina, and guided with a finger to the back of the vaginal canal where it readily slips over the cervix (the neck of the uterus). The cap stays firmly in place by gripping the cervix and forming a strong suction, and provides a physical barrier to the sperm, while the spermicide affords an additional chemical barrier.

"Because it is smaller and more compact than the diaphragm, the Prentif has several distinct advantages. There is no large spring rim to press on sensitive vaginal walls, making it far more comfortable than the diaphragm. Thus, it can be left in place for longer than the diaphragm. The FDA recommends keeping the cap on for no more than 48 hours, but many women have reported keeping it in for three or four days with no problems. The cap stays snugly on the cervix, requiring no extra applications of spermicidal cream or jelly until it is removed. Consequently, it is not messy. Some women still prefer to use the cap more or less like a diaphragm, inserting it anywhere from a few minutes to a few hours before they anticipate having intercourse and removing it sometime the next day. Others keep it in for longer periods, and especially like the convenience of being able to keep it in over the weekend."

Because of the cap's obvious advantages, many practitioners who fit the cervical cap now see it as the first choice among barrier methods, and only recommend the diaphragm if you cannot be fitted with a cap.

"Unlike the diaphragm," Chalker notes, "the cervical cap, with its greater freedom from spermicide applications and other inconveniences, can be associated with a greater enjoyment of sexuality. Of course, as I mentioned earlier, there is no perfect available birth control solution, and the cervical cap is no exception to that rule. The most vexing drawback associated with cervical cap use in the United States is that not everyone can be fitted with the four available sizes." According to Chalker, about 80 percent of women *can* be fitted: "If one of the four sizes fits you just right, then the cervical cap may be an excellent solution. In rare cases the cervical cap may develop an odor when left in place too long. Soaking for twenty minutes in water with 10 percent household bleach usually kills odor-causing bacteria. A well-fitting cap may occasionally dislodge. If you have repeated dislodgments, see your practitioner to reevaluate your fit."

About 200,000 women in the United States and Canada have been fitted with the cervical cap, and more than 2,000 practitioners are scattered across North America. Chalker notes that several new cap models are now being studied and should be on the market before the end of the century. To find the nearest practitioner, call Cervical Caps, Ltd. at (408) 395-2100.

The Diaphragm

The diaphragm is considered a barrier method of birth control, but it is actually the spermicidal cream or jelly that is used with it that kills the sperm and prevents them from entering the cervix. The diaphragm is a shallow cup made of soft latex rubber, with a flexible rim that fits neatly into the palm of your hand. Once very popular, the diaphragm was overtaken in the early sixties by the heavy promotion and the flood of research dollars behind the pill. The diaphragm is made in a variety of sizes, ranging from two to four inches (50 to 100 mm) approximately, so that it may be fitted in accordance with the length of the vagina. When in place, one part of the rim is lodged behind the pubic bone, while the opposite part cups underneath the cervix in the back of the vagina.

The diaphragm with spermicide can be inserted up to six hours before vagina-penis contact. Between a teaspoonful and a tablespoonful of the spermicide is put into the shallow cup and then spread around, with a thin ribbon around the rim. Then squatting, sitting on the toilet, standing with one foot raised, or lying down with your knees bent, spread the lips of your vagina and insert the diaphragm into the upper vagina with the spermicide facing up. Then push the lower rim until the diaphragm locks into place. You should be able to feel the outline of your cervix with your finger through the rubber cup of the diaphragm.

The diaphragm should stay in place for at least six hours after intercourse to insure that most of the sperm are killed. The maximum amount of time the diaphragm should be left in is twenty-four hours. In the event you have repeated intercourse while the diaphragm is in place, it is necessary that you place more spermicidal jelly or cream into your vagina with an applicator each time, leaving the diaphragm itself in place.

The standard for fitting the diaphragm is to use the largest size that is comfortable. But what is comfortable in the doctor's office or clinic may not be after a few hours. If you are experiencing discomfort from the diaphragm, don't just put it in your drawer. Go back to your practitioner and ask for a smaller size. Then try using the smaller one, checking placement both before and after intercourse for a month or so. If the diaphragm will not remain in place, you should consider another method.

The New Our Bodies, Ourselves recommends that when you have your doctor, nurse-practitioner, or other women's health care provider fit you for a diaphragm, you want to make sure that you are correctly putting it in and taking it out by practicing doing so before leaving the practitioner's office, so that she or he can tell if you are doing it right. Alternatively, you can practice at home and then return to the practitioner's office with the diaphragm in place.

The diaphragm has few health risks. There is effectively no risk of it going farther inside than its correct position; if it pushes back against the rectum, it may be the wrong size. However, in addition to killing sperm, spermicide may also kill off the lactobacillus in the vagina that keep yeast under control. To help counteract this, between diaphragm uses, you can bathe the vagina with a solution of water and lactobacillus acidophilus (available at most health food stores) using a douche nozzle, a squirt bottle, or a plastic speculum. If a particular spermicide causes irritation either to your vagina or to your lover's penis, switching to a different brand may help.

About 20 percent of diaphragm users have occasional or recurrent bladder infections. This may be because the rim bruises the urethra and makes it more susceptible to infection, or because the spermicide alters the normal environment of the vagina and allows harmful bacteria to grow. If you are using the diaphragm and begin having recurrent bladder infections, you should look for a different method. If you have a prolapsed or otherwise displaced uterus, vaginal fistulas, or a protrusion of the bladder through the vaginal wall, the diaphragm will not be an option for you.

As with other barrier methods, the diaphragm is only effective if you use it consistently and correctly. Studies have shown that the diaphragm is between 89 and 98 percent effective for women who use it during every session of intercourse (except during the menstrual period). However, the effectiveness of the diaphragm can be increased to nearly 100 percent by combining its use with condoms or with fertility awareness.

Your partner should not be able to feel the diaphragm, but if he does, it is usually only an awareness that something is there. Of course, using the diaphragm in no way compromises your fertility, and all you have to do should you choose to become pregnant is stop using it.

Vaginal Contraceptive Film

Another well-kept contraceptive secret is vaginal contraceptive film or VCF. This one-inch square of material, which looks like plastic but turns into a viscous liquid after five to fifteen minutes in the vagina, is 28 percent nonoxynol-9, the sperm-killing ingredient in commercial spermicides. The film was designed to be used alone and seems to be about 85 to 90 percent effective when used that way, but most practitioners recommend that it be used with a cervical cap, diaphragm, or condom. Combining VCF with these barriers should increase their effectiveness to nearly 100 percent. Some people find the higher dose of nonoxynol-9—about three times as strong as regular spermicide—irritating. If this is so, you will probably have to stop using it. The other disadvantage of VCF is that it is somewhat expensive and not yet widely available in the United States. On the other hand, it is less messy than normal spermicidal cream or jelly and provides a stronger dose of spermicide. To find out where VCF is sold in your area, call Apothecus at (516) 624–8200.

The Pill

Birth control pills contain either a combination of synthetic estrogen and progesterone, or progesterone only. In the first part of the menstrual cycle, higher-than-normal estrogen levels prevent the release of follicle-stimulating hormone (FSH). The absence of this hormone, manufactured in the pituitary, prevents an egg from developing inside the ovary. In the second part of the cycle, higher levels of progesterone thicken cervical mucus and inhibit the cyclic buildup of the uterine lining. If an egg were to be released or sperm were to get through the cervical mucus, the uterine lining would be too thin to support an implanted pregnancy. The combination pills interfere with ovulation, thicken cervical mucus, and interfere with the buildup of the uterine lining. Progesterone-only pills, called mini-pills, only thicken cervical mucus and interfere with the buildup of the uterine lining.

In theory the pill is an elegant solution to the age-old problem of preventing unwanted pregnancies, and it has some positive aspects. Many women like the pill because its use can be completely separated from sex, and there is no mechanical barrier to be aware of during sexual activity. Because the pill suppresses the menstrual cycle, its takers often experience less painful menstrual cramps, fewer PMS symptoms, and lowered risk of anemia. Women with endometriosis may experience a decrease in pain and other symptoms, and those who have a tendency to develop ovarian cysts are less likely to do so. Studies also show a lower incidence of pelvic inflammatory disease caused by gonorrhea, as well as of cancer of the uterine lining (endometrial cancer) and ovarian cancer. *(See chapter 9, Endometriosis, and chapter 5, Cervical Dysplasia, Fibroids, and Reproductive System Cancers).*

But the pill, even in its present low-dose formulation, has some significant drawbacks. Higher-than-normal levels of hormones not only have the desired effect of preventing pregnancy but travel through the bloodstream and affect other organs that have nothing to do with contraception, often precipitating or exacerbating serious underlying conditions. In addition, synthetic hormones can affect mood or exacerbate a tendency toward depression. They may decrease the desire for sex or cause hair loss or fatigue, a bloated feeling, or weight gain over time. Some women don't experience any of these symptoms and enjoy the freedom from contraceptive jellies and devices, but others say that they simply don't feel like themselves.

The biggest problem that women have today with the pill is fear that it may promote the growth of cancer. Medical studies on this issue are conflicting, but too many studies do show an increased cancer risk to dismiss this issue. Some doctors are now, begrudgingly, acknowledging an increased risk among pill users—at least in certain subgroups of women, and especially among women who have a mother or sister who developed cancer.

About 10 million women in the United States use the pill at any one time, but from 30 to 50 percent stop using it within a year because of undesirable side effects.

In the 1960s and 1970s, high-dose pills caused serious problems for many women and are known to have caused a small number of deaths as well. But high doses equaled high effectiveness. The pill got a reputation for being 98 percent effective. Today, most women take the progesterone-only mini-pill, which is only about 96 percent effective in normal use. This is still quite acceptable in terms of effectiveness, but it's not really much better than condoms, the cervical cap, or the diaphragm when these barrier methods are used consistently. Failures with the mini-pills occur when women forget to take them or decide not to take them because they cease to be sexually active for a time. You can't just take one pill and be protected; it takes several weeks for the hormones to build up in your system.

Other failures occur because of fluctuations in women's normal hormone levels. You must take the mini-pill at the same time each day to get maximum protection. If you miss a day or two, double up on pills for at least two days. If you miss more than two days, you will really need to use some other method such as condoms or vaginal contraceptive film.

There are numerous caveats you need to be aware of if you take birth control pills. You absolutely should not take the pill if you have heart disease, severe varicose veins, serious circulatory problems, liver disease, or breast cancer. You should seriously consider using another method if you have diabetes, hypertension, gallbladder disease, depression, epilepsy, migraines, irregular periods, or sickle cell anemia—the trait or the disease. You should stop taking the pill if you are planning surgery or if you must have your leg in a cast. The pill may interfere with the absorption of certain vitamins—including B1, B2, B6, B12, C, E, and folic acid—and may alter carbohydrate metabolism. A woman with these conditions may take the mini-pill safely, but should only do so after thoughtful consultation with her doctor. If you smoke, the pill becomes far more risky for you.

CONTRACEPTIVE TECHNOLOGY, a leading family planning handbook, has devised an easily remembered acronym, ACHES, to help you be aware of the danger signs of the pill:

    A = abdominal pain (severe)
    C = chest pain (severe), cough, shortness of breath
    H = headache (severe), dizziness, weakness, numbness
    E = eye problems (vision loss or blurring), speech problems
    S = severe leg pain (calf or thigh)

If you experience any of these signs, call your doctor immediately.

Sterilization

Many people are surprised to learn that surgical sterilization—tying, clipping or cutting the egg (fallopian) tubes in women, or cutting the vas deferens in men—is the most widely used form of contraception both in the United States and in the world. About 15 million people—women and men—use this method.

Although parts of the body are surgically altered through discrete snips and sutures, sterilization is the ultimate in "hands-off" birth control. Once the snips have healed, you never have to think about birth control again—unless, that is, you want to have a baby. Reversal rates for surgical sterilization are around 25 percent, depending on the type of procedure. There is a relatively low rate of success of reversal, and studies have found that regret is not uncommon among women and men who have this procedure. Moreover, the surgery, which is not normally covered by insurance, may cost $15,000 or more. Once again, no available form of birth control is without its drawbacks.

In women, the surgery is most often done through a small incision below the belly button. The abdominal cavity is inflated with carbon or nitrous oxide, and a laparoscope is inserted through the incision to allow the surgeon to see and manipulate the egg tubes with various instruments. This surgery is usually done on an outpatient basis, and a light general anesthesia or spinal block is commonly used. Most women have some abdominal discomfort for one to three days and feel fully recovered within a week.

Hot News

Breast-feeding after the birth of one baby is a natural and effective means of preventing a second pregnancy, a number of recent studies have shown, for at least six months, and perhaps up to two years. Several herbal extracts show promise for more natural birth control than is offered by the pill; flavones extracted from the plant *Striga lutea* have demonstrated significant antifertility activity in rats and mice, and a herbal medicine based on *Vicoa indica* has prevented conception without side effects. The daily urine assay method of birth control seems effective with perfect use, but prone to high levels of failure with faulty use, according to one study. The bad news in recent research is about the birth control pill; study after study has linked the pill to breast and cervical cancer, heart disease, and strokes.

LACTATIONAL AMENORRHEA

Prolonged breast-feeding can result in infertility for 2 or more years. The unplanned pregnancy rate associated with lactational amenorrhea, for the first 6 months, is under 0.5 percent.

P. W. Howie, "Breast-feeding: A Natural Method for Child Spacing," *American Journal of Obstetrics and Gynecology* 165, no. 6, pt. 2 (December 1991): 1990–91.

Lactational amenorrhea is 98 percent effective provided: (a) babies are not fed supplements for 6 months; (b) after delivery, mothers are still amenorrheic; and (c) mothers are using breast-feeding in an informed manner as a contraceptive method.

K. L. Kennedy, "Contraceptive Efficacy of Lactational Amenorrhea," *Lancet* 339 (January 25, 1992): 257–60.

A study of 101 women shows that lactational amenorrhea is effective as a contraceptive up to 12 months postpartum whether or not babies get supplements. Less than 2 percent of the subjects became pregnant within the first 6 months, 7 percent in the first 12 months, and 13 percent after 24 months.

R. V. Short et al., "Contraceptive Effects of Extended Lactational Amenorrhea: Beyond the Bellagio Consensus," *Lancet* 337 (March 23, 1991): 715–17.

Lactational amenorrhea is 98 percent effective for the first six months if used in the traditional manner.

"Breast Feeding and Fertility," *Lancet* 335 (June 2, 1990): 1334–35.

OVULATION METHOD

The daily urine assay method of birth control has a first-year probability of failure of 3.4 percent with perfect use and 84.2 percent with imperfect use. In one study, 22.5 percent of the women became accidentally pregnant with typical use during the first year.

J. Trussell and L. Grummer-Strawn, "Further Analysis of Contraceptive Failure of the Ovulation Method," *American Journal of Obstetrics and Gynecology* 165 (December 1991): 2054–59.

Three hundred healthy women in a study used self-examination of cervical mucus, and 3,393 cycles were observed. Twenty-nine pregnancies were reported.

M. Y. Wang, [Use-Effectiveness of Natural Family Planning by Ovulation Method], *Chung Hua Fu Chan Ko Tsa Chih* 27, no. 5 (September 1992): 281–83, 316.

The Indian modified mucous method Prajanan Jagriti (Fertility Awakening) was evaluated in 3,000 women with over 24,700 cycles, over 10 months. Forty-two pregnancies resulted.

K. Dorairaj, "The Modified Mucous Method in India," *American Journal of Obstetrics and Gynecology* 165, pt. 2 (December 1991): 2066–67.

HERBS/PLANT EXTRACTS

In guinea pigs, yeuhchukene (10mg/kg body weight/day) reduced pregnancies by 40 percent.

M. Hammarstrom et al., "Yeuhchukene–An Indole Derivative Interacting with Guinea Pig Reproduction," *American Journal of Chinese Medicine* 18, no. 1–2 (1990): 1–4.

Acacetin and luteolin, flavones isolated from the plant *Striga lutea*, were administered orally to rats from days 1 to 4 of pregnancy. Results showed dose-dependent anti-implantation activity: one dose at 10 mg/kg body weight on day 1, 2, or 3 of pregnancy was 100 percent effective in preventing implantation.

S. P. Hiremath and S. H. Rao, "Antifertility Efficacy of the Plant *Striga Lutea* (Scrophulariacae) on Rats," *Contraception* 42, no. 4 (October 1990): 467–77.

Petroleum ether and chloroform extracts from *Striga lutea* show significant antifertility activity in mice.

S. P. Hiremath et al., "Antifertility Activity of *Striga Lutea*–Part I," *Indian Journal Physiol. Pharmacol.* 34, no. 1 (January 1990): 23–25.

Vicoa indica (Banjauri), at a dose of 15 g once a day for 3 days, for 3 cycles, showed antifertility activity without side effects.

K. Dhall et al., "Phase I and II Clinical Trials with *Vicoa Indica* (Banjauri), an Herbal Medicine, an Antifertility Agent," *Contraception* 37, no. 1 (January 1988): 75–84.

Over 200 extracts/fractions from 70 traditionally used Ethiopian plants were evaluated, with 33 percent showing anti-implantation activity.

B. Desta, "Ethiopian Traditional Herbal Drugs, Part III: Anti-Fertility Activity of 70 Medicinal Plants," *Journal of Ethnopharmacology* 44, no. 3 (December 1994): 199–209.

BIRTH CONTROL PILLS: RISKS

Risks of birth control pills can include cerebral arterial thrombosis, peripheral arterial thrombosis, cerebral embolism, pelvic vein thrombosis, pulmonary embolism, thrombosis of the sinus agittalis, recurrent pancreatitis, and focal nodular hyperplasia of the liver, according to a report.

C. Piper and B. Mathias, "Orale Kontrazeptiva: Unerwunschte Wirkungen im Bereich der Inneren Medizin" [Oral Contraceptives: Undesirable Effects in Internal Medicine], *Med. Klin.* 84, no. 5 (May 15, 1989): 227–35.

The risk of breast cancer associated with oral contraception depends upon how long the method is used. But even less than 3 months of use may increase the relative risk to 2.0. The risk of breast cancer before age 45 for less than 10 years of birth control pill use is 2.0; for 10 or more years, the risk estimate is 4.1.

D. R. Miller et al., "Breast Cancer before Age 45 and Oral Contraceptive Use: New Findings," *American Journal of Epidemiology* 129, no. 2 (February 1989): 269–80.

Evaluation of 163 very young breast cancer cases (age 32 or less) showed that oral contraception increases breast cancer risk. The relative risk is 2.2 at 6 years of use.

M. C. Pike et al., "Oral Contraceptive Use and Early Abortion as Risk Factors for Breast Cancer in Young Women," *British Journal of Cancer* 43, no. 1 (January 1981): 72-76.

The relative risk of breast cancer associated with birth control pills is not modified by pattern of use (or intermittent use); it depends, rather, on total duration of use.

C. E. Chilvers and S. J. Smith, "The Effect of Patterns of Oral Contraceptive Use on Breast Cancer Risk in Young Women: The UK National Case-Control Study Group," *British Journal of Cancer* 69, no. 5 (May 1994): 922–23.

If oral contraceptives are used before age 20, the risk of breast cancer at an early age increases.

M. A. Rookus and F. E. van Leeuwen, "Oral Contraceptives and Risk of Breast Cancer in Women Aged 20–54 Years: Netherlands Oral Contraceptives and Breast Cancer Study Group," *Lancet* 344, no. 8926 (September 24, 1994): 844–51.

Liver cancer has been linked to long-term use of oral contraceptives. The relative risk of primary liver cancer for those who have ever used the pill is 1.6; for long-term users (over 10 years), the odds ratio is 2.0.

A. W. Hsing et al., "Oral Contraceptives and Primary Liver Cancer Among Young Women," *Cancer Causes Control* 3, no. 1 (January 1992): 43-48.

A study found that, of 9 cases of hepatocellular carcinoma, 8 (89 percent) had used birth control pills. In comparison, 16 of 45 controls (36 percent) had used birth control pills.

J. R. Palmer et al., "Oral Contraceptive Use and Liver Cancer," *American Journal of Epidemiology* 130, no. 5 (November 1989): 878–82.

Heart disease has been shown linked to oral contraceptive use.

J. B. Croft et al., "Adverse Influences of Alcohol, Tobacco, and Oral Contraceptive Use on Cardiovascular Risk Factors during Transition to Adulthood," *American Journal of Epidemiology* 126, no. 2 (August 1987): 202–13.

Oral contraceptive use has been linked to high fibrinogen levels, a major cardiovascular risk factor. Sixty percent of young female patients in a study with angiographically confirmed stenoses and occlusion took oral contraceptives and showed no other risk factor.

W. Holtmann and G. Berger, "Uber die Bedeutung des Risikofators bei Zerebrovaskularen Prozessen unter Ovulationschemmer-Eiinnahme" [The Importance of Risk Factors in Cerebrovascular Processes While Taking Oral Contraceptives], *MMW Munch. Med. Wochenschr.* 119, no. 49 (December 2, 1977): 1557–60.

The risk of cerebral thromboembolic attacks has been linked to low doses of oral contraceptives. The progesterone-only pill did not increase risk, however.

O. Lidegaard, "Oral Contraception and Risk of a Cerebral Thromboembolic Attack: Results of a Case-Control Study," *British Medical Journal* 306, no. 6883 (April 10, 1993): 956–63.

The risk of venous and arterial thromboembolic episodes increases with estrogen dose.

T. W. Meade, "Risks and Mechanisms of Cardiovascular Events in Users of Oral Contraceptives," *American Journal of Obstet. Gynecol.* 158, no. 6, pt. 2 (June 1988): 1646–52.

Myocardial infarction risk has been linked to oral contraception.

J. Bonnar, "Coagulation Effects of Oral Contraception," *American Journal of Obstet. Gynecol.* 157, no. 4, pt. 2 (October 1987): 1042–48.

Women who had ever used oral contraceptives showed an increased risk of stroke and fatal stroke, all other factors being adjusted for.

P.C. Hannaford et al., "Oral Contraception and Stroke: Evidence from the Royal College of General Practitioners' Oral Contraception Study," *Stroke* 25, no. 5 (May 1994): 935–42.

Oral contraceptives increase stroke risk in young women, a study showed.

J. F. Brick and J. E. Riggs, "Ischemic Cerebrovascular Disease in the Young Adult: Emergence of Oral Contraceptive Use and Pregnancy as the Major Risk Factors in the 1980s," *W. V. Med. J.* 85, no. 1 (January 1989): 7–8.

Ischemic colitis is uncommon in the young. But oral contraceptive use increases the risk by a factor of 6, researchers found.

D. G. Deana and P. J. Dean, "Reversible Ischemic Colitis in Young Women: Association with Oral Contraceptive Use," *American Journal of Surg. Pathol.* 19, no. 4 (April 1995): 454–62.

Cervical ectopia and cervical infection by *C. trachomatis, Neisseria gonorrhoeae*, herpes simplex virus, and cytomegalovirus have all been linked to oral contraceptives.

C. W. Critchlow et al., "Determinants of Cervical Ectopia and of Cervicitis: Age, Oral Contraception, Specific Cervical Infection, Smoking, and Douching," *American Journal of Obstet. Gynecol.* 173, no. 2 (August 1995): 534–43.

Oral contraceptive use doubles the risk of adenocarcinoma of the cervix, and the risk increases with duration of use.

G. Ursin et al., "Oral Contraceptive Use and Adenocarcinoma of Cervix," *Lancet* 344, no. 8934 (November 19, 1994): 1390–94.

Use of the birth control pill increases the risk of cervical cancer by 21 percent, with further increased risk associated with longer duration of use.

L.A. Brinton et al., "Oral Contraceptive Use and Risk of Invasive Cervical Cancer," *International Journal of Epidemiology* 19, no. 1 (March 1990): 4–11.

Recurrent vulvovaginal candidiasis can be attributed to birth control use in 11–12 percent of the cases.

A. Spinillo et al., "The Impact of Oral Contraception on Vulvovaginal Candidiasis," *Contraception* 51, no. 5 (May 1995): 293–97.

Oral contraception—used after conception—increases the risk of the baby's having congenital urinary tract anomalies fivefold.

D. K. Li et al., "Oral Contraceptive Use After Conception in Relation to the Risk of Congenital Urinary Tract Anomalies," *Teratology* 51, no. 1 (January 1995): 30–36.

4. BREAST CANCER

Breast cancer is the most frequently occurring cancer in women. We see 182,000 new cases a year and 46,000 fatalities. In 1950, one in twenty females were diagnosed with the disease; today, the number has risen to one in eight.

Causes

Dr. Michael Schachter, a complementary physician from Rockland County, New York, describes some of the key factors in the development of the disease:

ESTROGEN. "Women whose menstrual periods start when they are relatively young have an increased risk for developing breast cancer, as do women who have a late menopause," explains Dr. Schachter. "This suggests that a woman who has a longer exposure to female sex hormones during her lifetime is at greater risk for developing breast cancer, and that estrogen, the female sex hormone that stimulates cell growth, may play a role in its formation. Women who have no children, and also women who have children but do not breast-feed, also have an increased risk. This suggests that the other female sex hormone, progesterone, may have a protective effect.

"Other known and accepted risk factors include an increased alcohol intake, a diet high in fat, being overweight, and a family history of breast cancer. Some of the reasons for this is that fat tissue can make estrogen, and alcohol tends to stimulate its production. In summary, most risk factors seem to be associated with increased lifetime exposure to estrogen, decreased lifetime exposure to progesterone, or a combination of the two.

"Estrogen and progesterone tend to balance each other in the body. Excessive estrogen or reduced progesterone may lead to a condition known as estrogen dominance. The symptoms of estrogen dominance include water retention, breast swelling, fibrocystic breasts, pre-menstrual mood swings and depression, loss of sex drive, heavy or irregular periods, uterine fibroids, craving for sweets, and fat deposition in the hips and thighs.

"Estrogen tends to be transformed into two major metabolites in the body. They can be called the good and the bad estrogen, just as there is the so-called good and bad cholesterol. The bad estrogen, known as 16-alphahydroxyestrone, favors the development of breast cancer, whereas 2-hydroxyestrone seems to protect against it. Certain chemicals stimulate the formation of one or the other."

XENOESTROGENS. "Now that we've seen that the role of estrogen is very important," Dr. Schachter continues, "this leads to a discussion of something called xenoestrogens. *Xeno* means foreign, and xenoestrogens are chemical substances that are foreign to the body, but behave like estrogens. These substances mimic estrogen's actions. Some xenoestrogens can reduce estrogen's effects. These varieties, which are rapidly degraded in the body, usually occur in plant foods such as soy, cauliflower, and broccoli. They protect against the development of breast cancer. Other xenoestrogens, typically synthetic ones, appear to stimulate cancer growth.

"We are living in the petrochemical era. This period began in the 1940s as a result of technological advances in the procurement of oil, and the manufacture of its products. In 1940 one billion pounds of synthetic chemicals were manufactured; by 1950 the amount had increased to fifty billion pounds; and by the late 1980s, 500 billion pounds of synthetic chemicals were being produced annually. Many of these compounds are toxic, mutagenic, and carcinogenic. The majority have not been adequately tested for toxicity, let alone for their environmental and ecological effects.

"Approximately 600 chemicals have been shown to be carcinogenic in well-designed, controlled, and validated animal experiments. And within the scientific community, the overwhelming consensus is that chemicals carcinogenic to animals are also carcinogenic to humans. In large-scale epidemiological human studies, approximately twenty-five chemicals have been proven carcinogenic. For each of these twenty-five chemicals, animal research established carcinogenicity one to three decades earlier, making the animal studies all the more significant.

"Many synthetic chemicals behave as these bad xenoestrogens, particularly pesticides, fuels, and plastics. They do so in various ways. Some enhance the production of the so-called bad estrogens that I mentioned earlier, and others bind to estrogen receptors, inducing them to issue unneeded signals to increase cellular growth. Xenoestrogens may enter the body through animal fat, as they tend to accumulate in fatty tissue and tend to concentrate as you go up in the food chain.

"Xenoestrogens tend to be synergistic so that a mixture of tiny amounts of many chemicals may have dire effects. As an example, at Mount Sinai, in New York City, Dr. Mary Wolf found that levels of DDE, a relative of DDT, were higher in 58 women who developed breast cancer compared to those who had not. At Laval University, 41 women who had estrogen-responsive breast cancers had higher concentrations of DDE. And in a 1990 study of breast cancer and pesticides in Israel, a strong relationship between the two was shown. In the 1970s Israeli women had one of the highest breast cancer mortality rates in the world, but in the ten years that followed a 1976 ban on several organochlorine-type pesticides, the incidence of breast cancer declined 20 percent, while it increased in all other industrial nations, strongly suggesting that the pesticides had a major causal effect on the development of breast cancer. Prior to the ban in Israel, some dairy products there had pesticide residues as high as 500 percent above U.S. levels, and residues in human milk were 800 times that level."

POOR LYMPHATIC DRAINAGE. Dr. Schachter describes the relationship between xenoestrogens and poor lymphatic drainage: "When xenoestrogens cause breast cancer, they do so by accumulating in the fatty tissues of the breast. It is the job of the lymphatic system to drain toxic substances from the tissues. Poor lymphatic drainage may therefore play a role in breast cancer formation.

"The lymphatic system is a specialized part of the circulatory system that functions as a central component of the immune system. It consists of fluid called lymph, derived from blood and tissue fluid. The lymph moves through the lymph vessels, called lymphatics, back into the bloodstream. Lymph contains cell debris, nutrients, waste products from the cells, hormones, toxins, and many other substances. It is the microenvironment of the cells. Lymph flow does not move along like the blood through the contraction of the heart, but is dependent upon other factors, such as muscle contraction that massages the outside of the lymphatic vessels, breathing, which pulls lymph along with each inhalation, pressure from the pulsation of the arteries, changes in posture, and passive compression of soft tissues. Therefore, it is very sensitive to constricting external pressure that can impede its flow.

"This leads to practical implications. It may be somewhat surprising to learn that bras may play some role in lymphatic blockage and in the development of breast cancer. Over 85 percent of lymph fluid flowing from the breast drains to the armpit lymph nodes. Most of the rest drains to the nodes around the breast bone. Bras and other tight clothing can impede this lymphatic flow, thereby trapping toxic chemicals in the breast. The nature of the bra, its tightness, and the amount of time it is worn influences the degree of blockage.

"This was popularized recently by Sydney Ross Singer, Ph.D., a medical anthropologist, with the publication of his book, *Dressed to Kill: The Link between Bras and Breast Cancer*. In this book Singer describes an epidemiological study that he carried out, which shows a very strong link. This study is similar to the early studies that showed a relationship between smoking and lung cancer. In fact, its results were even stronger. Women who wore bras more than twelve hours daily had a nineteen times greater chance of developing breast cancer than those who wore bras less than twelve hours a day. And women who never wore bras seemed to have an even greater protection against breast cancer.

"The message to women is to wear bras as little as possible, and when wearing them to choose one that is least constricting. When a woman does not wear a bra, lymph flow through the lymphatics in the breast will be less impeded, thus promoting removal of toxic chemicals from the tissues of the breast," Dr. Schachter concludes.

X-RAYS. John Gofman, M.D., Ph.D., and Professor Emeritus of Molecular and Cell Biology at the University of California, Berkeley, sounds the alarm on the harmful effects of x-rays in his book, *Preventing Breast Cancer*.

The effects of x-rays take years, even decades, to manifest, which is why orthodox medicine does not pay attention to this danger. Indeed, x-rays are standard practice for medical diagnosis and treatment. "The incubation time is what has led organized medicine exactly in the wrong direction," says Dr. Gofman. "In the first half of the twentieth century, medicine looked at treatments in this way. If you gave someone poison, the effects would be seen in weeks or months. They did not think in terms of years or decades. What we have learned about x-ray-induced cancer is that a very small proportion occur in the first few years after the x-rays are administered. But most of them take ten, twenty, even fifty years. Women with breast cancer, who are forty-five, fifty, or sixty, are thinking, 'Why me? I haven't done anything wrong.' What these women are not thinking about is what they were exposed to early in life. In the early 1940s, for example, pediatricians in New York City, Rochester, and the Pacific Northwest were giving children fluoroscopic examinations twelve times a year for the first two years of life as part of their well-baby examination. Fluoroscopy is far worse than x-rays because the beam is left on for a long time. This laid the foundation for the development of breast cancer, and other forms of cancer, later in life. If you really want to know the story about breast cancer today, you have to ask yourself, What happened thirty, forty and fifty years ago?"

It is not the radiation itself that persists but chromosomal damage, Dr. Gofman says: "Inside the nucleus of every one of our cells is a string of DNA organized into forty-six chromosomes. That's a treasure. Damage to your chromosomes is going to be there for the rest of your life."

Dr. Gofman bases his claims on well-documented research published in the 1960s and 1970s, as well as his own work. "Ian Mackenzie, a great Nova Scotia physician, discovered the relationship between breast cancer and medical x-rays when he studied women who had been in tuberculosis sanitoria, and who had received a treatment known as pneumothorax. This was a wonderful treatment that injected air into the chest cavity to rest the lung. It saved many lives. Unfortunately, during the course of treatment, these women were given 100, 200, or even more fluoroscopic exams to check whether the air had been placed in the lungs. Twenty to thirty years later, Mackenzie's work showed a twenty-fold increase in breast cancer in these women. His results were published in 1965 in the *British Journal of Cancer*.

"Many people doubted his findings, saying that if he was correct we would have seen breast cancer in Nagasaki and Hiroshima. Turns out nobody looked to see if this was the case. So one of the members of the Radiation Research Foundation looked, and found exactly what Mackenzie had found.

"Arthur Tamplin and I raised a flag in the *Lancet* by saying that the Wanabo and Mackenzie studies suggest that breast cancer is one of the easiest cancers to induce by radiation. Today, everybody who is anybody in medical science knows that breast cancer is related to ionizing radiation, such as medical x-rays.

"A couple of years ago, I tried to answer this question—not whether x-rays cause breast cancer, but what part of all breast cancers are being caused by x-rays? My estimate was about 75 percent. Everybody said, 'Oh, that's too high. It must be much lower.' Since that time, I've done much more extensive work, and I have changed my numbers from 75 percent to better than 90 percent. Moreover, I now have enough data on a variety of other cancers to say that most cancers, not just breast cancer, are caused by medical x-rays."

Whether Dr. Gofman is 100 percent right or just partly right, whether medical x-rays are a primary cause of breast cancer and other types of cancer, or merely an important secondary factor that until now has been ignored by our government and the medical establishment—in either case, women need to recognize the seriousness of the problem and to insist that radiation exposures be as minimal as possible.

"If you have a serious problem and you are told you need an x-ray, I don't want to stand in the way of your getting that x-ray," says Dr. Gofman. "But I want to be very sure that you are not getting a dose that is two, four, eight, or twenty times higher than is needed. I think there is room for at least a three- to four-fold reduction in dose, possibly even a ten-fold reduction. Every community should insist that their radiological facilities produce evidence that their dose is low. Mammography is a lesson in what you can do when you are pushed to the wall to do it. In the 1970s, radiologists were giving 2, 5 and 10 rads per mammogram. When they were told that this would cause more cancers than it helped cure, they went to work and got the dose down to 3/10 of a rad or less. That is a twenty- to fifty-fold reduction in dose. Getting the dose down further should be a major national priority. If we do that, we are going to bring about the single most significant reduction in cancer incidence in this country. That's real prevention."

HIGH-FAT DIET. Earlier, Dr. Schachter gave one explanation why fat can cause breast cancer. Here, Dr. Charles Simone, director of the Protective Cancer Institute in Lawrenceville, New Jersey, gives another reason why fats generate disease: "We know that fatty foods actually convert normal cells into problematic cells. Consuming high-fat foods, particularly unsaturated fats, increases free radical production, damaging the cell membrane. At this point, the damaged cell has two choices. It can die. That's fine, because if it dies you make another one. Or it can repair itself. In the repair process, a cell can go awry and metamorphosize into a cancer cell. So fats cause free radicals which damage cells, which in turn try to repair themselves, and transform themselves into cancer cells."

Additionally, Dr. Simone cites these other two factors as leading contributors: "We know that tobacco is the number two cause of cancer in our country, and the number two cause of breast cancer as well. Regarding alcohol, we know that two to three drinks per week is enough to confer a two- to three-fold risk of getting cancer of the breast independently of everything else. So the number one, two, and three causes of breast cancer—high-fat diet, smoking, and alcohol consumption—are totally within our control."

Symptoms

Initial symptoms of breast cancer include thickening, a lump in the breast, or dimpled skin. Later on there may be nipple discharge, pain, ulcers, and swollen lymph glands under the arms.

Once breast cancer is diagnosed, the prognosis depends on the course of the disease. Dr. Schachter explains: "The staging of the breast cancer involves the size of the cancer in the breast, whether or not it has spread or metastasized to regional lymph nodes, and whether or not it has metastasized to distant organs. The more lymph nodes involved and the greater the size of the tumor, the worse the prognosis. Stage zero is limited to the topmost layer, and the five-year survival rate is about 90 percent. In stage four, in which cancer has metastasized to lymph nodes above the collar bone or has distant metastases to organs such as the liver, lungs or brain, the five-year survival rate drops to 10 percent."

Clinical Experience

PREVENTION
While the possibility of a positive diagnosis for breast cancer is terrifying, it is empowering to know that there are steps to take to prevent the condition, that minimally invasive treatments are often beneficial, and that it is possible to avoid a recurrence.

Dr. Tori Hudson, a naturopathic physician in Portland, Oregon, says, "I believe that breast cancer is a preventable disease. Just look around the world. Women in our culture have one of the highest—if not the highest—incidences of breast cancer, while women in Japan have the lowest.

"The reason is diet. To make a big story simple to understand, cultures that have a vegetarian diet, or are closest to a vegetarian diet, have the least breast cancer. That's how it all pans out no matter how you look at it. This implies that cultures that eat less fat, and less animal fat, have the least amount of breast cancer. So the big picture is really clear. Eat a lot of vegetables, fruits, and whole grains and beans. Those foods provide protection."

Letha Hadady, a herbalist and educator in New York City, visited China to learn why Chinese women had such a low incidence of breast cancer as compared to American women and those in other Western nations. While diet was a big part of the picture, she learned that other factors came into play. In order to prevent breast cancer, Asians build immunity through diet, cleansing herbs, and the avoidance of pollution, stress, negative emotions, smoking, alcohol, and radiation: "They have much cleaner habits than we do." In addition, Hadady made this important discovery: "I found it quite interesting that breast cancer is considered a disease of melancholy in China. That feeling of heaviness in the chest leads to poor circulation and excess phlegm. This leads to two conclusions. Increase circulation and you have a better chance of prevention. And reduce phlegm. The easiest way to reduce phlegm is to stay away from foods like cheese, chocolate, fried foods, and milk. You will not find dairy in the diet in China. Their diet tends to be grains and greens."

In his book, *Breast Health: A Ten Point Prevention Program*, Dr. Simone outlines the following plan for optimal breast health:
Optimize nutrition.
Take antioxidant supplements.
Avoid tobacco.
Avoid alcohol.
Avoid estrogens.
Exercise.
Minimize stress.
Become spiritually involved.
Increase awareness of sexuality.
Get a good regular physical examination, starting at age thirty-five.

REEXAMINING CONVENTIONAL ASSUMPTIONS

When a diagnosis of breast cancer is made, minimally invasive therapy may be just as effective as more intrusive standard medical approaches, according to Dr.

Robert Atkins, a well-known advocate of holistic medicine: "Women develop a lump in their breast and appropriately have a mammogram or biopsy which leads to the diagnosis. At this point the trouble begins. The doctor gives the patient two choices: a mastectomy or a lumpectomy with radiation. A paper just published on this reported a third option that was every bit as good regarding survival rate and life expectancy. That was simply to do a lumpectomy without the radiation."

Dr. Atkins goes on to say that unbeknownst to women, after diagnosis and treatment, there is much a woman can do to regain total health: "The biggest fallacy of all is when doctors tell patients after therapy that they've done all they can do and there is nothing left to do. This ignores the whole concept that people can get healthier by enhancing all their internal systems to make sure that the neoplasia, the process of forming cancer, no longer takes place. In other words, cancer is not the tumor itself; cancer is a process.

"Once you know that, you can ask, 'What can nutrition do?' You learn that it can help in multiple ways. First and foremost, free radicals trigger the formation of cancer, and the recurrence of cancer. Nutritional antioxidants can help to slow down the formation of free radicals. Additionally, plant foods have antioxidant and immune-enhancing properties."

YOUR DIET AND OTHER NUTRITION-BASED APPROACHES

ANTIOXIDANTS. To prevent and reverse free radical damage to breast tissue, Dr. Steven Rachlin, an internist in Syosset, Long Island, has his cancer patients follow this daily protocol:

Emulsified vitamin A (up to 50,000 IU)
Beta carotene (up to 100 mg)
B1 (400 mg)
B6 (500 mg)
Folic acid (3,200 mcg)
Vitamin C (up to 5 g)
Coenzyme Q10 (270 mg)
Flaxseed oil (1 tbsp)
Cat's claw (1800 mg)
Melatonin (up to 10 mg)
Shark cartilage (1 mg per kg of patient's weight)
Pycnogenol (150 mg)
Essiac (several ounces)
Pancreatic digestive enzymes (up to 40 g)
Aloe vera juice (9–12 ounces)

MINERALS. Dr. Schachter adds that trace minerals play a vital role in the prevention of free radical damage: "The body contains certain antioxidant proteins, such as SOD (super oxide dismutase), which helps neutralize oxidatively induced free radicals. SOD requires three minerals, zinc, copper, and manganese, to function properly. Deficiencies of any one of these minerals may predispose to oxidation damage, with a resulting increase of susceptibility to breast cancer.

"Adequate amounts of calcium and magnesium are also important. Considerable evidence exists supporting the role of selenium in preventing and treating cancer. A dosage of 200 mg daily is safe, and large amounts may be given with monitoring. Chromium and molybdenum may be supplemented as well, and these are also important.

"Recently I have begun to use the whole range of trace minerals in colloidal form as a supplement. That's a liquid form where the minerals are bound to organic chemicals. We use about seventy different minerals. Many of these minerals are in trace amounts, and have already been shown to be essential, and are probably lacking in our synthetically fertilized soil. I believe these colloidal trace minerals will play an important role in bolstering the immune system."

DIET. As mentioned earlier, a diet that is largely vegetarian and low in fat, mainly consisting of whole fresh foods, such as vegetables, fruits, whole grains, nuts, and seeds, protects against breast cancer. In addition, certain foods are medicinal in their ability to protect against breast cancer. They include:

Soybeans, soy products, and lima beans. Isoflavones and phytoestrogens found in soybeans, soy products, and lima beans protect against cancer. The low incidence of breast cancer among Japanese women is largely attributed to the widespread use of soybeans.

Flax. The omega-3 fatty acids in flax seeds and oil protects against breast cancer.

Fish. Fish high in omega-3 include salmon, tuna, sardines, mackerel, and herring.

Cruciferous vegetables. Vegetables such as broccoli, cauliflower, and Brussels sprouts contain cancer-fighting substances.

Mushrooms. Reiki, shiitake, and maitake mushrooms have strong anticancer properties.

Hot, spicy foods, oily foods, and stimulants such as coffee, black tea, drugs, and alcohol should be avoided. Water should be pure, free from fluoride, chlorine, pesticides, and other synthetic chemicals. Many urban and suburban water supplies cannot be trusted and need filtering. As some filters remove chemicals and chlorine but not fluoride, a reverse-osmosis type of water purifier is recommended.

HERBS. Natural herbal substances are a veritable gold mine for protecting women against breast cancer. Some herbs to know about are listed below:

Carnivora (Venus' fly trap). This powerful herb is popular in Europe but less known in the United States. In Germany, it is even used to wipe out cancer that already exists.

Essiac. This is a Native American herbal combination that has a synergistic effect in putting an end to cancer and in its prevention.

Cat's claw. This formula is used by the Peruvian Indians for the prevention and treatment of cancer.

Evening primrose, borage, and black currant seed oils. All these supply gamma linolenic acid, known for its strong anticancer activity.

Xiao Yao Wan. This combination of digestive herbs increases circulation, builds blood, and breaks apart fibroids. The Chinese say it prevents breast cancer caused by phlegm and feelings of melancholy, which impede circulation to the chest. Xiao Yao Wan is available in Chinatowns throughout America.

Dandelion. Helps prevents cancer by breaking up phlegm and eliminating it from the system. Excess phlegm can turn into tumors.

Astragalus. A wonderful immune-strengthening herb that can be used in cancer prevention or as an adjunct to cancer treatments. Letha Hadady says, "It has worked wonders for my friends on chemotherapy who take this between sessions for strength." Add one teaspoon of astragalus powder to some pure water, and drink once or twice a day. Or try Astra-8, a combination of astragalus and other immune-strengthening remedies in capsule form, found in health food stores.

OTHER DETOXIFICATION THERAPIES

EXERCISE. Dr. Schachter notes, "Any activity that removes accumulated toxins in the breast reduces the chance of women developing breast cancer. Studies show that aerobic exercise is associated with decreased cancer risk, as exercise promotes lymphatic drainage and sweating helps remove toxins from the tissues.

"Although I am not aware of any direct studies showing reduction of breast cancer with a detoxification program using saunas and certain nutrients as done with the Hubbard method of detoxification," says Dr. Schachter, "I do know that this procedure has been clearly shown to reduce pesticides and other toxic chemicals in the bloodstream and in fat tissues. Since high levels of these substances increase the risk of breast cancer in women, reducing them with this detoxification method should help to reduce the risk of breast cancer to women."

MASSAGE. Lymphatic detoxification is aided by manual lymphatic drainage (MLD), a simple method of massage, using light, slow, rhythmic movements to stimulate the flow of lymph in the body. Massage therapist James Kresse notes that this is especially important for women suffering from lymphedema, a condition that often occurs after a mastectomy: "When our lymph nodes are not functioning properly, or have been irradiated or removed, an excessive accumulation of stagnant waste occurs. The lymph system becomes overloaded, thus forming lymphedema.

"MLD should be applied directly after surgery, rather than when a massive edema has formed. This will guard against any possibility of a blockage in the system or alleviate any that exists. Studies in Europe show that severed lymph vessels regenerate with constant MLD therapy. The therapy makes the scars from the mastectomy more subtle, which increases the mobility of the arm. It also lessens pain from surgery and the uncomfortable sensitivity that occurs." *(For more on MLD, see subsection "Lymphedema," below.)*

IMMUNOAUGMENTIVE THERAPY (IAT). In the 1950s, Dr. Burton and a team of researchers discovered IAT, a nontoxic, noninvasive method of controlling cancer by restoring the patient's own immune system. Although the therapy demonstrated success, Burton left the United States after medical politics prohibited him from practicing here. In 1977 he opened the Immunology Research Center in Freeport in the Grand Bahama Islands, where thousands receive treatment for the disease.

Since Dr. Burton's death, Dr. John Clement, an internationally respected cancer specialist who studied with Dr. Burton, heads the center. Dr. Clement gives an overview of how the treatment works: "The intellectual basis of the treatment is that many cancers can be controlled by restoring the competence of the patient's immune system, as the body's complex immune-fighting system may well be the first, best, as well as last line of defense against many cancers.

"The method we use is similar in any type of cancer we treat, although each patient has her treatment tailored to the results of her own blood test. We do not deal with toxic chemicals in any way. We assay the blood for the factors we believe are aiding the patient's own cancer. By identifying these factors, we are able to control them, put them back into balance, and hopefully destroy the patient's cancer."

Regarding breast cancer, Dr. Clement says: "We have had patients with breast cancer who have had no other treatment other than IAT for upward of twenty years who have no recurrence of disease. While we are still claiming only to control their cancer, you will see that to all intents and purposes, by any kind of medical description, they have been cured."

Dr. Clement reports less success with patients who come to him after extremely arduous chemotherapy and those with advanced cancer where there is a loss of bone marrow and fluid collection in the abdomen or pleural effusions in the lungs.

Addressing other forms of cancer that affect women, Dr. Clement states that IAT is often successful with cancer of the cervix if it is caught early, even after surgery. Additionally, lung cancer, which is becoming more widespread among women, and which is generally untreatable by conventional methods, can be more successfully treated with IAT. "We have a good measure of control with adenocarcinoma of the lung and with squamous cell carcinoma. If fluid is present, however, which indicates a more severe type of disease, very often we do not have much control. Nor do we have much luck with the type of cancer that is associated with smoking, the small-cell lung cancer. This is because small-cell lung cancer grows rapidly. Tumors will double in size in just thirty days. Our treatment does not work quickly enough to do these patients much good." As for ovarian cancer, Dr. Clement states, "We have been lucky. We have been able to control this cancer in people even after metastases and recurrences of the cancer following operations and chemotherapy."

WORKING WITH MIND/BODY CONNECTIONS. Exploration into the effects of outlooks and emotions on health and disease processes has opened up an exciting area of science, known as psychoneuroimmunology. Researchers have discovered that the mind, nervous system, and immune system interact with one another at the cellular level. When we feel joy, we enhance our healing mechanisms. Conversely, when we feel fear or hopelessness, we generate disease.

Dr. Carl Simonton, medical director of the Simonton Cancer Center in California and coauthor of *Getting Well Again* and *The Healing Journey*, is one of the early pioneers in this field. In the late 1960s, as a radiation oncologist, he noticed that emotional factors and patient attitudes influenced the course of treatment. His research led him to an extensive body of literature, where he learned that the three biggest mental influences on cancer are a tendency to respond to stressful situations with hopelessness, bottling up of emotions, and perceived lack of closeness to parents. This understanding prompted Dr. Simonton to look at the influence of counseling on the course of treatment. He discovered that survival times doubled, quality of life improved, and there was a better quality of death in association with counseling efforts.

Dr. Simonton firmly believes that emotions drive healing systems and that the imagination and standard counseling can be used to increase a patient's will to live: "The emphasis of our approach is to focus on what is right with the individual. We ask, What are the person's goals and aspirations? What are their main sources of inspiration and creativity? What is their sense of purpose and destiny? As people become clearer and more connected to these concepts, they rediscover a strong desire to live. That in turn enhances their inherent healing mechanisms.

"As we explore these areas, we begin to address those things that interfere with achieving these very important aims. One primary culprit is unhealthy beliefs.

To demonstrate this, I would like to give an example of a patient that I have worked with for over twenty years. This thirty-six-year-old woman came to me in 1976 with metastatic breast cancer that had spread to her ribs and spine. Her father was a physician, and her husband's family had run a retail store for three generations. She was involved in helping her husband run the family business.

"Her religious and spiritual life were important to her. It was a great source of strength. She wanted more time to be involved in religious administration and spiritual counseling. As she began to pursue these areas, her beliefs about how she should be the good daughter, the good wife, the good mother, came into play. These beliefs were all quite rigid, allowing virtually no freedom for her own creativity. Over time, we helped her to make a shift in these beliefs and behaviors, which was central to her recovery.

"She has been free of disease for fifteen years. Currently, she is weller than well and runs marathons. The family store burned down about ten years ago. Now she works primarily in church administration, doing religious and spiritual counseling, which is what she always wanted to do."

Dr. Simonton emphasizes that there is a relationship between all types of cancer and rigid thinking: "Here we tend to be controlled by beliefs about how we should be or have to be. That allows very little room for the expression of the spirit. Becoming aware of the direction that our life force wants to go is essential for renewing vitality and healing power. It becomes important to listen to the voice within and to develop ways of enhancing that. This takes practice."

Dr. Simonton says the way we use our imagination can mean the difference between success and failure in treatment: "In our imagination, we must think about the things we do for ourselves that are helpful. There are three areas that we need to look at: our beliefs about treatment, our beliefs about the body's ability to heal itself, and our beliefs about the disease itself. When a person is first diagnosed with cancer, if she shares the common cultural perspective, she believes that cancer is strong, that the body is weak, and that treatment is harsh. In keeping with these beliefs, a person is going to experience much in the way of undesirable side effects and less benefit. As we look at those beliefs, we find that they are not at all compatible with reality; cancer is a weak disease composed of weak cells. It is important to remind ourselves that our bodies have always been able to recognize and destroy cancer cells since before we were born. Shifting those images helps healing to occur."

Patient Stories

MARYLOU

I have always been interested in holistic medicine, and I was a great fan of Carlton Fredericks. In 1989, when I discovered a lump in my breast, I sought help directly from a holistic doctor, Dr. Robert Atkins. I went to him before any diagnosis because I knew that if I had to have surgery, I wanted to see someone who was open-minded to alternative therapies.

The lump was malignant, and I had a modified radical mastectomy. Fortunately, my lymph nodes were clean, but the tumor was not a hormonal tumor and it was a very aggressive one.

I started therapy with Dr. Atkins, consisting of a low-carbohydrate diet. That meant absolutely no caffeine, and no sugar of any kind. I was also on a program of vitamins and nutrients targeted to my specific problem. Once a week, I was given an intravenous drip of an anticancer formula developed by Dr. Atkins, which was largely vitamin C.

Soon after surgery, I had a problem. The tumor grew back into the incision. Both the surgeon and Dr. Atkins advised radiation, which I was given for five weeks. While I was undergoing radiation, I did the IV weekly, and it alleviated any side effects of the radiation. I wasn't tired, and I was able to work half-days.

A month or so after the radiation, the tumor came back again in the area of the incision, and again it was removed. I continued Dr. Atkins's therapy. That was almost seven years ago, and I haven't had a problem since. I am still on the diet and the vitamin program. The intervals between the IVs have been extended to two months.

There is no question in my mind that Dr. Atkins saved my life.

RITA

I got breast cancer ten years ago, when I was thirty-nine. I had conventional surgery but would not undergo chemotherapy or radiation. Since I had no positive node involvement and no metastases after surgery, I was told that I was fine and that there was nothing else to do. But because it was a very large tumor, and an aggressive one, I was concerned about it. Since I had been involved with natural medicine for a long time and pretty well educated in it, I started to search for ways to prevent the return of the cancer.

I discovered a lot of things. I went on a one-year program of injections of a formula that was mostly mistletoe. I had to get the prescription for the vials and send away to Switzerland for the formula. I injected myself with the herbal formula.

I did a lot of reading, and I took courses in Chinese herbology. I learned about several herbalists, and studied with Letha Hadady over the years. I took several workshops with her, where I learned about Chinese herbs and the whole philosophy of Asian medicine as well as the Ayurvedic and the Tibetan systems. Over the years, I have taken formulas of Chinese and Western herbs.

The results are difficult to show concretely. All I can tell you is that I don't have cancer and that ten years later, after having had a very aggressive kind of tumor, I am still fine.

I believe in natural medicine. I also believe very firmly that it is important to have a practitioner, to not use the local health food store as your medical advisor. Everybody has to be examined individually.

SUSAN

When I was forty-six, my doctor found tumors in my breasts and my uterus. He screamed at me to see a surgeon, but I refused. The reason I said no is because of what happened to one of my best girlfriends, Kimberly. Kimberly was thirty-four, beautiful, and very sensitive, with a wonderful husband and three stepchildren. She found a lump on her breast and went to the doctor. Her mammogram was negative but they did a biopsy anyway and found that it was cancerous. Three days later, she had her breast lopped off. That was followed up with lots of chemotherapy. Her hair fell out and she vomited twenty-four hours a day. She couldn't keep any food down. Then they did radiation and her skin burnt up and two of her ribs broke. Most people don't know how dangerous radiation is. I had seen enough. I wouldn't touch any of that medicine with a ten-foot pole.

I decided that I was going to try to heal myself using entirely natural means. By the way, I was already in a stage 4 situation, and my doctor had given me two months to live. So I had this deadline. I had to get well by February 15th.

Norman Cousins, who wrote a bestselling book about healing through laughter, says that a doctor shouldn't tell a patient that he or she is terminally ill. When you tell someone they are going to be dead in eighteen months, they die in exactly eighteen months. To counter that, I gave my immune system the opposite message. I had to get well in two months. Otherwise, I would lose my breasts, my uterus, and probably my house and my studio too because I don't have health insurance. I believe in giving yourself a deadline in a positive way, rather than in a negative way. Giving your body a positive deadline sets a healing situation in motion because. And of course, the brain is the main master of the immune system, so what you tell yourself will influence what happens to your body.

I got a lot of books out of the library. One said to eat brown rice. Another said to visualize. Still another said to do psychological work on yourself. I decided that I needed a whole program covering every single aspect of my life. I called my program MOTEP, Marathon Olympic Tumor Eradication Program. It's a funny title, but it shows how hard I worked on it.

First of all, I joined a Y and swam one mile per day. While I was swimming, I would incorporate Dr. Carl Simonton's visualization technique. I had used it before to get rid of a lump in my neck that I got from using acrylic paint. So I did have some experience at "self-lumpectomy," and this is what I was attempting to do.

I started to talk to myself in a very positive way, visualizing the tumors as shrinking and going away. This occurred during the Gulf War, so I would visualize a Scud missile actually hitting my breasts, and little white particles of the tumor floating into the water. I would actually see this. Then when I would take a sauna after the swim, I would visualize the tumor as actually melting.

All day I would invent these very aggressive visualizations. When you visualize, you don't want passive imagery, such as snowflakes or Tinkerbell sprinkles. Those are ineffective. You want to use very aggressive imagery: sharks eating your cancer, or Pacman, or Scud missiles hitting your tumor. It helps to believe that you can conquer this disease. So I believed 100 percent in my program.

My program also consisted of special foods based on the macrobiotic diet. I ate whole grains and fresh juices, vegetables and fruits, and some fish. No meat and no dairy products were included. I had lots of carrot juice because the beta carotene is very healing. I also meditated and chanted to get rid of stress.

There are two major points in my program. One is to detoxify the body and the other is to de-stress because your body cannot heal if you are full of heavy-duty anxiety. You want to calm your body down with meditation, chanting, and other spiritual activities, such as white-light meditation, in which you visualize a white light cleaning out your body.

I also got myself into group therapy because this has been shown to extend the lives of cancer patients. Furthermore, I healed my relationships. People in good relationships with social support are the ones who live the longest. So you want to mend your relationships or get out of them. If a relationship is destructive, you don't want to be in it. A woman in my group is going through a terrible divorce and she has breast cancer. She decided to go away to Puerto Rico to Ann Wigmore's healing place for awhile. I think that's the best thing she can do. She needs to get away from her stressful situation so that her body can heal.

I broke up with a boyfriend and turned him into a friend because he was causing me a lot of distress. He was going out with other women and bringing out feelings of jealousy and anger in me. I cleaned out all those negative emotions from my body.

One month later, my body went through a horrible healing reaction, called inflammatory breast cancer. My breasts turned bright red and hard as a rock, and my left arm was totally paralyzed. Unfortunately, inflammatory breast cancer is not recognized as a healing reaction. If a surgeon cuts the body at that time, the patient dies immediately from the trauma. Women need to support their bodies at this time. Then they have a great chance of living through it.

I continued with my program throughout my healing crisis. Three weeks later—this is one week before my appointment—I knew I had won the battle. My yellow-green hue disappeared and natural color came back to my cheeks. Two days later, both tumors were gone. This was five days before my appointment. My body responded to my deadline.

My doctor was shocked not to find any lumps. He examined my breasts three times to be sure. He looked for my uterine tumor, but that was gone too. He finally said that I should make a video about my experience. That's when I decided to write my book, *Keep Your Breasts: Preventing Breast Cancer the Natural Way.*

Women around the country are using this program to get well without subjecting themselves to surgery or drugs. And we have had outstanding results. One woman changed her mammogram results in only ten days from the time she told them to clear, and she was high-risk. Another woman dissolved a lump in only two weeks. Once you have the information, it's easier to utilize than if you have to look here and there and try to piece it together like I did.

Hot News

Substances that have shown promise in preventing or delaying the development of breast cancer in recent studies include alpha-linolenic acid; genistein, an estrogenic component of soy; a new vitamin D3 analog; iscador, a mistletoe (*Viscum album*) extract; and epigallocatechin gallate (EGCG), a substance found in green tea. Researchers have found a strong inverse association between breast cancer deaths and fish oil; in one study, fish oil supplemented with ferric citrate proved to significantly protect mice against the spread of tumors. *(See "From the Medical Literature," at the end of this chapter.)*

Fibrocystic Breast Disease

Causes

Fibrocystic breast disease is caused by overcongestion from foods that clog the system, such as wheat, dairy products, refined foods, and fats. Caffeinated products, such as coffee, tea, chocolate, and soft drinks, are hard on the body and add to the problem, as does a sluggish thyroid, which makes metabolism more difficult and leads to constipation, causing a buildup of toxins. Toxic accumulations worsen congestion and can manifest as breast lumps (cysts). Stress further accelerates the condition.

Symptoms

Fibrocystic breast disease shows up as single or multiple breast lumps. Cysts are usually harmless, but are related to a higher-than-normal chance of breast cancer later on. Mammograms determine whether or not breast lumps are benign.

Clinical Experience

DIET AND NUTRITION
A diet high in complex carbohydrates can make a difference; fruits, vegetables, grains, beans, and some fish are recommended. Red hot peppers, cayenne pepper, and regular or daikon radishes cut through mucus and help to eliminate breast lumps.

SUPPLEMENTS. These nutrients offer extra help when combined with a cleansing diet:
Antioxidants. Selenium, and vitamins A, C and E.
Magnesium. Magnesium cleanses by entering cells and forcing out excesses of calcium and other minerals.

Iodine drops. Iodine speeds up the metabolism of the thyroid gland. As the metabolism perks up, breast lumps tend to disappear. Iodine drops from seaweed can be obtained in the drugstore in a saturated solution of potassium iodide or Lugol solution. There is also an Edgar Cayce remedy called Atomodine. In addition, health food stores sell iodine drops as liquid kelp. Before using iodine, a thyroid blood test should be done to check for thyroid antibodies. This ensures that there is no thyroiditis, an inflammation of the thyroid gland.

HERBS. Herbalist Letha Hadady recommends the following plant remedies to break up congestion in the chest, and release phlegm and mucus from the system before they lead to more serious problems:

Xiao Yao Wan. This formula is a combination of digestive herbs that increase circulation, build blood, and break apart fibroids. Xiao Yao Wan is available in Chinatowns throughout America.

Dandelion. Dandelion tea or capsules can be taken everyday to break apart fibroids.

EXTERNAL TREATMENTS

CASTOR OIL PACKS. According to medical psychic Edgar Cayce, stimulating liver circulation ends constipation. Substances that clog the body and form breast lumps are then eliminated. To do this, rub castor oil on the skin over the liver. Cover with a towel, and place a heating pad over it. Do this for twenty minutes each day.

PEPPERMINT OIL. Rubbing peppermint oil on breast lumps diminishes them by stimulating circulation.

PHYTOLACA OIL AND HYDROTHERAPY. Joseph Pizzorno has found success with this combination

treatment: "We have a woman put a hot compress on her breast so that it gets real warm. She then covers the area with phytolaca oil. Following the application, she covers it with a cold pack. We combine herbal medicine with hydrotherapy to help the cysts drain out of the breasts. I use that treatment with a lot of women, and have had quite a good response."

COLON CLEANSING. *(See "Colon Cleansing" in chapter 1, Aging.)*

YOGA

Gary Ross, M.D., a family physician and certified yoga instructor from San Francisco, California recommends yoga poses, meditation, and breathing exercises for alleviating fibrocystic breast disease brought on by stress and a sluggish thyroid. These three postures increase blood flow to the thyroid and chest area:

Shoulder stand. On a mat or thick blanket, lie flat on your back. You may choose to place a rolled towel under your neck. Raise your legs over your head so that your body is in a U formation. Rest the elbows firmly on the floor and support the back with both hands. Adjust your body so that it is completely vertical. Then press the chin against the chest. Hold still as you breathe slowly, concentrating on the thyroid gland. You may only be able to do this for several seconds at first, but work up to one minute. To come down, lower the legs slowly toward the head. Then lower the back to the floor one vertebra at a time. When the back is on the floor, continue to lower the legs gradually until you are once again flat on your back. Do this once in the morning and once in the evening. For full benefit, follow with the fish pose.

Fish pose. Lie on your back. Legs can be straight or folded. If straight, place hands under buttocks, with palms down. Otherwise, hold onto crossed feet. Resting on the elbow, arch the chest and neck back. The head should be on the floor, but do not apply pressure there. Support should come from your elbows. Do not bend the neck too far back as that can impede circulation. Focusing on the thyroid, breathe deeply in this position, holding for 30 seconds.

Cobra. Lie face down, with elbows and palms down to the floor or mat and palms beneath the shoulders. With a smooth, gradual motion, raise the eyes upward, then the head, neck, and spine, one vertebra at a time. Allow the area below the hips to remain on the blanket. Hold the pose and then come out of it using reverse motions that are equally slow and gradual. Breathe in as you come into the posture, hold the breath while in the cobra, and breathe out when coming down.

In addition to these yoga *asanas*, Dr. Ross advocates deep breathing exercises for bringing more energy into the chest area. Visualization creates a mindset that helps lumps to disappear. Further, meditation creates spiritual and mental tranquility conducive to healing.

Patient Stories

DR. ROSS ON HIS PATIENTS

A 24-year-old woman came to me with benign breast lumps on one breast. She had had a life-long history of severe constipation, requiring laxatives and enemas. On top of that, she basically lived on muffins, breads, and coffee.

The first thing we did was take her off all caffeine. That included coffee, tea, chocolate, and soft drinks. To eliminate the congestion, we asked her to stop eating muffins and bread.

This was a start, but it didn't address her constipation problem. I investigated that further and found that she had a mild case of subclinical hypothyroidism. This means that her blood tests for thyroid function were normal, but clinically she felt sluggish and constipated, with slightly dry skin, and a low body temperature. This condition is crucial to correct; when thyroid function is low, the body is unable to metabolize excessive amounts of congesting foods. I put her on a low dose of natural thyroid. That, coupled with dietary changes, antioxidants, magnesium shots, and castor oil packs, absolutely changed her life. The breast cysts and constipation went away. Her energy picked up. It was absolutely amazing.

Another excellent case involves a 29-year-old woman who also had breast lumps. In her case, this related to stress, heavy caffeine intake, and smoking. Of course, I advised her to cut out the caffeine and smoking right away, which she did. And I had her rub peppermint oil onto the actual breast lumps to stimulate circulation. As circulation increases, the body decongests, and the lumps tend to go away, as they did in this case.

A third case is a 33-year-old woman who was under a lot of stress. In her case, what seemed to work best was a combination of yoga, meditation, and breathing exercises.

Are breast implants really a problem? Going by news reports, the woman without medical training is bound to be confused. One report attests to their safety, while the next one says they are terribly damaging. Dr. Vicki Hufnagel, a gynecological surgeon and activist for women's health rights, offers the following view based on cases she has seen and her reading of the literature:

"I have seen plenty of women with breast implants who are dancers, actresses, or models, and I have seen terrible, terrible results. I have seen deformed breasts, and I have seen women who are fatigued, depressed, and in pain. Where their skin was once soft and supple, it is now hard and wrinkled. They look like they have aged twenty years.

"We did blood studies of women with implants and found antigens to the silicone. All their immunological studies were abnormal. To my mind, many of these women are experiencing a silicone reaction. It is real, not a figment of crazy women's imaginations."

Dr. Hufnagel adds that all implants cause damage from silicone, even those using saline: "A lot of women say, 'I'm going to have a saline implant and it is going to be safe.' That's a myth. All implants made are made of silicone. Saline is put in a silicone holding capsule."

Fragments of silicone react with tissue, even when the capsule remains intact. Dr. Hufnagel learned this after operating on a patient to remove saline implants and sending tissue to pathology for an analysis: "This was big news, and I flew to Washington with it. Here a woman with a saline implant, without a rupture, without a leak, with silicone only being used to hold her saline, gets silicone in all of her chest wall tissue. I reported it to the FDA two years ago, and they have still taken no action."

Removing implants to reverse the problem has never been a simple option. Women who consider this choice are often talked out of it by surgeons who tell them that their breasts are too stretched out and that they will look terrible afterward. "Women are too scared to do anything about it," Dr. Hufnagel says. "They are afraid that they are going to look worse than they did before the implants were put in, which probably was fine to begin with. A lot of this image issue about having breast implants is probably due to social problems that we have in our society."

Indeed, once the implants are removed, women's breasts cave in and become grossly deformed. This sad state of affairs prompted Dr. Hufnagel to devise new surgical methods for restoring breast appearance during breast implant removal.

Surgical Procedures That Conserve Women's Breasts

Dr. Hufnagel's challenge was in figuring out how to take implants out without having breasts cave in. She reports success using an argon beam: "I asked myself, 'How do we shrink the dead space that has been created in a woman's body from tissue being pushed out?' I use the argon gas to send a heat-fiber type of electricity in a spraylike manner. This will not burn the body but it will shrink tissue. We take the whole chest wall, where this envelope is, and we shrink it. That prevents massive deformity.

"We operated on two small, thin women who had large implants in very small chests. Normally, they would have been deformed had we removed their implants. But we have had good outcomes. We really think we've hit on something.

"Also by using the argon beam, we are ablating the reactive tissue and allowing new healthy tissue to grow in its place. This is breakthrough surgery." Dr. Hufnagel adds that ending the need for such operations depends on psychological and sociological factors. "The silicone problem is going to be with us as long as women don't like themselves."

PREPARING FOR SURGERY. Before surgery, Dr. Hufnagel advises women to learn as much about silicone as they can, to get a complete diagnostic workup, including a silicone antibody test, and to follow a good vitamin program. "Surgery is stressful to go through, so build up your body," she advises. "Not too much vitamin C for the first two weeks, as it will increase scar formation. You want higher amounts of A and E. Avoid C until two weeks after surgery.

"Learn everything. Ask questions. Ask to look at pictures of women who have had their implants removed. If they don't remove the capsule, be sure that they at least biopsy it and submit it for tissue analysis to look for silicone.

"Finally, report your case to the FDA. Every case should be reported. That doesn't mean that the government is going to take action. But if we have enough people, someone someday may stick their nose in the file and find out, 'My goodness, after the FDA retracted their announcement on silicone, they got all of these reports and still did nothing.'"

Lymphedema

Lymphedema, a swelling of the limbs due to collecting lymph fluid, affects 1 percent of the U.S. population. Health practitioner James Kresse explains, "There are two types of lymphedema. The first is primary lymphostatic lymphedema, an inherent condition that predominantly affects women in their mid-thirties but which can manifest at birth or during adolescence. The second is more common, and frequently occurs in patients who have had mastectomies or the removal of malignant tumors. The large increase in the incidence of breast cancer and subsequent mastectomy operations is one of the major reasons for the rise in lymphedema today. Secondary lymphostatic lymphedema can occur from six months to three years after the initial surgery."

Symptoms

Lymphedema appears as a swelling or skin thickening of a limb. It is important to detect the condition early, and this can be done in several ways. Kresse advises, "Notice any jewelry becoming

tighter over a short period of time on the affected limb. Or squeeze the affected limb for ten seconds. If an indentation is noticed, notify your surgeon immediately. Or measure your arm with a cloth tape measure around your wrist and forearm. If you notice an increase in the circumference of your arm, call your surgeon right away."

Clinical Experience

MANUAL LYMPHATIC DRAINAGE (MLD)
Lymphatic detoxification is aided by manual lymphatic drainage, a simple method of massage, using light, slow, rhythmic movements to stimulate the flow of lymph in the body. "This type of therapy is very, very light," says Kresse. "It's almost feather-like. We're working on the parasympathetic nervous system. A regular massage stimulates the sympathetic nervous system. That is our fight or flight nerve. The parasympathetic nervous system is our night nerve, our rest and relax nerve. This is the nerve that lymph drainage affects in order to calm the patient down."

COMPRESSION BANDAGING

In addition to MLD, compression bandaging is used to apply pressure around the affected limb. Exercises performed with the bandage enhance muscular contractions that help with lymph flow.

LIFESTYLE CHANGES

Kresse states, "If lymphedema is not brought under control with a combination of MLD, specific exercises, and a no-protein/sodium diet, along with combined decongestive therapy or the use of pneumatic pump, the affected limb can swell to an unsightly size and become life-threatening.

"There are dos and don'ts that a person should be aware of. Just to mention a couple, as far as the dos are concerned, the person needs to practice meticulous skin care with the use of pH-balanced lotions and creams to protect the skin. Following a good nutritional program consisting of lots of fruits and vegetables is helpful. Salt and fatty foods should be eliminated, and protein intake limited. It is important to maintain an optimum weight, as obesity contributes to lymphedema. Exercise such as swimming, walking, and stretching is excellent. Incorporating deep diaphragmatic breathing techniques, along with specific exercises taught by an MLD therapist, is good. While sleeping, the patient can elevate the limb by tilting the mattress or by placing pillows under the arm. Antibiotic solutions should be carried at all times, for incidental cuts, scratches, or bites. Infection should be treated at the first sign.

"Precautions to take include not subjecting oneself to extreme temperature changes, such as hot tubs, saunas, steam baths, or other thermal treatments. Care must be taken when using instruments on the infected limb, such as the instruments used in manicures and pedicures. Pets must be watched to see that they don't scratch or bite. Blood pressure readings, injections, vaccinations, or acupuncture should be avoided on the infected arm. Constrictive clothing and jewelry should not be worn. Heavy prostheses can cause excess pressure on the infected limb. Care must be taken when cooking, gardening, or doing daily chores. Finally, heavy objects must not be lifted. This can cause a lymphedema right away or somewhere down the line."

Other therapies that help lymphatic conditions include rebound exercise, ozone therapy, enzyme therapy, colon hydrotherapy, deep breathing exercises, and a good vitamin and herbal program.

Patient Story

SUSAN

I had been overexposed to the sun and wound up with a severe toxic reaction. It was sun poisoning that went one step further and became lymphedema. Instead of just having blisters on the surface of the skin with lymphatic fluid in them, my lymphatic fluid was backed up. The lymph nodes weren't clearing them up, and it wasn't coming to the surface the way it should. So, I wound up with a severe case of lymphedema. My ankles were the size of my knees, and I couldn't really walk. I let myself get dehydrated because I couldn t even take going to the bathroom. It was the most horrible thing I ever encountered.

I finally dragged myself to the Healing Center after three or four days of agony. That's when I began alternative treatments. I had a vitamin infusion, using 75,000 mg of vitamin C. I had lymphatic massage and was prescribed homeopathic remedies. I was also prescribed huge amounts of bioflavonoids, as well as quercetin, essential fatty acids, and lecithin.

I also used magnets, which were great. Not only did they help the lymphatic drainage, but they freed me from pain. I applied those to my legs—first ceramic magnets, and afterward electro-magnets. These really helped with circulation and healing.

I had great relief and was once again able to walk normally instead of dragging my feet.

NUTRITION

A study of 121 breast cancer patients found that a low level of alpha-linolenic acid in the content of fatty breast tissue was associated with metastases. Based on these findings, the authors suggest supplementation with alpha-linolenic acid may prevent or delay the development of breast cancer.

P. Bougnoux et al., "Alpha-Linolenic Acid Content of Adipose Breast Tissue: A Host Determinant of Risk of Early Metastases in Breast Cancer," *British Journal of Cancer* 70 (1994): 330–34.

A study looked at diet as it related to the risk of breast cancer in two Chinese populations with one-fifth the rate of breast cancer of that in the United States. Results showed a strong inverse correlation between consumption of vitamin C, carotene, and crude fiber and breast cancer. Women from the one Chinese group who consumed the most fat and least crude fiber had a risk of breast cancer almost three times that of those consuming high-fiber, low-fat diets.

J. M. Yuan et al., "Diet and Breast Cancer in Shanghai and Tianjin, China," *British Journal of Cancer* 71 (1995): 1353–58.

Eating a lot of vegetables, fruits, and olive oil is associated with a decreased risk of breast cancer. High intake of margarine, on the other hand, was seen to significantly increase breast cancer risk.

A. Trichopoulou, "Consumption of Olive Oil and Specific Food Groups in Relation to Breast Cancer Risk in Greece," *Journal of the National Cancer Institute* 87, no. 2 (January 18, 1995): 110–16.

The National Breast Cancer Screening Study in Canada found that the risk of dying from breast cancer increased 50 percent for every 5 percent increase in energy taken from saturated fat. High vitamin C and beta carotene consumption were both shown to have a significant inverse association with breast cancer mortality.

M. Jain et al., "Premorbid Diet and the Prognosis of Women with Breast Cancer," *Journal of the National Cancer Institute* 86, no.18 (Sept. 21, 1994): 1390–97.

Citing numerous studies on the relationship between diet and breast cancer, a review article makes the following observations: Consumption of whole wheat and soybeans may reduce the risk of breast cancer due to their each containing estrogen-reducing substances. Low-fat and high-fiber diets may also reduce the risks. Additional plant foods believed to decrease the risk include orange oil, onions, garlic, green tea, and cruciferous vegetables. Carotenoid and retinoid supplements have also been shown to prevent breast cancer, including beta carotene, apocarotenal, and canthaxanthion.

"Foods that May Prevent Breast Cancer: Studies are Investigating Soybeans, Whole Wheat and Green Tea, Among Others," *Primary Care and Cancer* 14, no. 2 (February 1994): 10–11.

Two-thirds of all animal studies on the effects of genistein-containing soy materials on the risk of cancer yielded results showing the risk to be significantly reduced by the soy.

S. Barnes, "Effect of Genistein on In Vitro and In Vivo Models of Cancer," *Journal of Nutrition* 125 (1995): 777S–83S.

Animals treated with genistein, an estrogenic component of soy, had a reduced level of breast cancer compared with controls.

C. A. Lamartiniere et al., "Neonatal Genistein Chemoprevents Mammary Cancer," *Proceedings of the Society for Experimental Biology and Medicine* 208 (1995): 120–23.

High-risk breast cancer patients were given 90 mg of coenzyme Q10 as well as antioxidants and fatty acids. Of the 32 receiving the treatment, 6 experienced partial tumor regression. In 2 patients who increased their doses of coenzyme Q10 to above 300 mg, tumors completely disappeared in 1 to 3 months.

K. Lockwood et al., "Partial and Complete Regression of Breast Cancer in Patients in Relation to Dosage of Coenzyme Q10," *Biochem. Biophys. Res. Commun.* 199, no. 3 (March 30, 1994): 1504–8.

Vitamin D was shown to work against the proliferation of breast cancer cells in humans.

R.V. Brenner et al., "The Antiproliferative Effect of Vitamin D Analogs on MCF-Human Breast Cancer Cells," *Cancer Letter* 92, no. 1 (May 25, 1995): 77–82.

A study showed that a low intake of dietary fiber was significantly associated with breast cancer patients, compared to controls. Breast cancer was significantly associated with low intake of cereal products as well.

P. Van't Veer et al., "Dietary Fiber, Beta-Carotene and Breast Cancer: Results from a Case-Control Study," *International Journal of Cancer* 45, no. 5 (May 15, 1990): 825–28.

Mice were injected with human breast cancer cells, and some were fed diets containing fish oil supplemented with ferric citrate. Compared to the controls, these mice received significant protective effects against the spread of tumors.

W. E. Hardman et al., "A High Fish Oil Diet Supplemented with Ferric Citrate Safely Inhibits Primary and Metastatic Human Breast Carcinoma Growth in Nude Mice," *Proc. Annu. Meet. Am. Assoc. Cancer Res.* 36 (1993): 679.

A review of studies supports the idea that melatonin acts as the body's own antioxidant, and that it has anti-cancer effects.

J. Waalen, "Nighttime Light Studied as Possible Breast Cancer Risk," *Journal of the National Cancer Institute* 85, no. 21 (November 3, 1993): 1712–13.

A study examined the effects of diet on breast cancer risk, comparing 107 cases of the disease to controls. Significant associations were seen between high intake of meats, alcohol, and cheese and increased risk. Decreased risk was associated with consumption of green vegetables, cucumbers, onions, and pears.

F. Levi et al., "Dietary Factors and Breast Cancer Risk in Vaud, Switzerland," *Nutrition and Cancer* 19, no. 3 (1993): 327–35.

A study demonstrated the efficacy of a new vitamin D3 analog in inhibiting proliferation of breast cancer cells.

J. Abe et al., "A Novel Vitamin D3 Analog, 22-oxa-1,25-Dihydroxyvitamin D3, Inhibits the Growth of Human Breast Cancer in Vitro and in Vivo without Causing Hypercalcemia," *Endocrinology* 129, no. 2 (August 1991): 832–37.

Reducing total calories obtained from fat and increasing fiber comsumption to 25 to 30 grams a day can reduce the risk of breast cancer.

D. P. Rose, "Diet, Hormones and Cancer," *Annual Review of Public Health* 14 (1993): 1–17.

A study of 590 middle-aged women without breast cancer found that after 15 years of follow-up, those who subsequently developed the disease had consumed more of their total calories from fats, as well as more total calories in general, than those women not developing the disease.

E. Barrett-Conner and N. J. Friedlander, "Dietary Fat, Calories and the Risk of Breast Cancer in Postmenopausal Women: A Prospective Population-Based Study," *Journal of the American College of Nutrition* 12, no. 4 (1993): 390–99.

A reduced risk of breast cancer has been linked to the consumption of high amounts of fruits, vegetables, folic acid, vitamin C, carotenoids, and beans.

L. A. McKeown, "Diet High in Fruits and Vegetables Linked to Lower Breast Cancer Risk," *Medical Tribune* (July 9, 1992): 14.

Low vitamin A is a risk factor for breast cancer. Supplementation with retinol and carotenoids offers a protective effect.

D. J. Hunter, "Antioxidant Micronutrients and Breast Cancer," *Journal of the American College of Nutrition* 11, no. 5 (October 1992): 633.

In a study of Chinese women with breast cancer, consumption of high amounts of red meat and animal protein was associated with an increased risk of the disease in premenopausal women. Associated with a decreased risk: high intakes of polyunsaturated fatty acids, soy proteins and total soy products, and beta carotene.

H. P. Lee et al., "Dietary Effects on Breast Cancer Risk in Singapore," *Lancet* 337 (May 18, 1991): 1197–1200.

In reviewing 12 case-controlled studies on the relationship between breast cancer and diet, scientists conclude that saturated fat intake is a definite risk factor for postmenopausal women. Data showed high intake of fruits and vegetables to have a protective effect and that vitamin C had the strongest inverse association with the risk of breast cancer in women of all ages. Based on their findings, the authors argue that 24 percent of all breast cancers in postmenopausal women and 16 percent in premenopausal women could be prevented through dietary modification.

G. R. Howe et al., "Dietary Factors and the Risk of Breast Cancer: Combined Analysis of 12 Case-Controlled Studies," *Journal of the National Cancer Institute* 82 (1990): 561–69.

A review of the literature on the relationship between breast cancer deaths and fish oil consumption found a very strong inverse association.

L. Kaizer et al., "Fish Consumption and Breast Cancer Risk," *Nutrition and Cancer* 12 (1989): 61–68.

Vitamin E should be considered a chemopreventive agent for breast cancer, some researchers assert, due to its prevalence in healthy breast adipose tissue and its high concentration in breast secretions.

N. V. Dimitrov et al., "Some Aspects of Vitamin E Related to Humans and Breast Cancer Prevention," *Adv. Exp. Med. Bio.* 364 (1994): 119–27.

Consumption of green vegetables is significantly associated with a decreased risk of breast cancer.

C. LaVecchia et al., "Dietary Factors and the Risk of Breast Cancer," *Nutrition and Cancer* 10 (1987): 205–14.

An epidemiologic survey conducted in 21 countries found that, in women over 45, high dietary intake of sucrose appears to be a significant risk factor for breast cancer.

S. Seely and D. F. Horrobin, "Diet and Breast Cancer: The Possible Connection with Sugar Consumption," *Medical Hypotheses* 11, no. 3 (1983): 319–27.

Dietary sugar has been shown to be positively associated with an increased risk of mortality from breast cancer, while breast cancer mortality is negatively correlated with the consumption of complex carbohydrates.

K. K. Carroll, "Dietary Factors in Hormone-Dependent Cancers," in M. Winick (ed.), *Current Concepts in Nutrition*, vol. 6, *Nutrition and Cancer* (New York: John Wiley & Sons, 1992).

Data from epidemiological studies suggest that dietary fiber may have a protective role against the risk of breast cancer due to its influence on estrogen metabolism and excretion or because of the endocrine effects of the lignans.

D. P. Rose, "Dietary Fiber and Breast Cancer," *Nutrition and Cancer* 13, nos. 1 and 2 (1990): 1–8.

HERBS/PLANT EXTRACTS

The Greek herbal combination IBV-BK, Aristolochia, and Iska has been shown to have an anti-breast-cancer effect.

I. E. Voloudakis-Baltatzis et al., "Experimental Applications of Herbs of Greek Flora with Anticancer Properties in Breast Cancer in Vitro and in Rats in Vivo," *Anticancer Research* 12, no. 6A (1992): 1883–992.

A study examining the effects of a mistletoe extract on breast cancer patients found an immune-enhancing effect.

J. Beuth et al., "Vergleichende Untersuchungen zur Immunaktiven Wirkung von Galaktosid-Spezifischem Mistellektin. Reinsubstanz Gegen Standardisierten Extrakt" [Comparative Studies on the Immunoactive Action of Galactoside-Specific Mistletoe Lectin: Pure Substance Compared to the Standardized Extract], Arzneimittelforschung 43, no. 2 (February 1993): 166–69.

Iscador, a mistletoe (*Viscum album*) extract, was shown to have an anti-breast-cancer effect.

T. Hajto, "Immunomodulatory Effects of Iscador: A *Viscum Album* Preparation," *Oncology*, 43, supp1. (1986): 51-65.

Breast cancer patients in a study were administered a single infusion of iscador, an extract of mistletoe (*Viscum album*) intravenously. While immune response decreased significantly after 6 hours, it then significantly increased 24 hours later.

T. Hajto and C. Lanzrein, "Natural Killer and Antibody-Dependent Cell-Mediated Cytotoxicity Activities and Large Granular Lymphocyte Frequencies in *Viscum Album*-Treated Breast Cancer Patients," *Oncology* 43, no. 2 (1986): 93–97.

In a placebo-controlled study, the effects of a mistletoe preparation were examined in advanced breast cancer patients. Those receiving the treatment showed significantly higher white blood counts and leukocyte levels compared to controls following the fourth cycle of chemotherapy.

B. M. Heiny, [Adjuvant Treatment with Standardized Mistletoe Extract Reduces Leukopenia and Improves the Quality of Life of Patients with Advanced Carcinomas of the Breast Getting Palliative Chemotherapy], *Krebsmedizin* 12 (1991): 3–14.

The treatment of lymphocytes with an eleutherococcal preparation in vitro resulted in an immune-enhancing effect in breast cancer patients as well as in healthy controls.

V. I. Kupin and E. B. Polevaia, [Stimulation of the Immunological Reactivity of Cancer Patients by Eleuterococcus Extract], "Povyshenie Immunologicheskoi Reaktivnosti Onkologicheskikh Bol'nykhs Pomoshch'iu Ekstrakta Eleuterokokka," *Vopr. Onkol.* 32, no. 7 (1986): 21–26.

A case-controlled study found that ginseng consumption has a significant protective effect against cancer in humans, supporting previous results seen in animal studies. Ginseng powder and extract proved to be more effective than juice, tea, or freshly sliced ginseng.

T. K. Yun et al., "A Case-Control Study of Ginseng Intake and Cancer," *International Journal of Epidemiology* 19, no. 4 (1990): 871–76.

Administration of lentinan to advanced breast cancer patients resulted in lengthened survival times.

A. Kosada et al., "Effect of Lentinan Administration on Adrenalectomized Rats and Patients with Breast Cancer," *Gan to Kagaku Ryoho* 9, no. 8 (1982): 1474–81.

Coumarin was shown to inhibit tumor growth.

E. von Angerer et al., "Antitumor Activity of Coumarin in Prostate and Mammary Cancer Models," *Journal of Cancer Research and Clinical Oncology* 120, suppl. (1994): S14–S16.

Results of a study suggest that garlic possesses anticancer effects, acting on tumor cell metabolism by inhibiting the initiation and promotion phases of cancer and by modulating immune response in the host.

B. Lau et al., "*Allium Sativum* (Garlic) and Cancer Prevention," *Nutrition Research* 10 (1990): 937–48.

Numerous studies provide evidence of the anticarcinogenic properties of green tea. Epigallocatechin gallate (EGCG) is singled out as being the main physiologically active polyphenol in green tea, which is most likely responsible for such effects.

A. Komori et al., "Anticarcinogenic Activity of Green Tea Polyphenols," *Japanese Journal of Clinical Oncology* 23, no. 3 (1993): 186–90.

Pure lapachol given in daily doses to 9 patients with various cancers was shown to reduce pain and shrink tumors in all patients, with complete remissions occurring in 3 patients.

C. F. Santana et al., "Preliminary Observations with the Use of Lapachol in Human Patients Bearing Malignant Neoplasms," *Revista do Instituto de Antibiotics* 20 (1980/81): 61–68.

Taxol and cisplatin, given together, may be useful for the management of breast cancer.

S. Kodali et al., "Taxol and Cisplatin Inhibit Proliferation of T47D Human Breast Cancer Cells," *Biochemical and Biophysical Research Communications* 202, no. 3 (August 15, 1994): 1413–19.

Taxol was administered intravenously continuously for 24 hours every 21 days to 28 breast cancer patients who had not received prior chemotherapy. Results showed objective responses in 16 of the patients, 3 of them being complete reponses and 13 partial responses.

B. S. Reichman et al., "Paclitaxel and Recombinant Human Granulocyte Colony-Stimulating Factor as Initial Chemotherapy for Metastatic Breast Cancer," *Journal of Clinical Oncology* 11, no. 10 (October 1993): 1946–51.

EXERCISE

Researchers found that women exercising at least 4 hours per week had a risk of breast cancer almost 60 percent lower than women who did not exercise.

B. Jancin, "Exercise Study May Point to Hormones as the Breast Cancer Culprit," *Family Practice News* (November 1, 1994): 5.

A study of newly diagnosed cases of breast cancer found that the average number of hours spent exercising per week from menarche up to a year before diagnosis was a significant predictor of breast cancer risk reduction. Women who exercise 3.8 hours or more a week had an odds ratio of breast cancer of 0.42 relative to those women who did not exercise.

L. Bernstein et al., "Physical Exercise and Reduced Risk of Breast Cancer in Young Women," *Journal of the National Cancer Institute* 86, no. 18 (1993): 1403–8.

TRADITIONAL CHINESE MEDICINE

Breast cancer patients treated with the traditional Chinese medicine *Juzentaiho-to* (JTT) experienced lowered rates of bone marrow suppression from chemotherapy.

I. Adachi and T. Watanabe, [Role of Supporting Therapy of *Juzentaiho-to* (JTT) in Advanced Breast Cancer Patients], *Gan To Kagaku Ryoho* 16, no. 4, pt. 2-2 (April 1989): 1538–43.

ACUPUNCTURE

Cancer patients suffering from late-onset radiation injuries of soft tissues and skin were treated with acupuncture, which was shown to improve lymph flow and to be beneficial for patients experiencing edema and pain as a result of these injuries.

M. S. Bardychev et al., [Acupuncture in Edema of the Extremities Following Radiation or Combination Therapy of Cancer of the Breast and Uterus], *Vopr. Onkol.* 34, no. 3 (1988): 319–22.

BIOFEEDBACK

Thirteen breast cancer patients who had recovered from modified radical mastectomies received relaxation, guided imagery, and biofeedback training. The treatment produced significant immune-enhancing effects when these patients were compared to controls.

B. L. Gruber et al., "Immunological Responses of Breast Cancer Patients to Behavioral Interventions," *Biofeedback Self Regulation* 18, no. 1 (March 1993): 1–22.

MASSAGE

Six breast cancer patients recovering from radiotherapy reported less symptom distress, higher degrees of tranquility and vitality, and less tension and fatigue following treatment with gentle back massage, relative to controls.

S. Sims,"Slow Stroke Back Massage for Cancer Patients," *Nursing Times* 82, no. 13 (1986): 47–50.

HYPNOSIS

In a study of women with breast cancer, subjects were treated in group therapy with or without hypnosis as a means of coping with the stress and pain resulting from the cancer. Both approaches provided significant positive results relative to controls; however, the hypnosis patients experienced the greatest amount of pain reduction and the greatest improvements in mood.

D. Spiegel and J. R. Bloom,"Group Therapy and Hypnosis Reduce Metastatic Breast Carcinoma Pain," *Psychosomatic Medicine* 45 (1983): 333–39.

RELAXATION

A study provided evidence supporting the use of cognitive-behavior interventions involving relaxation and visualization techniques as a means of coping with the physical pain and distress that accompanies metastatic breast cancer.

D. Arathuzik, "Effects of Cognitive-Behavioral Strategies on Pain in Cancer Patients," *Cancer Nursing* 17 no. 3, (1994): 207–14.

RISK FACTORS

Having menstrual cycles of extreme length at ages 25–29 increases a woman's breast cancer risk twofold. Women with less than 150 or more than 350 cumulative cycles have an increased risk as well.

E. Whelan et al., "Menstrual Cycle Patterns and Risk of Breast Cancer," *American Journal of Epidemiology* 140, no.12 (1994): 1081–90.

A review article on the risks of breast cancer argues that 55 percent of cases can be explained by recognized risk factors, and identifies the following as examples: socioeconomic status, reproductive behavior, familial susceptibility, and menstrual characteristics. The authors also make the following observations: breast-feeding may reduce the risk, as might physical activity and increased consumption of vitamins A, C, E, and fiber. Oral contraception appears to be a risk factor for early onset of the disease. A 50 to 80 percent increased risk has been documented in those using menopausal estrogens.

L. A. Brinton, "Ways that Women May Possibly Reduce Their Risk of Breast Cancer," *Journal of the National Cancer Institute* 86, no.18 (Sept. 21, 1994): 1371–72.

A case-control study on newly diagnosed breast cancer cases in women between the ages of 40 and 85 found a significant inverse association between breast-feeding and the risk of the disease.

J. L. Freudenheim et al., "Exposure to Breast Milk in Infancy and the Risk of Breast Cancer," *Epidemiology* 5 (1994): 324–31.

There is a significant inverse association between the risk of breast cancer and age of first lactation in premenopausal women. Increasing duration of lactation was also significantly associated with a decreased risk in premenopausal women.

P. A. Newcomb, "Lactation and a Reduced Risk of Premenopausal Breast Cancer," *New England Journal of Medicine* 330, no. 2 (January 13, 1994): 81–87.

MAMMOGRAMS

The advent of mammagragraphy is leading to overtreatment of ductal carcinoma in situ (DCIS), some researchers feel. Most of these milk-duct cancers are too small to be felt, and show up only on x-rays. Because more are being found through mammography, thousands of women undergo mastectomies every year after being diagnosed with DCIS. The problem is that a lot of these cancers, if left alone, would never progress to a dangerous stage; in a previous study of milk-duct cancers that went untreated, only 7 out of 25 progressed to invasive cancer within a decade. Also, this type of tumor is quite common: 6 to 18 percent of women who die of causes other than breast cancer are discovered, upon autopsy, to have DCIS. More research is needed to distinguish between harmless and life-threatening tumors.

V. L. Ernster et al., *Journal of the American Medical Association,* March 27, 1996.

A study showed that 99.85 percent of premenopausal women screened by mammography obtain no benefit from the screening.

M. Shaffer, "Breast Cancer Screening under 50 Called Opportunistic and Immoral," *Medical Tribune* (March 26, 1992): 4.

To prevent or postpone 1 breast cancer death, 5,000 women had to be screened in a New York HIP trial. Also, the risks of false positives and unnecessary surgery have to be taken into account.

P. Skrabanek, "Mass Mammography: The Time for Reappraisal," *International Journal of Technological Assessment Health Care* 5, no. 3 (1989): 423–30.

U.S. breast cancer detection study results: Ten-year survival rates were not significantly higher when mammograms detected tumors rather than when physical examinations or a combination of mammograms and physical exams detected the tumors.

I. Mittra, "Breast Screening: The Case for Physical Examination without Mammography," *Lancet* 343 (February 5, 1994): 342.

Thirteen studies showed no reduction in breast cancer mortality in women getting mammograms from ages 40 to 49 after 10- to 12-year follow-up.
K. Kerlikowskie et al., *JAMA* 273, no. 2 (January 11, 1995): 149–54.

Mammography, especially in younger women, may result in radiation-induced cancer; the sensitivity of young women's breast tissue makes radiation-induced cancer more likely in this group. Three hundred thousand women screened annually between age 40 and 50 received x-ray doses high enough to increase breast cancer risk by 20-30 percent.
S. Epstein, "The Cancer Establishment," *International Journal of Health Services* 22, no. 4 (1989): 747–49.

Based on National Institutes of Health data (in 1986), from 150 to 1000 radiogenic (radiation-induced) breast cancers may be expected from screening 1 million women annually after age 40. The projected number of radiogenic breast cancers varied depending on the mammographic system and the screening schedule used.
J. K. Gohaga et al., "Radiogenic Breast Cancer Effects of Mammographic Screening," *Journal of the National Cancer Institute* 77, no. 1 (July 1986): 71–76.

A study reported that mammography combined with physical exams found 3,500 cancers, 42 percent of which could not be detected by physical exam. However, 31 percent of the tumors were noninfiltrating cancer. Since the course of breast cancer is long, the time difference in cancer detected through mammography may not be a benefit in terms of survival.
I. Mittra, "Breast Screening: The Case for Physical Examination without Mammography," *Lancet* 343 (February 5, 1994): 342.

PHYSICAL BREAST EXAMS

Women who have discovered benign lumps through self-exam are 3 times more likely to stop performing self-exams than those who never found a lump. On the other hand, women who had the lump discovered by a physician, nurse, or mammogram are two times more likely to start doing self-exams than women who never had a lump.
"Discovery of Breast Lump May Stop Exams," *American Medical News* 33, no. 4 (October 26, 1990): 18.

A survey of 302 women over 35 showed that 40 percent do not perform self-exams. Sixty-five percent of women who do not perform self-exams think a yearly mammogram or breast exam by a doctor is enough.
"Women Uncertain about Mammograms and Breast Health," *Cancer Biotechnology Weekly* (July 3, 1995): 4.

BREAST SURGERY

Breast-conserving surgery is just as effective as modified radical mastectomy for T1 breast cancers. However, a review of the Colorado Central Cancer Registry records over 5 years shows that 72 percent of T1 breast cancer patients in Colorado chose modified radical mastectomies. The reason appears to be surgeon bias.
B. Tarbox et al., "Are Modified Radical Mastectomies Done for T1 Breast Cancers Because of Surgeon's Advice or Patient's Choice?" *American Journal of Surgery* 164, no. 5 (November 1992): 417.

From 1977 to 1990, Dr. Roger Poisson falsified lumpectomy research data. His results were part of the research that in 1985 led to the acceptance of the effectiveness of lumpectomies for early stages of breast cancer. However, Poisson's falsification does not undermine the value of lumpectomies since—even if his data are not considered—the remaining data support the current acceptance of lumpectomies.
R. A. Badwe et al., "Timing of Surgery During Menstrual Cycle and Survival of Premenopausal Women with Operable Breast Cancer," *Lancet* 337 (1992): 1261.

The best time for surgery may be the middle of the menstrual cycle. The results of a 12-year study of 44 women who had breast surgery shows that those who had operations between 7 and 20 days after the start of their last period were four times less likely to have cancer reoccur in comparison to those who had surgery at the very end or beginning of the menstrual cycle. Progesterone levels are high and estrogen levels low at the beginning and end of the menstrual cycle, and studies have shown that cancer cells grow faster at those levels.

"Timing Is Everything in Breast Cancer Operations," *Edell Health Letter* 9, no. 3 (March 1990): 7.

A study of 249 women who had breast cancer surgery showed 10-year survival rates of 54 percent for those whose last menstrual period was 12 days before surgery and 84 percent for those whose last menstrual period was either 0 to 2 days or 13 to 32 days before surgery.

R. A. Badwe et al., "Timing of Surgery during Menstrual Cycle and Survival of Premenopausal Women with Operable Breast Cancer," *Lancet* 337 (1992): 1261.

5. CERVICAL DYSPLASIA, FIBROIDS, and REPRODUCTIVE SYSTEM CANCERS

CERVICAL DYSPLASIA

Cervical dysplasia is an abnormal growth of cervical tissue caused by the sexually transmitted human papilloma virus (HPV), the same virus that is responsible for cervicitis, genital warts, and possibly cervical cancer. These conditions can be detected with a Pap smear.

Causes

The likelihood of a woman contracting cervical dysplasia increases with intercourse at an early age, having unprotected sex with several male partners, smoking, birth control pills, and weak immunity. Dr. Tori Hudson explains, "Women who have intercourse at an early age are more vulnerable to getting genital warts and cervical dysplasia because the cells of the cervix at that age are more susceptible to being infected by the virus.

"Smoking is the biggest factor in acquiring cervical dysplasia and cervical cancer. If you smoke, and you are exposed to the virus, you are much more likely to develop dysplasia, and you are much more likely to develop cervical cancer from your dysplasia. We know that the nicotine itself actually lodges in the glands of the cells of the cervix. When exposed to the virus, the DNA can change to take on more abnormal features. If you have genital warts and you smoke, it is much more likely that they will turn cancerous as well.

"Oral contraceptives are known for creating a folic acid deficiency, and folic acid deficiency is associated with acquiring cervical dysplasia, and having the disease progress to cancer."

Symptoms

Dr. Hudson describes cervical dysplasia as a progressive syndrome that develops over time: "After initial exposure to the virus, there is no indication that anything has changed. Later, immune changes may occur. Warty tissue may develop, then mild dysplasia, moderate dysplasia, severe dysplasia, carcinoma in situ, and then invasive cancer." Since these symptoms are not evident upon physical examination, Pap smears are necessary.

Clinical Experience

PREVENTION

Since HPV is sexually transmitted, the conditions associated with it are preventable. Notes Dr. Hudson, "Cervical dysplasia, genital warts, and cervical cancer are all sexually transmitted diseases. That should make an impression on all of us, because it really dictates how we should protect ourselves.

"Obviously, we shouldn't smoke. We should protect ourselves by having safe sex and a healthy immune system. If you take birth control pills, it is advisable to take folic acid. A good maintenance dose would be 800 mcg daily. Those are the main ways to protect against cervical dysplasia and genital warts." Additional preventive daily supplementation may include 1,000 mg vitamin C and 25,000 units of beta carotene.

To catch the condition early, Dr. Hudson stresses yearly Pap smear exams. Statistics show that the longer women wait between Pap smears, the higher the incidence of cervical dysplasia and cervical cancer.

DIAGNOSIS

Before treatment, it is essential to get fully diagnosed to determine the stage of the illness. If a woman has an abnormal Pap smear, her partner needs to be examined by a urologist for warty tissue. Otherwise, they will be passing the virus back and forth and reinfecting each other. Diagnosis by a licensed, well-trained, alternative practitioner will determine if a woman is a candidate for natural treatments only or whether she needs to integrate these approaches with conventional methods.

CONVENTIONAL TREATMENTS

Conventional medicine usually does nothing to treat mild dysplasias and genital warts. "Basically, they wait to see if it gets worse," says Dr. Hudson. "Often the body can reverse mildly abnormal states to normal on its own, as the body has an extraordinary ability to heal itself. But when it can't, then the disease progresses, and the downside of waiting becomes apparent."

In the later stages, aggressive measures may be taken. The preferred conventional treatment is known as LEEP (loop excisional electrosurgical procedure), which uses an electrical wire to cut out abnormal tissue. This is less expensive and less traumatic than the method of treatment previously used, called cone biopsy or conization. In advanced disease states, a hysterectomy may be needed to save a woman's life.

NATUROPATHIC TREATMENTS

Women with cervical dysplasia often have excellent results using naturopathic approaches. Dr. Hudson notes, "In the results of a research study that I conducted at the College of Naturopathic Medicine in Portland, we treated forty-three women with varying degrees of cervical dysplasia. Through my treatment protocol, thirty-eight of the forty-three reverted to normal, three partially improved, and two had no change, meaning they didn't get better and they didn't get worse."

Dr. Hudson's protocol consists of three parts: systemic, local, and constitutional treatment. An overview of her therapy is outlined below:

SYSTEMIC TREATMENT

Beta carotene. 150,000 IU daily.
Vitamin C. 3,000–6,000 mg daily.
Folic acid. 2.5–10 mg daily.
Note: High doses of folic acid must be prescribed by a naturopathic physician. After three months, the amount of folic acid is decreased.
Immune herbal formulation

LOCAL TREATMENT

Vitamin A suppositories
Herbal suppositories

CONSTITUTIONAL TREATMENT

Dietary changes
Use of condoms
Avoidance of smoking
An optimal immunity diet is low in fat, and high in whole grains, vegetables, and fruits. Immune system inhibitors such as coffee, sugar, alcohol, and fat are omitted.

At the end of three months, it is very important to follow up again with a health practitioner, and to obtain another Pap smear. Sometimes a biopsy is also needed.

IMMUNOAUGMENTIVE THERAPY (IAT)

Treating cervical cancer by restoring the patient's own immune system has also proven successful at John Clement's Immunology Research Center in Freeport in the Bahamas. Dr. Clement specifies that success can occur if the treatment is begun early, even after surgery. *(See chapter 4, Breast Cancer.)*

FIBROIDS AND UTERINE BLEEDING

Fibroids are growths, composed of muscle tissue and usually benign, that attach themselves to the inner or outer wall of the uterus. One in five women over thirty-five has them; the majority of these women are African-American. These tumors grow in response to estrogen levels. Medically, they are also referred to as *fibromyoma uteri* and *leiomyoma uteri*.

Causes

Complementary physician Dr. Robert Sorge says that fibroids are nature's way of encapsulating toxins that result from an unhealthy diet and lifestyle: "Most of our patients with this condition consume tremendous amounts of coffee. As far as I'm concerned, this is something that every person concerned about their health must stop drinking. Diet sodas, greasy fries, pizza, potato chips, dough-nuts and danishes, and other devitalized foods add to the problem."

Registered nurse and licensed acupuncturist Abigail Rist-Podrecca, of New York City and Kingston, New York, adds that Oriental medicine sees fibroids as the result of blockage to the uterine area: "This can be caused by anger, emotional upsets, or a history of problems with menstruation, where it is either late or prolonged. Sometimes, after an abortion, the endometrial wall will still have some cells from that particular pregnancy. Further down the line, that can develop into fibroids."

Symptoms

Small fibroids are symptomless, but when they grow, they may result in painful periods, bladder infections, and infertility. Uterine bleeding is another common symptom, explains Rist-Podrecca: "If the fibroid is located on the inside of the uterus lining, then you will have this uterine bleeding, which usually sends women to the gynecologist, where they opt for hysterectomy. If the fibroid is located on the muscle wall, then there is not so much bleeding, but the fibroid will continue to grow."

Dr. Sorge adds that bleeding is the body's attempt to restore balance, according to naturopathic medicine: "Circulation and oxygenation of the uterine muscles and blood vessels is diminished, and metabolic waste products begin to build up. Bleeding is the sign of a highly toxic condition attempting to correct itself."

Clinical Experience

CONVENTIONAL APPROACH

Small fibroids that do not cause problems are sometimes removed by a procedure known as a myomectomy. This procedure removes the fibroid only and does not interfere with a woman's ability to have children.

For larger tumors, or fibroids that cause heavy bleeding, hysterectomies are standard treatment. Dr. Herbert Goldfarb, a gynecologist and assistant clinical professor at New York University's School of Medicine, reports that the majority of these operations are unnecessary, as well as dangerous: "Each year 750,000 hysterectomies are performed, and 2,500 women die during the operation. These are not sick women, but healthy women who go into the hospital and do not come out. Surgical procedures have morbidity, which means complications, and they have mortality, which means death."

In addition, hysterectomy can be psychologically destructive: "Some women want the operation and are all right about it, but most women feel like lambs being led to slaughter. They really don't want to have this procedure done, but their physicians give them no alternative.

"A new laser procedure, called myoma coagulation, has the potential to end the use of hysterectomy for fibroids once and for all, but most people don't know about it. My book, *The No Hysterectomy Option,* was written in response to my frustration at having a technology to help women avoid hysterectomies, but women not knowing about it. Sometimes women need hysterectomies, but often they are told they need them for frivolous reasons. My book is designed to help women understand when it is needed and when other options are available. I always like to say that hysterectomy may be indicated, but it may not be necessary. Our best customer is an informed consumer.

"We could avoid hysterectomies in well over 50 percent of the patients now having them. Breaking it down, somewhere between 10 and 20 percent are done for cancer. At this point, I am not going to say that these can be avoided, although some of the ones done for precancerous conditions of the cervix can. But hysterectomies for conditions like endometriosis are not needed. Endoscopic, laparoscopic procedures, and judicious use of alternative medications will control these conditions. Regarding fibroids and bleeding, we can take care of this with myoma coagulation if the condition is caught early enough."

Dr. Vicki Hufnagel, using the new technique of Female Reconstructive Surgery (FRS), has been successful in removing uterine fibroids no matter the size or number of tumors, limiting both blood loss and surgical complications.

MYOMA COAGULATION

Dr. Goldfarb lectures extensively to doctors on this new technology, which has enabled him to successfully prevent hysterectomies in hundreds of women with fibroids and uterine bleeding. Here he describes how he discovered the technique and why it works: "Approximately five years ago, on a trip to Europe, I observed a technique where a fibroid was being pierced with a special type of laser which destroyed the fibroid tissue, and subsequently shrunk the tumor.

"When I returned to the United States, I performed the first myoma coagulation. (Other physicians call it myolysis.) A young woman with a fibroid tumor was undergoing a tubal sterilization. I pierced the fibroid with a laser fiber, and lo and behold, the fibroid disappeared. Five years later, this woman is functioning perfectly well. The fibroid is gone, and she has absolutely no symptoms.

"Subsequent to that, I have performed this technique in well over 300 patients. A number of my colleagues also perform the procedure. I travel from coast to coast, north to south, lecturing and teaching. Physicians are uniformly performing it."

The typical candidate for this procedure is the woman uninterested in reproduction, since the uterine wall may become too weak to support pregnancy. Also, the size of the tumor must be 10 cm or less (approximately 6 inches). If the fibroid exceeds this size, it can be reduced with the medication Lupron: "Lupron reduces estrogen levels in the body, and temporarily reduces the size of fibroids. With Lupron, we get a 30 to 50 percent reduction in size."

Once the tumor has become smaller, coagulation can be performed, which shrinks it another 50 to 75 percent and puts an end to the problem: "When we do this procedure, we literally undermine the tumor by destroying its blood supply. As we put needles around the fibroid, it turns blue, showing that the blood supply has been interrupted. Fluid and blood go out, and the tumor shrinks. It becomes stringy tissue and just sits there, becoming very small, which eliminates the need for removal. The patient has no symptoms and can go about her life without the need for further surgery."

The cost of myoma coagulation is equal to other operations, but cost-effective in the long run: "The good news is that patients come into the hospital in the morning, have the procedure done, and go home in the afternoon. That saves the insurance company significant amounts of money. Also, these patients go back to work within a week so that there is very little cost in terms of disability."

DIET AND EXERCISE

Since fibroids grow in response to estrogen, nutritionist Gracia Perlstein advocates the natural lowering of estrogen, through diet and exercise, as a first-line defense against fibroid growth:

DIET. "Research shows that an over-fatty diet increases estrogen in the diet, and we know overweight women produce more estrogen. So the first approach would be dietary.

"The best diet for a woman attempting to decrease the size of her fibroids, or at the very least keep them from getting any larger, consists of whole foods, and is semivegetarian or vegetarian. The best protein sources are from vegetables and include whole grains, especially millet, amaranth, quinoa, buckwheat, whole grain oats, and brown rice. A wonderful way for cooking whole grains is to put one part grain to four parts water in a slow cooker. Before going to sleep, turn the cooker on low or automatic shift, which starts high and lowers. When you wake up in the morning, you have a creamy, delicious whole-grain cereal. That's a wonderful way to eat whole grains every day.

"Eat small quantities of legumes daily. Soybeans and foods made from soy, in particular, contain isoflavones that discourage tumor growth. Foods made from soy include tofu, fortified soy milk, miso, and tempeh. A variety of other beans can be used to make wonderful ethnic dishes and include black beans, adzuki, pinto beans, chickpeas, mung beans, lentils, and lima beans. Grains and beans are your best source of proteins.

"If you eat meat, I recommend eating only small quantities of it, no more than 3 ounces per day. Three ounces fits into the palm of your hand. It should be only from animals that are free-range and grass-fed, with no hormones or antibiotics. A good way to get animal protein is to make soup stock with chicken or fish bones. Simply put them in pure water and simmer, with a little organic cider vinegar, for a couple of hours or overnight. Red meat, poultry, and conventional dairy products, which are fed hormones, should be avoided entirely.

"The liver detoxifies excess estrogen, so you want to support liver function by avoiding all recreational drugs, alcohol, fried foods, coffees, and any processed or refined foods. Be sure to drink at least two quarts of pure water a day to help your bowels and kidneys. You are trying to remove excess estrogen from the system, and this is supported when your organs of elimination work properly."

EXERCISE. "Regular exercise will reduce excessive estrogen levels. Most people are familiar with the fact that hard-training women athletes sometimes reduce their estrogen levels to the point where they stop menstruating. We are not after that kind of effect, but regular exercise is very beneficial and helps the body remove excess estrogen."

SUPPLEMENTS. For further uterine support, Perlstein recommends the following supplements and herbs:

Balanced oil supplement. One tablespoon daily. Balanced oil supplements are a mixture of flax, borage, and other unrefined, natural, organic oils.
Multiple vitamin/mineral supplement.
Iron and herb supplement. This should be taken if there is anemia from heavy bleeding. Avoid high doses of iron as they are implicated in cancer and heart disease.
Vitamin E. 400 units, twice daily.
Silica supplement.
Vitamin C with bioflavonoids. 1,000 mg, five times daily divided over the course of the day.
Evening primrose oil. 100 mg, three times daily.
False unicorn root. Fifteen drops of the tincture in a small amount of water can be taken every hour when there are acute uterine problems.
Shepherd's purse. Fifteen drops of the tincture in a small amount of water, three times a day, may stop excessive bleeding.
White ash may reduce size of fibroids.

Perlstein asserts that such a comprehensive program of diet and lifestyle changes, geared toward reducing excess estrogen, gives the body the tools it needs to shrink fibroids or keep them from growing any larger. In addition, the side effects of such a program are wonderful: "You will be slimmer and have more energy than you would using conventional methods, which have harmful effects."

WESTERN NATUROPATHIC TREATMENTS

NATURAL HYGIENE. Complementary physician Dr. Anthony Penepent recommends fasting for excessive uterine bleeding, short of life-threatening situations where the woman needs hospitalization: "This condition signals liver poisoning. During the course of the month, a little fasting might be in order, in addition to a very strict hygienic regimen, to straighten out the condition. I have had patients with all forms of dysfunctional uterine bleeding, and to my recollection, I cannot remember any woman who followed my instructions who did not have a good result."

OIL-SOLUBLE LIQUID CHLOROPHYL. Dr. Joseph Pizzorno, N.D., president of John Bastyr College of Naturopathic Medicine, says this old natural therapy can quite effectively put an end to abnormal uterine bleeding. Oil-soluble liquid chlorophyl is available in capsules. Two to three are usually taken two to three times a day.

Dr. Pizzorno says that for some unknown reason, the chlorophyl seems to relieve this condition: "Many people think this works because it improves clotting, but it turns out that women with abnormal uterine bleeding do not have clotting abnormalities. So why it works is not clear. But the bottom line is, it works quite well."

ORIENTAL NATUROPATHIC TREATMENTS

HERBS. Rist-Podrecca says the following herbs are good to stop dysfunctional uterine bleeding when taken under the supervision of a Chinese herbal practitioner:

Poo wha. Made from bee pollen.
Er jow. From the hide of an animal.
Chuan xiong (*Ligusticum wallichi*). Regulates bleeding by the amount taken. Too much causes uterine bleeding, and too little stops it.
Han lian cao (warrior's grass). Helps tone the spleen and uterine and stops intense uterine bleeding.

ACUPUNCTURE. Acupuncture points that relate to the uterus are found on the ankle. Rist-Podrecca explains how electrical acupuncture to this area helps reduce fibroids: "We use a small electrical current. This makes the uterus contract and expand. It palpates the area slightly to get the body to recognize that the fibroids are there, to increase circulation, and to start vibrating them so that they are released."

HOMEOPATHY
Consider the following remedies for uterine bleeding and fibroids:
Ipecac. Dr. Marjorie Ordene, of Brooklyn, New York, recommends this remedy to stop acute hemorrhaging with bright red blood. "When given in the 200 potency, every fifteen minutes, ipecac slows down the bleeding. That's two pellets under the tongue, until the bleeding actually stops. I have had success with a number of patients, and other physicians have reported this as well."

Dr. Ken Korins says the two remedies to think of first for heavy bleeding are shina and sabina.
Shina. This is for heavy, dark, blood that forms clots and leads to debility and exhaustion.

Sabina. Also for clots, but here the blood is bright red. When large clots are being expelled, there is a laborlike pain that radiate from the sacrum to the pubis.

In addition, these are other formulas to consider:

Secale. Women who need secale have dark blood that is almost black. Periods are profuse and prolonged.

Phosphorus is indicated when there is bright red blood with no clots.

Trillium. Bleeding is very heavy and bright red. The person characteristically feels faint and dizzy after bleeding. Periods occur biweekly, and are worse with any slight movement.

The following remedies are specifically for fibroids:

Aurum muriaticum. This remedy is for fibroid, when there are no other symptoms. There is no heavy bleeding and no particular discomfort. It may help reduce their size of the fibroids.

Hydrastinum muriaticum. Has been known to cure large fibroids, especially when they seem to be on the anterior wall of the uterus, pushing on the bladder and causing symptoms of urinary frequency and pain.

REPRODUCTIVE SYSTEM CANCERS

Women are susceptible to ovarian cancer and carcinomas of the uterine cervix, either cervical or endometrial cancer. Of the three, ovarian cancer occurs most often, and is growing in frequency. It usually manifests after menopause, especially in women who have few or no children, who were unable to conceive, or who gave birth later than the average age. Other factors that place women at risk include a past history of spontaneous abortions, endometriosis, type A blood, radiation to the pelvic region, or exposure to cancer-causing chemicals, such as asbestos.

Cervical cancer is associated with promiscuity at an early age, a genital herpes infection, and multiple pregnancies, while endometrial cancer is related to a history of infertility, failure to ovulate, the use of drugs containing estrogen, and uterine growths.

Symptoms

Uterine cancers are easier to detect in the beginning stages, and tend to be more treatable, whereas ovarian cancers are rarely discovered early on, and are terribly damaging to the individual's quality of life.

Abnormal bleeding in the vaginal area, especially after menopause, is the chief sign of endometrial cancer. Sometimes there is pain in the lower abdomen or back. A Pap smear does not always catch endometrial cancer early on, but it can be detected with a surgical exam of the uterus.

In the early stages of cervical cancer, symptoms are usually absent, although there may be a watery, vaginal discharge or spotty bleeding. Signs of advanced cervical cancer include dark, odorous vaginal discharges, fistulas, weight loss, and back and leg pain. One's chance of survival increases with early discovery through yearly Pap tests.

Women should look for these early indications of ovarian carcinomas: abnormal vaginal bleeding, weight loss, and changes in patterns of urination and bowel movements. While a Pap smear will not detect ovarian cancer in the beginning stages, it may be discovered through annual pelvic exams.

Clinical Experience

Contemporary treatments for ovarian cancer are a disappointment in that while they can make cancers disappear for weeks or months at a time, they will, in fact, fail in the end, as the cancer returns with a vengeance to finish the job. In fact, orthodox survival rates for ovarian cancer patients are only between 5 and 10 percent. Cancers of the uterine cervix initially exhibit higher success rates with surgery, which may involve the removal of the uterus (hysterectomy), as well as both ovaries and the fallopian tubes (salpingo-oophorectomy), in addition to x-ray and hormone therapies. But there is no guarantee that the cancer will not return. Gar Hildebrand, president of the Gerson Research Organization in San Diego, California, says that more patients would triumph over reproductive system cancers if a combination of approaches were employed. He states, "No one should be treated by a single specialty, and then watched in hopes that the cancer will not come back. It's not scientifically justifiable, nor is it acceptable to the patient. Sitting and waiting just causes horrible, immune-suppressing anxiety." Here Gar Hildebrand informs us about multiple modalities that work best for patients with ovarian and uterine cancers:

NUTRITION

"Let's say a woman with an ovarian cancer has just been admitted to Memorial Sloan Kettering Cancer Center. The first thing the doctors will do is a laparotomy. She will be opened up, and a surgeon will get the bulk of the tumor out. I have no problem with that.

"But the second step would definitely not be to use drugs that kill tumors. Tissue damage always accompanies cancer; unless it is addressed, the cancer is sure to reappear. In other words, throughout the body, tumor toxins cause cells to lose potassium, and to swell with extra salt and water. This state is worse around the tumor itself. Often times a treatment that goes into the bloodstream fails to penetrate to a tumor effectively because the tissue next to the tumor has no immunity. What's really needed, then, is for the patient to be stabilized physiologically. The ideal treatment would be for the person to receive nutritional salt and water management, a diet that nourishes and corrects the water retention in the cells. We're going to feed the whole body to try to get the tissues back to normal functioning."

Hildebrand recommends a diet that detoxifies and stimulates cells back to health. "Doctors have long been aware that most cancer patients have an aversion to meat. They'll smell it and gag; that's a self-defense mechanism. It's absolutely essential for these people to stop taking in heavy proteins—animal proteins and sometimes even heavy vegetable proteins, like legumes—for a while, just to clear up. The tumor's converting that stuff into caustic chemicals, related to the ammonia we use in our laundry machines. It's those chemicals that create damage systemwide.

"We can also detoxify the body by supplying oodles of plant chemicals, called phytochemicals. These foods can be eaten cooked or raw, and should include vegetables of all sorts, fruits, and a few whole grains. Fruit and vegetable juices are especially important. You have to flood the system with nutritious fluids, such as carrot and green leaf juices. Apple juice should always be added because apples contain a material that is very good for cellular energy. If you put those juiced phytochemicals into the body every hour, these cancer patients will have their cellular enzyme systems speeded up so that the individual cells can spit up toxins.

"Eating an excess of empty calories and proteins creates toxicity that causes the immune system to overproduce white blood cells that aren't very adept at what they do. Once you restrict protein and calories and get the nutrient level up, these patients' immune systems become intelligent again. They stop making excess stupid white cells, and create more lymphocytes interested in more types of challenges. In other words, you get a very lean, mean immune system."

In addition to changes in diet, most patients need additional arms in their fight for survival. Hildebrand explains why the following therapies are so important:

COFFEE ENEMAS. "These enemas have been used by thousands of cancer patients, outside the realm of traditional medical care, because they work. Boiled coffee in retention enemas stimulates the liver's enzyme system, which in turn causes great relief from pain in cancer patients. The liver has more than a thousand documented medical functions. When we help it to work better and faster, the cancer patient's overall physiological condition changes, sometimes within hours, and certainly within the first several weeks of treatment. You have a whole different person. People come off gurneys and out of beds, excruciating chronic pain is eased, and addiction to morphine is broken.

"Every three minutes, all the blood in our bodies goes through our liver. Our livers and small intestine walls have an enzyme system with a fancy name that we will call GST for short. This enzyme system naturally responds to cancer in the body by going up, and the coffee enema has been shown in laboratory experiments with rats, and in later experiments with humans, to produce increased liver bile flow, and to stimulate the GST enzyme system. In fact, it's raised to 700 percent of normal levels of activity. When the GST system is running that fast, it can effectively remove tumor toxins from the bloodstream. And it doesn't take very long. The effects of these coffee enemas will last for sometimes four, six, or eight hours before a feeling of discomfort and pain around the tumor returns. They're that effective.

"You have to know how much coffee to use: a quart of water with three tablespoons of coffee boiled in it. That's cooled and strained, not filtered, because a filter would remove some of the molecules that stimulate the GST enzyme system. The coffee is safely taken into the colon, while the person is lying on his or her right side, retained for 10 to 15 minutes, and then released. Patients doing this without the supervision of a physician should know that anything cooler than 100 degrees is going to cause cramping in the intestines."

HYPERBARIC OXYGEN. "We're also going to try to increase circulation with full-body-immersion oxygen therapy. Hyperbaric oxygen treatment is given in a diving chamber that used to be used to treat the bends. There's been a lot of fascination with ozone in cancer treatment in the alternative field. But what we found is that ozone applications only raise tissue oxygen by 25 to 50 percent, whereas hyperbaric oxygen can predictably raise oxygenation by 800 to 1000 percent. This means that tissue around the tumor, which doesn't have enough oxygen to function, can get sufficient oxygen for energy production. This will also allow the tissue to repair itself by producing a high-potassium, low-sodium environment, so that this edema can come out of the tissue."

COLEY'S TOXINS. Hildebrand states that this treatment has the most glorious record of any treatment in the cancer literature, especially when combined with the Gerson diet program, consisting of hourly glasses of fresh juice and coffee enemas: "I am hopeful that much interest will be sparked in this therapy because, right now, the only reports I've seen of long-term survival for ovarian cancer patients have been from a combination of these approaches.

"The word toxin is a little confusing, because Coley's toxin is not really a poison. It refers to a bacterial endotoxin that is an immune stimulant. I would put that directly into the abdominal cavity once the tissue around the tumor has been stabilized.

"Coley was a physician who searched the literature for cancer treatments after a heartbreaking experience of losing a child patient to the disease. Much to his surprise, he found a skin infection called erysipelas. Erysipelas is caused by a streptococcus that causes a skin fever of 105 to 106 degrees. This fever causes an inflammatory infection which interferes with tumor action.

"Coley constructed a live erysipelas vaccine, which was too toxic at first. Some patients died, but others experienced a tumor regression. He went through a lot of trial and error, and eventually settled on something which we now call *Serratia marsecians.* He mixed the serratia and the strep in a ratio of 1,500 cells to one, and then crushed the mixture through a microfilter to liberate the internal toxins of the bacteria. This liberated antigens, which would in turn cause the immune system of the patient to think that there was a chronic infection that had to be fought.

"Coley's toxins seem effective due to the fact that the immune system, when turned on, can cause a lot of dust to rise. These patients need to be put into an intensive care unit, and hooked up to monitors, just in case of a problem, although there have never been any heart attacks or kidney failures reported in the 900 cases that have been thoroughly studied. Then a tiny amount of toxins is administered intravenously for four hours through a drip. About two hours into the process, the immune response begins. The patient will develop chills and shaking and that last for about half an hour to ninety minutes, followed by a rise in temperature of about a degree every ten minutes. Once that temperature hits 105 or 106, the ICU staff lies them down or puts in a suppository of Tylenol to stop it.

"The reaction is the immune system's response. This is not a poison. This is not a toxin. It's not like chemotherapy making your hair fall out or causing bone marrow suppression. The Coley's toxins are much more like what happens when your immune system decides to cure you of an infection. So the symptoms are more flulike, without the nausea and vomiting. After the second or third IV application, patients usually get sleepy and actually nod off. The fever lessens progressively. In other words, there's a honeymoon period.

"Coley himself said that if you don't keep these up for at least three or four months, in booster dosages, you won't get a permanent response. The literature reveals that gains are lost when Coley's toxins are given in lower concentrations or for shorter durations. But when properly used, there is an extraordinary 50 percent cure rate in advanced, inoperable uterine and ovarian cancers."

THE BENEFITS OF AN OVERALL APPROACH. Gar Hildebrand reemphasizes the importance of utilizing any and every cancer protocol that works: "We believe that it's time we stopped living in an either/or world, where orthodoxy is over on one side and the marginalized alternative professions are in the trenches and foxholes, and nobody talks. We believe it's time to get the doors and windows of communication open, so that we can find the context for each of these treatments and the way they fit together. Our own experience reveals that using the nutritional approach takes a toxic load off of the immune system and speeds up intracellular enzymes, so that they can repel toxins and pull them from the blood rapidly. Calorie and protein restrictions, and a diet high in nutrients, can lead to sensitization of the tumor. Years of experience shows that diet therapy alone can produce monthly fevers. And tumors may or may not regress through those fevers. But if you stimulate the immune system when those fevers are hitting, you have a much greater chance of tumor reduction. That's why we suggest the marriage of these disciplines, and the respectful recognition of the role of every aspect of anticancer medicine that's ever been developed."

Patient Stories

MORGAN ON HER EXPERIENCE WITH CERVICAL CANCER:
I still have cervical cancer, but I am working on overcoming it through a number of approaches. I watch my diet very carefully. I feel that my condition is in an early enough stage where I can handle it nutritionally. But it's not just nutrition that I have to deal with. I have to deal with all the emotions that help to create disease in the body. It's also a matter of detoxing. I do colonics and a lot of juicing. I take supplements. And I do meditation, and exercise.

The major reason I started to see a nutritionist was, of course the wake-up call, the cervical cancer, which was just diagnosed three months ago. But I had also had ulcerative colitis for almost twenty years.

I feel like I now have energy again. I exercise at least several times a week, which was literally impossible before. I even had trouble getting up a flight of subway steps without feeling exhausted at the top. So I have several different things that I am working with: nutrition, meditation, and detoxification. I'm working on it.

Now I have to find a gynecologist who is holistically oriented because my primary care physician dropped me after I refused to have a hysterectomy. I feel very lucky. I feel that someone else trying to deal with this would have followed the recommended course of action and would have given up their reproductive rights, allowing themselves to be mutilated, and always fearful of having the cancer reappear.

Also, I feel that the cancer is nothing more than a wake-up call. Your body is saying, "Hey, something is wrong here. You're out of balance. You need to address this, this and this." If you don't, disease is the end result. Now I am vegetarian and doing a lot of things differently. If I didn't, I might not be alive now. I might be at a higher risk for the cancer to spread throughout more of the body. This doesn't mean that I am 100 percent there. I still have a lot of work to do. But I feel very hopeful.

GAR HILDEBRAND ON AN OVARIAN CANCER PATIENT'S RECOVERY:
The ability of diet therapy to produce tumor regression in ovarian cancer is best illustrated by the experience of a woman named Leslie. This is a woman that had an omentectomy, a bilateral salpingo-oophorectomy, and a complete hysterectomy. She had tumors all over the inside of the back wall of the abdomen, on the pelvis, and on other organ structures, which were left for chemotherapy. But she declined the chemo and tried dietary therapy.

Several weeks later, this woman had a sudden fever response. It hit fast and was so debilitating that she could not even move. This is a classic reaction to diet therapy that patients sometimes have. Her husband put her to bed; he stopped measuring her temperature and started icing her down at 105 degrees. Leslie had this fever for twenty-four hours. When it was gone she said, "I know I'm going to be okay. I know I'm going to be fine." Today, Leslie is alive and well, and living in Florida with her husband.

Hot News on Cervical Dysplasia

Factors shown to increase the risk of cervical dysplasia in recent studies are oral contraceptives and a low calcium-phosphorus ratio. Substances that show promise in treating dysplasia include an ointment made from the flowers of the plant *Filipendula ulmaria*, which has resulted in regression of dysplasia in both humans and mice; cis-unsaturated fatty acids (c-UFAs), which have killed drug-resistant cervical cancer in in vitro studies; and iscador, an extract of mistletoe (*Viscum album*) tissue, which, combined with local irradiation, proved highly effective in eliminating tumors in mice; and a traditional Chinese medicine called Sanpin preparations. *(See "From the Medical Literature on Cervical Dysplasia," below.)*

Hot News on Fibroids

Smoking has been strongly linked to the development of ovarian cysts. Among the natural herbal substances that have been found helpful in treating fibroids are kelp, used in the East for ovarian problems; saw palmetto berry, a general reproductive system tonic; wild cherry, which is rich in bioflavonoids; *dong quai*, a Chinese herb that may relieve cramps from fibroids; red raspberry, an antihemorrhagic; and the common plants lady's mantle, yarrow, white dead nettle, partridge berry, goldenseal, and ginger. *(See "From the Medical Literature on Fibroids and Uterine Bleeding," below.)*

DIET/NUTRITION

An in vitro study indicates that cis-unsaturated fatty acids (c-UFAs) can kill drug-resistent cervical cancer.

N. Madhavi and U. N. Das, "Effect of n-6 and n-3 Fatty Acids on the Survival of Vincristine Sensitive and Resistant Human Cervical Carcinoma Cells in Vitro," *Cancer Letters* 84 (1994): 31–41.

Dietary factors increasing the risk of cervical changes include low levels of vitamins A, C, and E, as well as low levels of folic acid, selenium, zinc, and beta carotene. Lifestyle factors increasing the risk of cervical changes include sex at an early age, more sexual partners, testing positive for viruses such as genital herpes and warts, oral contraceptive use, underactive thyroid, smoking, passive exposure to smoking, giving birth in the teens, stress, and having sexual partners who work with chemicals, such as tar, machine oil, dust, asbestos, coal, and metals, if hygiene is poor.

A. McIntyre, *The Complete Woman's Herbal* (New York: Henry Holt and Co., 1993): 238–39.

Garlic has been shown to markedly reduce the risk of methylcholanthrene-induced cancer of the cervix in mice.

S. P. Hussain et al., "Chemopreventive Action of Garlic on Methylcholanthrene-Induced Carcinogenesis in the Uterine Cervix of Mice," *Cancer Letters* 49 (1990): 175–80.

Iscador, an extract of *Viscum album* tissue, increases immune reactivity in—and prolongs the life of—tumorous mice. In vitro, Iscador was shown to be toxic to tumor cells. Combined with local irradiation, it is a highly effective treatment. Local irradiation combined with Iscador resulted in tumor disappearance in over 65 percent of animal subjects.

M. Jurin et al., "Antitumorous and Immunomodulatory Effects of the *Viscum Album* L. Preparation Iscador," *Oncology* 50 (1993): 393–98.

In a study of 80 women with cervical dysplasia compared to 34 controls, those with dysplasia were found to have lower levels of vitamin C.

C. L. Romney et al., "Plasma Vitamin C and Uterine Cervical Dysplasia," *American Journal of Obstet. Gynecol.* 151, no. 7 (April 1, 1985): 976–80.

Lower intakes of vitamin C were shown to increase the risk of cervical dysplasia in a case-control study.

T. Liu et al., "A Case Control Study of Nutritional Factors and Cervical Dysplasia," *Cancer Epidemiol. Biomarkers Prev.* 2, no. 6 (November–December 1993): 525–30.

In a study, those women with the highest levels of vitamin C were 4 to 5 times less likely to have cervical cancer than those with the lowest levels.

J. Van Eenwyk, "The Role of Vitamins in the Development of Cervical Cancer," *Nutrition Report* 11, no. 1 (January 1993): 1, 8.

Insufficient intake of ascorbate increases the risk of cervical dysplasia, as does insufficient intake of riboflavin.

T. Liu et al., "A Case Control Study of Nutritional Factors and Cervical Dysplasia," *Cancer Epidemiol. Biomarkers Prev.* 2, no. 6 (November–December 1993): 525–30.

Average levels of folic acid decreased in cases of uterine cervix dysplasia, it was found in a case-control study.

R. Grio et al., "Antineoblastic Activity of Antioxidant Vitamins: The Role of Folic Acid in the Prevention of Cervical Dysplasia," *Panminerva Med.* 35, no. 4 (December 1993): 193–96.

Lower levels of folic acid increase the risk of papilloma virus, which is a risk factor for cervical cancer. Folic acid doses of 10 mg/day for 3 months produced better biopsy scores for oral contraceptive users with mild or moderate dysplasia.

C. E. Butterworth, "Folate Status, Women's Health, Pregnancy Outcome and Cancer," *Journal of the American College of Nutrition* 12, no. 4 (1990): 438–41.

Folate deficiency increases the risk of cervical dysplasia. Also, insufficient intake of vitamin A increases the risk, according to a case-control study.

T. Liu et al., "A Case Control Study of Nutritional Factors and Cervical Dysplasia," *Cancer Epidemiol. Biomarkers Prev.* 2, no., 6 (November–December 1993): 525–30.

Women who test positive for human papilloma virus type I6 are 5 times more likely to have cervical dysplasia if their folate is low.

C. D. Butterworth et al., "Folate Deficiency and Cervical Dysplasia," *JAMA* 367, no. 4 (January 22, 1992): 528–34.

Lower intake of folacin is linked to the presence of cervical dysplasia, a case comparison study of 159 women showed.

R. S. McPherson, "Nutritional Factors and the Risk of Cervical Dysplasia," *Dissertation Abstracts International* 51, no. 4 (1990): 1769.

Beta carotene deficiency may play a role in the development of cervical intraepithelial neoplasia (CIN) or cervical cancer.

P. Palan et al., "B-Carotene Levels in Exfoliated Cervicovaginal Epithelial Cells and Cervical Intraepithelial Neoplasia and Cervical Cancer," *American Journal of Obstetrics and Gynecology* 167, no. 6 (December 1992): 1899–1903.

Lower intake of lycopene appears to be associated with the presence of cervical dysplasia.

R. S. McPherson, "Nutritional Factors and the Risk of Cervical Dysplasia," *Dissertation Abstracts International* 51, no. 4 (1990): 1769.

High levels of serum ferritin play a protective role against cervical intraepithelial neoplasia (CIN).

C. F. Amburgey et al., "Undernutrition as a Risk Factor for Cervical Intraepithelial Neoplasia: A Case-control Analysis," *Nutrition and Cancer* 20, no. 1 (1993): 51–60.

A low calcium-phosphorus ratio was shown to increase the risk of cervical dysplasia.

T. Liu et al., "A Case Control Study of Nutritrional Factors and Cervical Dysplasia," *Cancer Epidemiol. Biomarkers Prev.* 2, no. 6 (November–December 1993): 525–30.

RISK FACTORS

Lifestyle risk factors for cervical intraepithelial neoplasia (CIN) include having multiple sex partners, possibly being married to a man who had multiple sex partners, and cigarette smoking. Also, human papilloma virus infection is a risk factor.

J. Van Eenwyk, "The Role of Vitamins in the Development of Cervical Cancer," *Nutrition Report* 11, no. 1 (January 1993): 1, 8.

Women testing positive for human papilloma virus (HPV) are 5 times more likely to have cervical dysplasia if their folate level is low.

C. E. Butterworth et al., "Folate Deficiency and Cervical Dysplasia," *JAMA* 367, no. 4 (January 22, 1992): 528–34.

Oral contraceptives appear to double the risk of adenocarcinoma of the cervix, judging by a study of 195 cases compared to 386 controls. The increased rate of this disease in young women over the past 20 years may be due, in part, to oral contraceptive use.

G. Ursin et al., "Oral Contraceptive Use and Adenocarcinoma of the Cervix," *Lancet* 344 (November 19, 1994): 1390–94.

HERBS/PLANT EXTRACTS

Forty-eight cases of cervical dyplasia were treated with an ointment made from *Filipendula ulmaria*. A positive response was seen in 67 percent of the cases, and 52 percent experienced a complete regression of dysplasia. At follow-up, 10 out of the 48 patients were completely cured and had no recurrence within 12 months. When tested on mice, drugs prepared from the flowers of this plant produced a 39 percent decrease in squamous-cell carcinoma of the cervix and vagina.

A. P. Peresun'ko et al., [Clinico-Experimental Study of Using Plant Preparations from the Flowers of *Filipendula Ulmaria* (L.) Maxim for the Treatment of Precancerous Changes and Prevention of Uterine Cervical Cancer], *Vopr. Onkol.*, 39 (1993): 291–95.

Gota kola has been used around the world for skin, blood, and nervous system diseases, including cervicitis.

D. B. Mowrey, *The Scientific Validation of Herbal Medicine* (New Canaan, CT: Keats Publishing, 1986): 193.

TRADITIONAL CHINESE MEDICINE

The traditional Chinese medicine called Sanpin preparation has been shown effective in reducing hypertrophic cervices to normal size, in treating cervical erosion (cure rate 84 percent), and in treating cervical neoplasms (cure rate 92 percent).

N. H. Xiong [Clinical and Experimental Studies on Sanpin Therapy for Chronic Cervical Diseases], *Chung Kuo Chung Hsi I Chieh Ho Tsa Chih* 13, no. 1 (January 1993): 3.

Kelp is used in China, Malaysia, and Japan for ovarian problems. Also, a nutritive tonic based on saw palmetto berry is used for almost all reproductive system diseases.

D. Mowrey, *The Scientific Validation of Herbal Medicine* (New Canaan, Conn.: Keats Publishing, 1986): 154.

Smoking is antiestrogenic, linked with the occurrence of ovarian cysts and with the earlier occurrence of such cysts, according to a study of over 5,000 women, aged 21 to 80. Women who smoke, or who have smoked, are about one and a half times as likely to get ovarian cysts as are nonsmokers.

G. Wyshak et al., "Smoking and Cysts of the Ovary," *International Journal of Fertility* 33, no. 6 (November–December 1988): 398-404.

NUTRITION

A cleansing and detoxification diet may retard or inhibit fibroid growth; some recommend fasting on fruit or vegetable juice or raw foods only, followed by a maintenance diet based on foods that normalize estrogen.

C. Cabrera, "Holistic Treatment of Fibroids," *Medical Herbalism* 5, no. 3 (Fall 1993).

A plant-based, low-fat, high-fiber diet is optimal for fending off fibroids, especially if the diet is rich in soy products. Soy foods are rich in phytoestrogens called bioflavonoids; they normalize estrogen levels in the body. Citrus fruits and berries are also helpful. They're rich in vitamin C, which helps normalize estrogen levels. Another nutritional factor in this problem may be vitamin A. A study showed that women with excessive menstrual bleeding, a common symptom with fibroids, had low levels of A, and that supplementation is effective in returning bleeding patterns to normal. Beta carotene sources include sweet potatoes, carrots, and romaine lettuce.

S. Lark, "Fending off Fibroids," *Vegetarian Times* 193 (September 1993): 100.

Supplements recommended for treating fibroids include B complex, E, and lipotropic factors.

C. Cabrera, "Holistic Treatment of Fibroids," *Medical Herbalism* 5, no. 3 (Fall 1993).

HERBS/PLANT EXTRACTS

Wild cherry is rich in bioflavonoids, and may be helpful in treating fibroids at a dose of 1 to 4 capsules daily or one dropperful of tincture 1 to 3 times daily. Also, *dong quai*, a Chinese herb, is a rich source of phytoestrogens and a smooth-muscle relaxant; it may relieve cramps from fibroids (500 to 1000 mg/day).

S. Lark, "Fending Off Fibroids," *Vegetarian Times* 193 (September 1993): 100.

Red raspberry *(Rubus idaeus)* is an astringent antihemorrhagic and a general toner and strengthener of uterine tissues. Other herbs that have been recommended by holistic practitioners for treating fibroids: lady's mantle *(Alchemilla vulgaris),* a strong antihemorrhagic, with tissue specificity for the uterus; yarrow *(Achillea millefolium),* antihemorrhagic, with volatile oils that promote blood flow to the pelvic basin; white dead nettle *(Lamium album),* which increases pelvic circulation and is an antispasmodic for the uterus; partridge berry *(Mitchella repens),* rich in tannins and saponins; goldenseal *(Hydrastis canadensis)*—reduces bleeding, improves integrity of tissue, reduces pelvic congestion; motherwort *(Leonurus cardiaca),* a general uterine tonic; stone root *(Collinsonia canadensis),* a pelvic decongestant and diuretic; and ginger *(Zingiber officinalis),* which stimulates pelvic circulation.

C. Cabrera, "Holistic Treatment of Fibroids," *Medical Herbalism* 5, no. 3 (Fall 1993).

TRADITIONAL CHINESE MEDICINE

Keishi-bukuryo-gan (KBG) is a traditional Chinese medicine used to treat gynecological disorders. In premenopausal patients with uterine myomas, it improved over 90 percent of cases of hypermenorrhea and dysmenorrhea, and it shrank uterine myomas in 60 percent of cases.

S. Sakamoto et al., "Pharmacotherapeutic Effects of *Kuei-chi-fu-ling-wan (keishi-bukuryo-gan)* on Human Uterine Myomas," *American Journal of Chinese Medicine* 20, nos. 3–4 (1992): 313–17.

A study on urinary tract fibrosis showed that the Chinese medicine Sairei-to was more effective than other drugs.

K. Shida et al., [Clinical Efficacy of *Sairei-to* in Various Urinary Tract Diseases Centering on Fibrosis], *Hinyokika Kiyo–Acta Urologica Japonica* 40, no. 11 (1994): 1049–57.

ACUPUNCTURE

A study found acupuncture to be highly effective in treating hysteromyoma.

H. Yan and J. Wang, [The Clinical Study on Hysteromyoma Treated with Acupuncture], *Chen Tzu Yen Chiu* 19, no. 2 (1994): 14–16.

CONTROVERSY OVER HYSTERECTOMY

Fibroid tumors are the most common reason for hysterectomies in the United States, although fibroids are a common, non-life-threatening problem. Doctors often argue that the operation should be performed when the fibroids are still small, to avoid surgical complications. It should be noted, though, that fibroid growth is influenced by estrogen production in the body, and fibroids tend to get smaller after menopause unless estrogen therapy is undertaken (in which the size tends to increase). A study shows that women with a uterus enlarged by fibroids to the size of a 12- to 20-week pregnancy are no more likely to suffer surgical complications than those with smaller uteri.

"Fibroid Tumors Need Not be Treated," *Health Facts* 17, no. 162 (November 1992): 1.

6. DEPRESSION

Depression is on the rise as the world becomes ever more technological and less personal. Dr. Michael Gallante, a complementary physician in Suffern, New York, notes that it is difficult for many people to adjust to modern life: "We don't get the smile, we don't get the wave, we don't get the 'Hello,' especially in the bigger cities. In a way, we don't give each other energy. We're out there doing battle to make a living to pay the taxes. It just gets to be too much." Often women bear the brunt of the depressive tendencies in both families and other societal groups, since women still tend to be in the care-giving roles.

Causes

Depression tends to run in families and can be due to genetic factors or lifestyle habits, such as poor diet, that get passed down from generation to generation. Women may become depressed after taking birth control pills over a long period of time, as these drain their body of vitamin B6 or pyridoxine. Certain individuals become depressed in the darker winter months, a condition known as Seasonal Affective Disorder (SAD).

Symptoms

Depression can be mild or severe, and is characterized by prolonged feelings of sadness, dejection, low self-esteem, lack of motivation, and physical slow-down. Chronic depression is associated with higher incidences of other types of disease, including heart disease and cancer.

Clinical Experience

CONVENTIONAL APPROACH

Orthodox treatments for depression range from counseling and psychotherapy to medication and electroshock therapy.

NATURAL APPROACH

DIET. When vitality is low, a diet that supplies optimal energy is especially important. Short juice fasts, from one to three days, can help women maintain their mental health, followed by a simple diet consisting mainly of fruits and vegetables.

It goes without saying that lifeless, processed foods, such as devitalized white bread, should not be eaten. Hard-to-digest and toxic foods, such as meat, processed foods, sugar, and alcohol, should be avoided. These create an imbalance, and remove energy instead of creating it. Additionally, sugar stresses the adrenal glands, causing the mind to race and scatter. It causes an initial high followed by a sustained low. Meat consumption can result in sleep disturbances, anger, and irritation. And alcohol damages the brain.

EXERCISE. Physical exercise is another key to lifting depression among women, especially when accompanied by a nutritious diet, meditation, and vitamin and mineral supplementation. According to Dr. William J. Goldwag, the medical director of the Center for Preventive/Holistic Medicine, in southern California, exercise is one of the most profound aids in the treatment of depression: "One of the major errors in the thinking of patients and therapists is the notion that in order to be active, you have to feel better. This is exactly contrary to our approach.

"We recommend that you do first, and then the feeling comes later. In other words, you must do what you have to do regardless of how you feel. This aids in feeling better. You can't wait until you feel good to do something, because in depression that may take days, weeks, months, or even years. You want to accelerate the process.

"Of course, women who exercise regularly have had days when they just didn't feel like it. That's the way depressed people feel about everything. They just don't feel like it. They don't have the energy, the motivation, the stimulation to go and do even the ordinary things. When it's severe, you may not even have the will or desire to get out of bed in the morning.

"The exercise may consist of very, very simple things, like just getting out and walking, getting up and doing some simple movements, some mild calisthenics, any kind of physical movement that gets the body in action. For some people just getting out of bed and getting dressed is a big accomplishment. That may be the first step.

"It is important for women who are depressed to get up and get dressed. They should not walk around in pajamas or nightgowns because this maintains that connection to the bed, and the bed means inactivity. That's the thing you're trying to overcome. Exercise may take the form of walking, walking the dog perhaps, or going outside to do some simple gardening. These are all very important for overcoming that feeling of lassitude that is so characteristic of depression.

"Another benefit of exercise is a feeling of accomplishment. Even doing a little bit of exercise will make you feel more energized later on. Finishing an exercise routine, even one that's fatiguing, after a brief period of rest will give you a feeling of revitalization, of energy, and a psychological feeling of accomplishment. It gives a feeling of, 'I've done it. It's completed.' For the depressed woman, the boost to self-esteem that this can give is important."

ACUPUNCTURE. Acupuncture frees blocked energy, and in so doing naturally lifts depression. Look at what Laura has to say about her experience: "When I was in my twenties, just after finishing college, I would go into a depression whenever I was about to get my period. It came on so suddenly that it was frightening. I went to see a doctor about it and was given a referral to an acupuncturist.

"After being in treatment for six months, my practitioner and I sat down to talk about how I was feeling. I realized then that the depression was gone.

"That was twelve years ago. I've stayed in treatment, although not as regularly as when I first started. It's my primary form of health care. My eating habits and sleeping patterns have become totally regulated. I have been able to lose forty pounds and to maintain my weight without dieting. I also quit smoking without ever trying. I never get sick anymore. I never get colds or flus. In general, I'm much more balanced.

"The whole experience of being brought into harmony keeps me from going to extremes. I don't work too hard, I don't play too hard, I don't rest too hard. I manage to stay pretty much in the center of my life. It's a huge improvement. I often wonder how people live without going through a treatment process like I did."

YOGA AND MEDITATION. Dr. Gallante overcame his own depression in adolescence by learning how to center his energy using these modalities: "When I was in my late teens, I went through a period of depression, where my energy was low. My whole being was unhappy. My parents and others I loved thought I should try seeing a psychiatrist for a while. I went a few times, but that wasn't satisfying to me. I thought nutrition might help so I started drinking raw vegetable juices and became vegetarian. I started eating to detoxify myself and to get myself back to feeling stronger again.

"Then I got into meditation and kundalini yoga. I learned about energy centers and started to learn how inner energy flows through the system. I began to sense blockages, and to identify emotions and limiting thoughts that were holding me back. Through practice, I was able to center energy into the emotional center in the chest and into the abdomen where stabilizing rootedness can occur. That started to awaken inner energies and to strengthen me.

"The important thing is to not get too hung up in the head, where we have all these conflicts. Our center is the lower abdomen, where a baby grows in a woman. The Japanese call this the *hara*. In Zen we concentrate the mind and the whole being there. That's the hub of the wheel. The mind can be clearer when you do that, and you don't get hung up living in the realm of thought.

"Set aside ten to twenty minutes daily to quiet the mind, to let tensions drain, to open up, and to resonate with the environment. Everyone does it in a different way. You can do it with meditation or biofeedback. You can do it with music, yoga, a hobby, it doesn't matter what. Anything that takes you to a creative, quiet place, allows you to recharge. Learn to take the time to express your inner needs.

"I like to ask my patients the question, 'Why do we have a physical body?' My answer is always that we exist as a physical entity to carry around our minds and our hearts, in a sense our spirits, so that we can fulfill ourselves. We can then learn and grow and do what we need to do in life. We are nothing without our emotions. Yet we neglect and suppress our feelings. We don't consider nourishing ourselves in a spiritual way. We need some sort of daily practice.

"We have a lot of outward pressures. We have rules made by corporations which are fulfilling needs of profits and ruining resources. There is a huge lack of wisdom across the board. The only thing that can make you happy is looking inwardly. Bring your mind and energies inside. Sometimes, when you start out, all you see is unhappiness and tension. But if you keep at it, sitting down, breathing quietly, not moving, and slowly bringing the mind inside, you will start to feel a sense of peace, relaxation and buoyancy. That is recharging your battery. That is the most profound thing you can do to bring your energy up."

HOMEOPATHY. Homeopathic remedies can be quite effective in lifting depression. Dr. Gennaro Locurcioas, a homeopathic physician in New York, New Jersey, and London, says that while money does not create happiness, the king of remedies for treating depression is gold—also known as aurum metallicum. Here he describes this and other remedies for treating depression:

Aurum metallicum. This is for the perfectionist woman who has set high goals for herself but is unable to meet them. At first, she will become irritable, a state that can last for several months. She feels as if she has lost the love of those around her and that it is her fault. This leads to feelings of frustration, accompanied by a strong sense of guilt, which may push her to suicide in extreme cases. Dr. Locurcioas observes, "At first sight, this woman appears perfect and polished. When we start talking to her, we get the idea that there is an abnormal focus on career and achievement. Being a workaholic just covers up the emptiness inside."

Arsenicum. This remedy is for depression accompanied by anxiety. The woman is restless day and night. She is constantly on the phone, calling her friends, for fear of being alone. She wakes up at night and walks around the room thinking about her fears and anxieties. She is afraid of a poverty-filled future and of death. "Arsenicum is from arsenic," says Dr. Locurcioas. "If we give that to a person, they die. But giving homeopathic arsenic to a person is completely safe and better than Xanax."

Ignatia. This helps depression associated with grief. A woman has lost her child or her mother, or has been disappointed by a romantic relationship. The patient may exhibit physical characteristics, such as a tic on the face, numbness, a lump in the throat, or sighing. "According to the homeopathic literature, if the patient says that she gets aggravated when she eats sweets, and she improves by traveling, these are signs that ignatia is indicated," notes Dr. Locurcioas.

Sepia is a good example of how homeopathic remedies use substances that relate to a person's symptoms: "This remedy is made from a black mollusk that emits a black ink. Black is the ink from which the remedy is prepared. And black is the color the depressed woman sees around herself. She sees black in her future. This little sea creature, at some point in its life, will deposit about 300 eggs, which are incredibly big for the size of this little animal, and then it will die. This is the housewife who had a job, and had to come home and prepare dinner for the husband and children. For years, she gives the best of her energy to her family and children. Now she is 40, 45, or 50. The children are gone, and she feels as if her mission in life is over. She sees no purpose in her life anymore. She does not hate her husband, but feels indifferent toward him. She does not want to be touched sexually, and cries many times during the day without knowing why. Inside she feels despair and isolation. Physically, she has a dull, inexpressive face, and the muscles of the body have lost their tone. The woman has varicose veins, constipation. *Sepia* is a remedy for the exhausted housewife."

SUPPLEMENTS. Nutrients that enhance brain function, such as the ones listed below, can improve mental and emotional states in depressed women:

Acetyl-L-carnitine. This nutrient crosses the blood brain barrier and provides the brain with more energy. This is a gentle, not jittery, energy, and it is especially important for older people, who tend to lose brain cells due to a lack of energy. Between 500 and 1,500 mg should be taken on an empty stomach.

Liquid zinc. According to Dr. Alexander Schauss, a clinical psychologist, certified eating disorder specialist, and researcher in Tacoma, Washington, "In our eating disorder studies, we used a multidimensional design, and evaluated the affective or mood state of our patients for five years. One of the first things to improve in patients treated with liquid zinc was the degree of depression that they were experiencing based on psychometric instruments such as the Beck Depression Scale, the profile of mood scales, and other depressive indices. This suggests that we might consider using zinc as an antidepressant. There is a growing concern among many patients, and even therapists, that antidepressant drugs, such as Prozac, might not be safe, and we are looking at viable alternatives. We have discovered this antidepressive effect and have documented it in patients under blind conditions."

Phosphatityl serine. This nutrient is produced by the body but lessens with age. Taking 200 to 500 mg improves the ability of brain cell membranes to receive signals and function better. That, in turn, can elevate mood levels, help overcome winter depression, and enhance short-term memory.

Herbal Pharmacy

Plants containing chemicals with antidepressant properties, in order of potency:

Pastinaca sativa (parsnip)
Myrciaria dubia (camu-camu)
Malpighia glabra (acerola)
Lactuca sativa (lettuce)
Amaranthus sp. (pigweed)
Portulaca oleracea (purslane)
Nasturtium officinale (berro)
Chenopodium album (lamb's-quarters)
Cichorium endivia (endive)
Spinacia oleracea (spinach)
Brassica chinensis (Chinese cabbage)
Brassica oleracea (broccoli)
Lycopersicon esculentum (tomato)
Avena sativa (oats)
Raphanus sativus (radish)
Anethum graveolens (dill)
Phaseolus vulgaris (black bean)
Cucurbita foetidissima (buffalo gourd)
Corchorus olitorius (Jew's mallow)

Patient Story

MARIA

Depression and anxiety are very difficult. You get up and do the things you feel you have to do. But you don't feel like you are in the flow of life. My conditions were probably not that apparent to the rest of the world, but I experienced them as very uncomfortable, and they took away from my quality of life. I felt stressed much of the time. And I had difficulty concentrating. At times I would forget things. Someone would ask me to do something, and I would forget to do it. I knew there wasn't something wrong with my mind. I felt my lack of focus was due more to my being so hyped up and tense.

I felt overwhelmed by ordinary, everyday demands, and I felt exhausted by the end of the day. Many times, after lunch, I would feel really tired, almost like I needed to have a nap. Anxiety and depression seemed to gobble up my energy very quickly. By the end of the day, I was not in the mood for recreational activities. Work wore me out. I would just go home and bug out in front of the boob tube. And I wanted more than that.

Once in a while, I would have a drink and notice a difference; I would be able to focus much better. The reason was that the drink helped me to relax. But I didn't want to relax that way. I wanted to find an alternative that would really work for me and help me to feel more joy in my everyday experience.

I went to several physicians, and they prescribed various medications for me. But I couldn't take medicines. They had all kinds of strange side effects, which were just as bad as the anxiety or the depression. The drugs masked my conditions, but underneath they were still there. All they did was make me feel very sleepy much of the time. I would be sitting at a meeting, dozing off, and I couldn't afford to do that. So I only took medications briefly.

I was looking for help when I happened to hear a Gary Null lecture at the Learning Annex. I was very impressed with some of the things I heard about limiting belief systems, and how difficult it is to see beyond them. I liked the talk on vegetarianism as well. As a result, I went to see Dolores Perri and was very impressed.

Dolores went over my history and concerns. I really enjoyed talking to Dolores because, unlike most physicians that I've encountered, she was very relaxed. I didn't get a sense that we were limited by time; we were done when we were done. Basically, I asked my questions and expressed my concerns. It was a very good experience. After we talked, she recommended certain foods, herbs, and supplements.

I have been following a nutritional routine for about two and a half months now, and I have definitely noticed a very dramatic shift. In particular, my hypoglycemia has disappeared. That's mostly from getting rid of refined sugars and processed foods. I used to feel very restless and nervous if I didn't eat. That's been stabilized, and I feel much calmer now.

My energy level is much, much better with a vegetarian regime, supplements, and herbs. The aloe I've been using is outstanding at perking me up at the beginning of the day.

I feel clearer as well. There are subtle differences in my ability to concentrate. And when I go through the day, I feel much calmer. A couple of days ago, I was late for a meeting, through no fault of my own. I had to be late for something I thought was very important. Normally, I would be a complete wreck about it. But because of my new regime, I was calm and centered, and I didn't run up the stairs. I just walked in, explained what had happened, sat down, and joined in.

In the past, I would have been practically shaking from anxiety. This is a real departure, which I attribute largely to my change in diet as well as to my holistic orientation.

I think it's important to know that it's not only a shift in diet that has helped me. I became involved in meditation to clear my mind and help me reach that stillness. I do that in the morning before anything else. In addition, I take a greater interest in the holistic world and participate in seminars. All these different elements help to enhance my well-being.

Hot News

Studies have shown again and again that there is a relationship between nutrition and depression, particularly in geriatric patients, whose ability to absorb nutrients from their diet may be compromised even if the diet itself is acceptable. Specifically, a link with amelioration of depression symptoms has been established regarding vitamins B1, B2, B6, zinc, and the elimination of caffeine and sugar. The efficacy of exercise has also been shown to be significant. Two other promising therapeutic approaches that spare the patient the side of effects of drug medication are light therapy and music therapy. (*See below.*)

NUTRITION/DIET

Epidemiological studies from around the world have shown a correlation between a low intake of omega-3 fatty acids and depression.

J. R. Hibbeln and N. Salem, "Dietary Polyunsaturated Fatty Acids and Depression: When Cholesterol Does Not Satisfy," *American Journal of Clinical Nutrition* 62 (1995): 1–9.

A double-blind, placebo-controlled study examined the relationship between intake of 10 mg each of vitamins B1, B2, and B6 and depression in geriatric patients. Results indicated that subjects taking vitamins suffered from less depression and had improved cognitive functions compared to controls.

I. Bell et al., "Brief Communication: Vitamins B1, B2 and B6 Augmentation of Tricyclic Antidepressant Treatment in Geriatric Depression with Cognitive Dysfunction," *Journal of the American College of Nutrition* 11, no. 2 (1992): 159–63.

Low zinc levels have been linked to mood disorders.

I. J. Mcloughlin et al., "Zinc in Depressive Patient Disorder," *ACTA Psychiatr. Scand.* 82 (1990): 451–53.

A study showed that nimodipine significantly reduced depression scores in 10 outpatients with recurrent depressive episodes.

J. Walden et al., "A Calcium Antagonist for the Treatment of Depressive Episodes: Single Case Reports," *Journal of Psychiatric Research* 29, no. 1 (1995): 71–76.

Elimination of caffeine and sugar from the diets of subjects suffering from major depression yielded significant improvements in terms of all measures of the illness.

L. Christensen and R. Burrows, "Dietary Treatment of Depression," *Behavior Therapy* 21 (1990): 183–93.

A placebo-controlled study showed that the administration of acetyl-L-carnitine to subjects with depression led to significant improvements relative to controls.

M. Gecele et al., "Acetyl-L-Carnitine in Aged Subjects with Major Depression: Clinical Efficacy and Effects on the Circadian Rhythm of Cortisol," *Dementia* 2 (1991): 333–37.

In a placebo-controlled study of geriatric patients with depression, one month of treatment with acetyl-L-carnitine provided significant benefits when the patients were compared to controls.

E. Tempesta et al., "L-Acetylcarnitine in Depressed Elderly Subjects: A Cross-Over Study Versus Placebo," *Drugs, Experimental and Clinical Research* 13, no. 7 (1987): 417–23.

There were negative consequences for depression patients when L-tryptophan was removed from the market. A number of case studies show the efficacy of this substance in treating depression, and many contend that because L-tryptophan is effective it should be left on the market.

I. N. Ferrier et al., "Relapse in Chronic Depressives on Withdrawal of L-Tryptophan," *Lancet* 336 (August 11, 1990): 380–81.

In a double-blind, placebo-controlled study, depressed patients were treated with SAMe (S-Adenosyl-L-Methionine). Results showed the treatment to be safe and effective and to have a relatively rapid onset of action.

B. L. Kagan et al., "Oral S-Adenosyl-L-Methionine in Depression: A Randomized, Double-Blind, Placebo Controlled Trial," *American Journal of Psychiatry* 147, no. 5 (May 1990): 591–95.

Results of a study showed significant improvement in patients with major depression who received SAMe twice daily.

J. F. Rosenbaum et al., "Antidepressant Potential of Oral S-Adenosyl-L-Methionine," *ACTA Psychiatr. Scand.* 81 (1990): 432–36.

In a cross-over, double-blind, placebo-controlled study, 21 Parkinson's disease patients suffering from depression were treated with SAMe. SAMe significantly improved the depression relative to controls.

P. B. Carrieri et al., "S-Adenosyl-L-Methionine Treatment of Depression in Patients with Parkinson's Disease," *Current Therapeutic Research* 48, no. 1 (July 1990): 154–59.

HERBS/PLANT EXTRACTS

In a double-blind, placebo-controlled study, 160 mg of *Ginkgo biloba* extract were given daily for 6 weeks to 60 patients with cerebral insufficiency manifesting in depressive mood. Overall improvements were significant in those taking the *Ginkgo biloba*.

F. Eckmann, "Hirnleistungsstorungen–Behandlung mit Ginkgo-biloba-Extrakt. Zeitpunkt des Wirkungseintrits in einer Doppelblindstudie mit 60 stationaren Patienten" [Cerebral Insufficiency–Treatment with Ginkgo-Biloba Extract. Time of Onset of Effect in a Double-Blind Study with 60 Inpatients], *Fortschr. Med.* 108, no. 29 (October 10, 1990): 557–60.

A placebo-controlled, randomized, double-blind study examined the effects of a St. John's wort extract, LI 160, on patients suffering from moderately severe depression. While 66 percent of those receiving treatment responded positively, only 27 percent of the controls did so.

U. Schmidt and H. Sommer, "Johanniskraut-Extrakt zur ambulanten Therapie de Depression. Aufmerksamkeit und Reaktionsvermogen bleiben erhalten" [St. John's Wort Extract in the Ambulatory Therapy of Depression: Attention and Reaction Ability are Preserved], *Fortschr. Med.* 111, no. 19 (July 10, 1993): 339–42.

A study compared the antidepressive and anxiety-relieving effects of a valerian root and St. John's wort extract to those of amitriptyline. Results showed the herbal extract to be as effective as the amitriptyline, prompting the authors to argue for the use of phytomedicines (plant-derived medicines) in the treatment of depression and mood disorders.

K. O. Hiller and V. Rahlfs, "Therapeutische Aquivalenz Eines Hochdoserten Phytopharmakons mit Amitriptylin bei Angstlich-Depressiven Verstimmungen - Reanalyse einer Randomisierten Studie unter Besonderer Beachtung Biometrischer und Klinischer Aspekte," *Forsch-Komplementarmed* 2, no. 3 (1995): 123–32.

In a randomized, double-blind, placebo-controlled study, 300 mg of the hypericum extract LI 160 was administered to patients with mild depression 3 times daily for 4 weeks. The treatment group showed significant improvement compared to controls, with 70 percent showing no symptoms after 4 weeks.

W. D. Hubner et al., "Hypericum Treatment of Mild Depressions with Somatic Symptoms," *Journal Geriatr. Psychiatry Neurol.* 7, suppl. (October 1994): 12–14.

Siberian ginseng has proven effective in numerous studies in treating psychological ailments such as depression, insomnia, hypochrondria, and various neuroses.

N. R. Farnsworth et al., "Siberian Ginseng (*Eleutheroccocus senticosus*): Current Status as an Adaptogen," *Econ. Med. Plant Research* 1 (1985): 156–215.

EXERCISE

A significant association was found between low levels of physical activity and the risk of depression. That risk can be decreased by increasing exercise levels.

T. C. Camacho et al., "Physical Activity and Depression: Evidence from the Alameda County Study," *American Journal of Public Health* 134, no. 2 (1991): 220–31.

Since lifelong exercisers suffer less from depression than do nonexercisers, numerous studies support exercise as an effective means of preventing and treating depression.

E. W. Martinsen, "Benefits of Exercise for the Treatment of Depression," *Sports Medicine* 9, no. 6 (1990): 380–89.

All women participating in a water exercise program who suffered from depression experienced an improvement after 8 weeks.

C. R. Weiss and N. B. Jamieson, "Women, Subjective Depression, and Water Exercise," *Health Care Women Int.* 10, no. 1 (1989): 75–88.

Depressed women participating in an aerobic exercise program for 10 weeks reported greater decreases in their depression than did those participating in a relaxation program and those receiving no treatment at all.

I. L. McCann and D. S. Holmes, "Influence of Aerobic Exercise on Depresssion," *Journal of Personality and Social Psychology* 46, no. 5 (May 1984): 1142–47.

A review of the interaction of exercise and depression concludes that there is clearly an inverse relationship between the two. The author argues that exercise should be considered a promising approach to treating the disorder.

E. W. Martinsen, "Benefits of Exercise for the Treatment of Depression," *Sports Medicine* 9, no. 6 (June 1990): 380–89.

LIGHT THERAPY

Fifty-four depressed patients with seasonal affective disorder were exposed to cool-white fluorescent light from 6:00 to 8:00 a.m. for 2 weeks. Depression scores dropped significantly as a result.

R. W. Lam, "Morning Light Therapy for Winter Depression: Predictors of Response," *ACTA Psychiatr. Scand.* 89 (1994): 97–101.

A study gave 2 hours of green light per day for a week compared to a week of red light therapy to 20 patients with seasonal affective disorder. Results showed that the green light resulted in stronger antidepressant effects than did the red light.

D. A Orem et al., "Treatment of Seasonal Affective Disorder with Green Light and Red Light," *American Journal of Psychiatry* 148, no. 4 (April 1991): 509–11.

A double-blind controlled study showed that morning light was significantly superior to evening light in reducing depressive symptoms. Based on these findings, the authors suggest that bright light therapy provides an earlier secretion of melatonin, which is responsible for the treatment's positive effects on winter depression, since these patients tend to have delayed circadian rhythms.

R. L. Sack et al., "Morning vs. Evening Light Treatment for Winter Depression: Evidence that the Therapeutic Effects of Light are Mediated by Circadian Phase Shifts," *Archives of General Psychiatry* 47 (April 1990): 343–51.

MENTAL IMAGERY

A study demonstrated a significant relationship between the use of guided mental imagery and a decrease in anxiety and depression levels relative to controls.

J. L. Rash, "The Use of Guided Mental Imagery in Its Effect on Anxiety and Depresson in the Cancer Patient," *Dissertation Abstracts International* 52, no. 3 (1991): 1735.

Relaxation with guided imagery significantly improved self-esteem and decreased anxiety and depression symptoms in women who had just given birth for the first time.

B. L. Rees, "Effect of Relaxation with Guided Imagery on Anxiety, Depression, and Self-Esteem in Primiparas," *Journal of Holistic Nursing* 13, no. 3 (September 1995): 255–67.

MUSIC THERAPY

It was shown that 8 weeks of music therapy significantly improved scores on tests of depression, distress, self-esteem, and mood in older adults suffering from minor depression. Benefits were maintained up to 9 months following treatment.

S. B. Hanser and L. W. Thompson, "Effects of a Music Therapy Strategy on Depressed Older Adults," *Journal of Gerontology* 49, no. 6 (November 1994): 265–69.

The effectiveness of 8 weeks of music therapy on patients with senile depression who were on antidepressive drugs was shown. Patients receiving the music therapy and drugs reported more benefits than those treated with drugs only. What's more, they experienced the benefits within a week, as opposed to those on drugs only, who did not start feeling better until 3–4 weeks into the trial.

X. Chen, [Active Music Therapy for Senile Depression], *Chung Hua Shen Ching Ching Shen Ko Tsa Chih* 25, no. 4 (August 1992): 208–10, 252–53.

7. DIABETES

Diabetes mellitus is a serious condition that claims over a quarter million lives a year, a number that, unfortunately, has grown over time. Today diabetes is the second leading cause of death in the United States and a primary cause of new cases of blindness, renal disease, and nontraumatic amputations. Dr. Robert Atkins, a complementary physician from New York City, says, "In 1960, 1 percent of the American population was diabetic, but now it is 3 percent. Diabetes has tripled in the last thirty-five years. In addition, certain subsegments of the population are more often affected; African-Americans, for example, are disproportionately affected." Women taking oral contraceptives may also be increasing their risk of diabetes, since oral contraceptives have been associated with lower vitamin B levels, which can lead to glucose intolerance.

Causes

Diabetes is closely associated with heart disease, and the incidence of both conditions increased when Americans began to change their diet patterns. "There is a wonderful book written about twenty-five years ago," Dr. Atkins continues, "called *The Saccharine Disease,* by Dr. Cleave. He made observations, one of which was the law of twenty years, which says that after you introduce refined carbohydrates into a culture, two illnesses emerge twenty years later, diabetes and heart disease. We know that a Third World diet, without the refined carbohydrates, leads to no heart disease and no diabetes. When one illness emerges, so does the other. Studies of this sort have linked diabetes with heart disease. We know that a woman who is diabetic is three times more likely than women in the general population to get heart disease."

Under normal circumstances, insulin is released by the pancreas in response to elevated levels of sugar in the blood. It promotes transport and entry of glucose to muscle cells and various tissues, thus lowering blood sugar levels. In the diabetic, part of the process is interrupted due to either a deficiency, resistance, or insensitivity to insulin:

Insulin deficiency. For many years, it was thought that diabetes was purely and simply a deficiency syndrome, in which the body did not produce sufficient quantities of insulin for proper glucose metabolism and assimilation. More recently, it has been learned that many diabetics do produce enough insulin, but their cells do not take it in. The problem is then due to insulin insensitivity or resistance.

Insulin insensitivity. Insulin enters cells at points known as receptor sites. When these receptor sites become plugged up by fat, cholesterol, inactivity, and obesity, insulin cannot enter. As a result, glucose stays in the blood and creates hyperglycemia or high blood sugar. This excess sugar is diagnosed as diabetes. In these cases, there is not a need to increase insulin production but a need to enhance insulin sensitivity. The person needs to work at making their own insulin more efficient, and simply increasing the amount of insulin will not do that.

Insulin resistance. This is a closely related phenomenon, in which there is also a sufficient or even overabundant supply of insulin. Here, allergic responses prevent insulin from doing its job. Usually, allergies to specific foods suppress the activity and efficiency of insulin. Different factors may be responsible for a disordered carbohydrate metabolism in different people. Wheat, for instance, may create symptoms of high blood sugar in one woman and corn may affect another. Offending substances can be determined on an individual basis with food allergy tests.

Different factors are responsible for the two main types of diabetes:

Juvenile or type I diabetes is the most serious form of the disease; it usually manifests itself in childhood or teenage years. This form of diabetes is characterized by a true insulin deficiency. It apparently results when the pancreas is damaged from some exotic viral infection or even a highly toxic state. The disease may also be a genetic condition. Since juvenile diabetics have an insulin deficiency, they have to receive insulin regularly, and generally for life.

Maturity-onset or type II diabetes is more of an acquired disease. It is often precipitated by chronic excess weight from poor diet and/or lack of exercise. It may also be brought on by overconsumption of stressor foods or other allergens that are insulin resistors. This form of the disease is characterized by complications of insulin resistance and insulin sensitivity rather than, in most cases, a true deficiency of insulin. For this reason, maturity onset diabetes can frequently be non-insulin-dependent.

Symptoms

Often there are no symptoms present, especially in the beginning stages of type II diabetes. The prediabetic state can be accompanied by obesity, especially when it is centered at the waistline and just above the waistline. Classical diabetic symptoms are more often experienced by type I diabetics and include frequent urination, especially at night, great thirst and hunger, fatigue, weight loss, irritability, and restlessness. Progressively, the eyes, kidneys, nervous system, and skin become affected. Infections and hardening of the arteries commonly develop. In type I diabetes, coma from a lack of insulin is an ongoing danger.

Clinical Experience

TRADITIONAL APPROACHES

INSULIN. Before the development of insulin in the 1920s, diabetic patients had a bleak prognosis. Sufferers saw the condition rapidly go from bad to worse as complications such as blindness, gout, and gangrene developed. Overall life span was drastically shortened.

In the beginning, insulin appeared to be a miraculous drug, and in fact it probably was. The life span of diabetic children was extended from months to decades. Today, many of these children live normal, productive lives.

The problem with insulin is that it is prescribed to all diabetics, not just those with true insulin deficiencies. While insulin addresses the immediate crisis by lowering blood sugar levels, it does little to correct long-range problems. In fact, many adverse effects can be heightened by aggressive insulin therapy. Insulin stimulates the development of antagonists in the body that counteract its blood-sugar-lowering effects. When a diabetic receives insulin, the person's blood sugar begins to fall. The body immediately responds to the falling levels of blood sugar by stimulating growth hormones and epinephrine. These hormones keep blood sugar levels elevated because the brain needs sugar.

The result of aggressive insulin therapy is a rebounding effect. Blood sugar is high, so insulin is injected. This makes the level plummet as the blood sugar is forced down by the insulin. But that drop cues the insulin antagonists to quickly raise blood sugar again to meet what the body perceives as a life-threatening situation.

This constant fluctuation of blood sugar levels leads to a wide range of long-term disorders. In fact, clinical experience shows that diabetics treated aggressively with insulin have a 40 percent greater incidence of eye problems than those treated moderately. Despite this finding, it is still common for diabetics with worsening eye problems to be treated more and more aggressively.

Insulin may also contribute significantly to inner arterial wall damage, which is a major problem among diabetics. The incidence of heart attacks and strokes is five to eight times greater among diabetics. About 75 percent of all diabetic mortality is due to heart disease brought on by hardening of the major arteries.

Other complications that may involve insulin use are related to the damage done to the microvascular vessels, particularly those leading to the eyes, kidneys, and peripheral nerves. As these arteries become thickened and brittle, they become less and less functional, and it becomes increasingly difficult for blood to pass through. In the eyes, sudden surges of blood sugar put extra stress on the retinal blood vessels. If the stress is repeated, as it frequently is in diabetics, the vessels will hemorrhage and break. Over time, many hemorrhages will occur and blindness will result. After glaucoma, this is the most common cause of blindness in older people.

In the kidneys a similar succession of events frequently results in a renal insufficiency and in an inability to eliminate nitrogen waste from the body efficiently.

Insulin's interference with proper blood circulation, involving both large and small vessels, is also responsible for a high incidence of neuritis and gangrene, which frequently lends itself to peripheral tingling in the fingers and toes, a loss of feeling, and amputation. Sexual dysfunction is also related to this. Most of these complications occur after repeated exposure to fluctuating blood sugar levels.

Many of the secondary problems associated with diabetes, then, result from the indiscriminate overuse of insulin and the failure of the medical profession to employ natural, noninvasive, and efficacious methods of holding diabetic symptoms in check. Although 90 percent of diabetics are type II, they have been lumped together with type I as being able to benefit from insulin treatment in cases where blood sugar remains consistently and dangerously high. Type II, maturity-onset diabetics can be non-insulin-dependent in most instances, and should not be treated with aggressive insulin programs prescribed for type I juvenile diabetics, who are, generally, insulin dependent. A great many people who need insulin can drastically reduce the amount needed by incorporating a wider spectrum of treatment approaches beyond just maintaining blood sugar levels.

ORAL HYPOGLYCEMIC MEDICATIONS AND HEART ATTACKS. Insulin is not the only culprit in traditional diabetes treatment; there is also a group of oral hypoglycemic medications that stimulate the secretion of more insulin and thus lower the blood sugar level. Some even act peripherally; that is, they awaken and increase the number of sensitive receptor sites so that there are more locations for glucose to enter the cell. This peripheral action, in effect, makes insulin go further. It extends its potential efficacy more than it could by merely increasing its presence in the bloodstream.

These oral agents—which include Orinase, Diabinase, Tolinase, and other pharmaceuticals—are a cause for concern because of their potential adverse side effects. They have been shown to greatly increase heart disease and death due to heart attack. What we are looking at is a disease in which heart disease is a risk factor being treated with drugs that drastically increase the likelihood of premature heart attacks.

CURRENT DIETARY RECOMMENDATIONS. Although insulin has been at the center of traditional diabetes treatment, some attention has also been given to dietary modification. Unfortunately, the greatest part of the dietary advice given is not well founded and may contribute to a worsening condition.

There are several shortcomings associated with the standard diabetic diet. First, the diabetic is told to avoid all carbohydrates, since these foods eventually break down into glucose. But no distinction is made between simple sugars and complex carbohydrates. Fiber is also denigrated because it is considered a carbohydrate, which it is not. In addition, there is no attempt to relate allergic responses to specific foods. The dietary advice commonly given only worsens the diabetic's condition and is responsible for many side effects and complications.

Unlike simple sugars, complex carbohydrates are beneficial. Although both are broken down into glucose, the latter do not go directly into the bloodstream. While simple sugars immediately enter the blood, complex carbohydrates go through a long process of digestion and only very gradually release sugar into the blood. Therefore, they do not then contribute to the high blood sugar levels, as do simple carbohydrates. Instead, they stabilize and improve health.

While diabetics are told to stay away from potatoes and rice, they are advised to eat more protein. They are, in effect, being told to jump from the frying pan into the fire. First, protein is high in fat and cholesterol, especially when it is derived from animal sources. Fat accumulates in the blood and sets the patient up for cardiovascular disease. In addition, it clogs receptor sites, which thus become more desensitized or resistant to insulin. Blood sugar inevitably rises, causing the doctor to prescribe more insulin or oral medication in an attempt to stabilize the blood sugar.

Large amounts of protein are also related to accelerated kidney damage. This is because protein must be immediately processed by the body; it cannot be stored. This puts a great stress on the nephron cells, which filter the body's toxins. Many diabetics suffer from kidney deterioration as a result and must receive dialysis or a kidney transplant. Studies show that the elimination of meat from the diet is often enough to reverse kidney damage.

THE NATURAL APPROACH

Despite its severity, diabetes need not be as debilitating as it usually is. While there is currently no cure, there are ways of enhancing the body's natural defenses through nutrition, avoidance of allergy-producing substances, and exercise. A healthy lifestyle and alternative approaches to treatment can decrease the amount of insulin or oral medications needed by some persons; others may be completely weaned off these substances. The goal of treatment can and should be to build up the body's ability to function as independently as possible.

When changing to a more holistic approach to treatment, it is important not to immediately discontinue any medication, including insulin. Instead, a preventive medicine physician should assist in the gradual transition. With a doctor's guidance, an insulin dependency may be reduced or completely eliminated with time. Complete elimination, however, is not always possible.

Physicians who practice alternative approaches to treating diabetes for the most part employ a program combining exercise and dietary modification aimed both at better nutrition and at weight loss, where indicated. Insulin and medications are used only as second- and third-line approaches. This sort of program usually controls the disease and its ancillary complications in a less invasive, more efficacious manner, in a short period of time.

While maturity-onset diabetics respond most dramatically, even juvenile diabetics may be able to reduce their insulin dependency. More importantly, they are able to alleviate many of the insidious complications that have come to be thought of as intrinsic to diabetes.

DIET. Since diabetes and heart disease are so closely related, Dr. Atkins recommends that some people with diabetes follow a Dean Ornish program, in which they drastically cut down on dietary fats. The best diet consists of organic vegetarian foods, eaten raw, sprouted, steamed, baked, or stir-fried with little or no oil. Those who have a true insulin disorder will not fare well on a high-carbohydrate diet, since diabetes is a carbohydrate metabolism disorder. "It is important to know who needs carbohydrate restriction versus who needs fat restriction," Dr. Atkins says. "To determine that, there are a variety of tests, including a cholesterol profile in which we look at the ratio between the triglycerides and the HDL. When a person has a blood sugar disorder leading to a lipid disorder, the ratio is extremely high. To be really safe, the number should be approximately the same, or the HDL should be higher than the triglycerides. It is perfectly appropriate to spend five or six weeks on one diet and then get all of your parameters checked again, and then five or six weeks on the other diet, and get them checked again. In that way, you can make an intelligent decision."

EXERCISE. An exercise regimen is crucial for burning calories and normalizing metabolism, and is especially important for overweight adults who tend to be inactive.

Exercise also heightens the body's sensitivity to insulin. By lowering cholesterol, it lowers triglyceride levels in the blood, making cells more available for glucose assimilation. This is why the insulin requirements of diabetic athletes always drop while they're engaged in swimming, soccer, and other sports. Athletes also notice an increase in their insulin requirements when they cease their physical activities for any extended period of time.

Athletes are not the only ones to benefit from exercise. Ten to twenty minutes of light exercise after each meal helps to reduce the amount of insulin necessary to keep blood sugar levels under control. A brisk walk gets the body's metabolism working a little bit faster so that the absorption of food is more easily distributed. That prevents blood sugar from rising too high.

An exception to the rule is for diabetics with heart disease. In these patients, exercising after eating may precipitate an angina attack because of the transfer of blood from the intestines to the legs and other parts of the body.

ALLERGY TESTING. Testing for food allergies can determine which foods are responsible for insulin resistance. Clinical experience has shown that this approach to treatment is the most useful way to get to the root of adult-onset diabetes and to reverse the condition. Patients can usually be weaned off insulin, since an insulin deficiency is not the cause of the problem. Eliminating allergy-producing foods may also foster weight loss. This occurs because people crave foods when they are allergic to them. When these foods are taken out of the diet, the desire for them eventually stops.

To determine whether a specific food is causing hyperglycemia, a doctor can monitor a patient's blood sugar before and after a specific food is eaten. Foods that raise the blood sugar cause allergic reactions and should be eliminated.

SUPPLEMENTS. In addition to diet and exercise, the following supplements are important to know about:

Chromium picolinate. Chromium helps normalize glucose levels in insulin-dependent diabetics.

Magnesium and *potassium* help to maintain a glucose tolerance level.

Zinc is essential for normal insulin production.

Enzymes. Digestive protylase, amylase, and lipase.

Vanadyl sulfate may be the most important mineral for diabetes. It was discovered in France in the late 1800s and used to control diabetes before insulin appeared. It works at the cellular level and is most effective when taken three times a day.

TOPICAL TREATMENT FOR DIABETIC ULCERS. Diabetic ulcers plague many patients with this disease and cause a condition that is often serious enough to warrant amputation. This tragedy can be averted with a simple solution. According to clinical studies, raw, unprocessed honey is an ideal dressing agent for almost every type of wound or ulcer. It sterilizes the area, and often works even after antibiotics fail.

HOMEOPATHY. The remedy Mucokehl, from Germany, may actually reverse diabetic neuropathy. People using this remedy get feeling back in their extremities, and their eyesight improves.

CHELATION THERAPY is known to reduce diabetic retinopathy and foot ulcers. *(See description in chapter 1, Aging.)*

Herbal Pharmacy

Plants containing phytochemicals with antidiabetic properties, in order of potency:

Cichorium intybus (chicory)
Rauvalfia serpentina (Indian snakeroot)
Thymus vulgaris (common thyme)
Arctium lappa (gobo)
Carthamus tinctorius (safflower)
Passiflora edulis (maracuya)
Opuntia ficus-indica (Indian fig)
Taraxacum officinale (dandelion)
Tetrapanax papyriferus (rice-paper)
Canavalia ensiformis (jack bean)
Linum usitatissimum (flax)
Pueraria lobata (kudzu)
Hordeum vulgare (barley)
Inula helenium (elecampane)
Althaea officinalis (marsh mallow)
Oenothera biennis (evening primrose)
Avena sativa (oats)
Triticum aestivum (wheat)
Medicago sativa (alfalfa)
Panicum maximum (guinea grass)

Plants containing phytochemicals with insulin-sparing properties, in order of potency:

Cocos nucifera (coconut)
Plantago major (common plantain)

Hot News

Recent studies have suggested that supplementation can provide clear assistance in the management of diabetes. For example, chromium supplementation can improve the ability of the body to maintain glucose levels with a lower output of insulin. Barley is a good natural source of chromium. Other types of supplementation that have been shown to help in recent studies include vitamin E, magnesium, biotin, powdered fenugreek seed, and the juice, seeds, or dried fruit of bitter melon. Yoga and biofeedback therapy have also been shown to help. *(See below.)*

NUTRITION/DIET

Diabetes mellitus is the third leading cause of death in the United States and is responsible for 12 percent of all new cases of blindness, 25 percent of all cases of end-stage renal disease, and 40 percent of all non-traumatic amputations of the feet and legs among adults. Studies have shown that vitamin B6 levels are significantly decreased during periods of hyperglycemia and that B6 deficiency can reduce pancreatic and circulating insulin levels. Deficiency of B6 can result in reduced liver glycogen levels, abnormal glucose tolerance, abnormal gluconeogenesis, reduced serum and pancreatic insulin levels, degenerative changes in B-cells, reduced growth hormone levels, reduced insulin response to glucose load, and reduced lactate dehydrogenase. Oral contraceptive intake has been associated with lowered vitamin B levels, leading to glucose intolerance. Vitamin B6 deficiency is also seen in cases of pregnancy-related insulin resistance. Low vitamin B6 has also been shown to cause high levels of xanthurenic acid, which is believed to be a factor in gestational diabetes and glucose intolerance. One hundred mg of pyridoxine administered daily for two weeks has been shown to reduce levels of xanthurenic acid.

K. S. Rogers and Chandra Mohan, "Vitamin B6 Metabolism and Diabetes," *Biochemical Medicine and Metabiologic Biology* 52 (1994): 10–17.

Results of a placebo-controlled study suggest that guar gum might improve glucose control in diabetics and reduce the risk of heart-related complications.

Helena Vuorinen-Markkola et al., "Guar Gum and Insulin-Dependent Diabetes: Effects on Glycemic Control and Serum Lipoproteins," The *American Journal of Clinical Nutrition* 56 (1992): 1056–60.

A study found that diabetic patients consuming between 14 and 26 g of guar per day had less glycosuria and required less insulin than did controls. Patients with diets consisting of at least 40 percent complex carbohydrates experienced the best results with guar supplementation.

D. J. A. Jenkins, "Diabetic Diets: High Carbohydrates Combined with High Fiber," *American Journal of Clinical Nutrition* 33 (1980): 1729–33.

Twenty mg of zinc gluconate was given to healthy subjects the evening before and 30 minutes following glucose tolerance samplings. Results showed that zinc increased glucose assimilation and effectiveness.

J. F. Brun et al., "Effects of Oral Zinc Gluconate on Glucose Effectiveness and Insulin Sensitivity in Humans," *Biological Trace Element Research* 47 (1995): 385–91.

A study found that soluble B-glucans consumed via an oat extract for five weeks reduced glucose responses and insulin responses in patients with moderately high cholesterol concentrations.

Judith Hallfrisch et al., "Diets Containing Soluble Oat Extracts Improve Glucose and Insulin Responses of Moderately Hypercholesterolemic Men and Women," *American Journal of Clinical Nutrition* 61 (1995): 379–84.

Taurine may lead to a decrease in diabetic complications, a study showed.

Flavial Franconi, "Plasma and Platelet Taurine are Reduced in Subjects with Insulin-Dependent Diabetes Mellitus: Effects of Taurine Supplementation," *American Journal of Clinical Nutrition* 61 (1995): 1115–19.

Vitamin C in doses of 100–600 mg per day was administered to 54 young adults between 19 and 34 years of age, 9 of whom had insulin-dependent diabetes mellitus. Within 30 days of supplementation, red blood cell sorbitol levels were normalized in the insulin-dependent diabetic patients.

J. L. Cunningham, "Vitamin C: An Aldose Reductase Inhibitor That Normalizes Erythrocyte Sorbitol in Insulin-Dependent Diabetes Mellitus," *Journal of the American College of Nutrition* 13, no. 4 (1994): 344–50.

A study done with vitamin C suggests that this vitamin may retard the progression of chronic diabetic complications.

"Vitamin C Reported to Cut Glycosylation," *Medical Tribune* (February 27, 1992): 27.

Researchers found that levels of vitamin C within cells were 33 percent below average in a group of insulin-dependent adult diabetics compared to controls. These results raise the possibility that some of the degenerative complications of diabetes may be due to intracellular scurvy.

J. Cunningham et al., "Reduced Mononuclear Leukocyte Ascorbic Acid Content in Adults with Insulin-Dependent Diabetes Mellitus Consuming Adequate Dietary Vitamin C," *Metabolism* 40 (1991): 146–49.

A review article explains that 13 out of 15 studies on chromium and glucose tolerance showed that chromium supplementation provides benefits by maintaining glucose levels with a lower output of insulin and that a deficiency in chromium causes insulin resistance, which supplementation can improve.

"Chromium: The Best Kept Secret for Diabetes," *Nutrition Report* (March 1994): 23.

Barley contains approximately 5.69 mcg of chromium per gram and, in fact, barley bread is a common Iraqi treatment for diabetes due to its ability to modulate glycemic response to carbohydrate ingestion, and slow excessive water consumption and weight loss. A study fed diabetic rats diets containing either barley, starch, or sucrose. Only the rats receiving barley showed any improvements on diabetic parameters and it's suggested that the chromium content of the barley was responsible for these results.

G. Mahdi et al., "Role of Chromium in Barley in Modulating the Symptoms of Diabetes," *Annals of Nutrition and Metabolism* 35 (1991): 65–70.

A review article outlines the benefits of chromium for diabetic patients. Examples include this element's role in regulating insulin's action and maintaining normal glucose tolerance. The author believes that chromium should be thought of primarily as a preventive measure for diabetes rather than as a treatment, yet still recommends its use in patients already suffering from the disease.

R. A. Anderson, "Chromium, Glucose Tolerance and Diabetes," *Biological Trace Element Research* 32 (1992): 19–24.

The biological functions of chromium and insulin are closely associated, since most chromium-induced reactions are dependent on insulin. Studies have shown that adequate chromium nutrition—dependent on organic rather than synthetic versions of this mineral—may improve blood lipid profiles and decrease the need for insulin.

R. A. Anderson, "Nutritional Role of Chromium," *Science Total Environ.* 17, no. 1 (January 1981): 13–29.

Researchers in Sweden have shown that prior to diagnosis, insulin-dependent diabetic children eat more foods containing nitrates, nitrites, and nitrosamines relative to controls, and that as much as 70 percent of total nitrate exposure may come through drinking water. In line with these findings, a Colorado study of nitrate concentrations in different water districts found a significant relationship between nitrate in the water and an increased risk of insulin-dependent diabetes in children.

"Low Level Nitrates May Promote Diabetes," *Medical Tribune* (December 24, 1992): 24.

Vitamin E appears to be useful in improving insulin action and reducing oxidative stress.

G. Parolisso et al., "Pharmacologic Doses of Vitamin E Improve Insulin Action in Healthy Subjects and in Non-Insulin-Dependent Diabetic Patients," *American Journal of Clinical Nutrition* 57 (1993): 650–56.

A study examined the effect of vitamin E supplementation in non-insulin-dependent diabetics with proliferative retinopathy. Vitamin E was found to inhibit ADP-induced platelet aggregation in a dose-dependent manner. Significantly more inhibition was observed in diabetic platelets than in the control platelets when vitamin E was supplemented in amounts small enough to be considered physiological doses in vivo. Such findings, the authors argue, indicate platelet function and prostaglandin metabolism in diabetes mellitus may be improved by supplementation with vitamin E, thus reducing vascular complications.

M. Kunisaki et al., "Effects of Vitamin E Administration on Platelet Function in Diabetes Mellitus," *Diabetes Research* 14, no. 1 (May 1990): 37–42.

Non-obese diabetic mice were given vitamin E beginning at 3 weeks old up through 30 weeks to examine this vitamin's effects on pancreatic beta cells leading to type 1 diabetes. Results showed that vitamin E significantly delayed the onset of the disease but did not reduce its incidence.

P. E. Beales et al., "Vitamin E Delays Diabetes Onset in the Non-Obese Diabetic Mouse," *Hormonal Metab. Res.* 26, no. 10 (October 1994): 450–42.

In a study, 4 g of evening primrose oil, 200 mg of vitamin E, and 2.4 g of sardine oil were given to 7 non-insulin-dependent diabetic patients for 4 weeks. Results suggest that abnormal lipid and thromboxane A2 metabolism in diabetics can be improved by such oil treatments.

R. Takahashi et al., "Evening Primrose Oil and Fish Oil in Non-Insulin-Dependent Diabetes," *Prostaglandins, Leukotrienes and Essential Fatty Acids* 49 (1993): 569–71.

Eating small amounts of food throughout the day can be a good nutrition strategy for diabetics. A study compared the effects of a "nibbling diet" and a more standard diet in non-insulin-dependent diabetes mellitus patients. For one day, patients consumed the same diet either broken down into 13 snacks throughout the day or in 3 meals and one snack. Results: The nibbling diet proved more effective than the 3-meal diet, with reductions reported in blood glucose, serum insulin, insulin concentrations, serum triglycerides, and C-peptide concentrations.

D. Jenkins et al., "Metabolic Advantages of Spreading the Nutrient Load: Effects of Increased Meal Frequency in Non-Insulin-Dependent Diabetes," *American Journal of Clinical Nutrition* 44 (1992): 461–67.

Arguing that magnesium balance is critical for insulin homeostasis in patients suffering from insulin-dependent diabetes, the authors suggest diabetics be periodically measured for magnesium levels in the blood and supplemented if necessary.

G. Saggese et al., "Hypomagnesium and the Parathyroid Hormone-Vitamin D Endocrine System in Children with Insulin-Dependent Diabetes Mellitus: Effect of Magnesium Administration," *Journal of Pediatrics* 118 (1991): 220-25.

A review article on the relationship between magnesium and glucose homeostasis notes that magnesium is a second messenger for insulin action, that insulin helps regulate intracellular magnesium accumulation, and that it is common to see low intracellular magnesium levels in diabetes patients. Studies have shown that supplementation with daily doses of magnesium between 240 and 480 mg in insulin-dependent diabetics improves beta-cell response and insulin action. One study in which non-insulin-dependent patients were supplemented with 3 g a day of magnesium for 3 weeks demonstrated an improvement in glucose and arginine-induced insulin secretion and in insulin sensitivity.

G. Paolisso et al., "Magnesium and Glucose Homeostasis," *Diabetologia* 33 (1990): 501–14.

Nicotinamide was given to 6 of 13 diabetics; those receiving the treatment showed an increase in insulin secretion, as opposed to controls, who showed a decrease. Based on these findings, it is suggested that nicotinamide repairs beta-cell function in high-risk diabetics without preexisting severe damage.

R. Manna et al., "Nicotinamide Treatment in Subjects at High Risk of Developing Insulin Dependent Diabetes Improves Insulin Secretion," *British Journal of Clinical Practice* 46, no. 3 (Autumn 1992): 177–79.

A placebo-controlled study examined the effects of psyllium fiber on glucose and insulin levels in non-insulin-dependent diabetics. When psyllium (sugar-free Metamucil) was ingested prior to a meal, it did significantly reduce postmeal levels of glucose and insulin.

J. G. Pastors et al., "Psyllium Fiber Reduces Rise in Postprandial Glucose and Insulin Concentrations in Patients with Non-Insulin Diabetes," *American Journal of Clinical Nutrition* 53 (1991): 1431–35.

The high-fat diets conventionally used to treat diabetes result in higher insulin requirements than do diets high in complex carbohydrates. Fiber is cited as an antidote to high levels of fasting triglycerides. A diabetic diet containing 35 to 40 g of fiber per 1,000 calories and relying on carbohydrates to make up 70 percent of total energy has been shown to decrease plasma glucose levels and insulin or sulfonylurea requirements. Such a diet can also produce a reduction in triglyceride and serum cholesterol levels in those suffering from hypertriglyceridemia.

J. W. Anderson, "High-Fibre Diets for Diabetic and Hypertriglyceridemic Patients," *Canadian Medical Association Journal* 123, no. 10 (November 22, 1980): 975–79.

A study of the influence of antioxidants and trace elements on diabetics found that a mixture of multivitamins including trace elements provided significant protection for diabetics against the damaging effects of free radicals.

V. Holecek et al., "Vyznam Podavani Multivitaminove Smesi a Stopovych Prvk-u u Diabetu" [Administration of Multivitamin Combinations and Trace Elements in Diabetes], *Cas Lek Cesk* 134, no. 3 (February 1, 1995): 80–83.

It has been shown that a legume-rich, high-carbohydrate diet leads to an across-the-board improvement in all measures of diabetic control.

H. C. R. Simpson et al., "A High Carbohydrate Leguminous Fibre Diet Improves All Aspects of Diabetic Control," *Lancet* 1 (1981): 1–5.

Supplementation with 16 mg per day of biotin significantly improved the control of glucose levels in diabetics.

A. Reddi et al., "Biotin Supplementation Improves Glucose and Insulin Intolerances in Genetically Diabetic KK Mice," *Life Sciences* 42 (1988): 1323–30.

Lower calorie intake results in lowered insulin needs. It was found that insulin doses can be reduced by half in diabetics when they are on a 500- to 800-calorie/day diet, and by another 10 percent after a week.

"Pre-Planned Decrease in Insulin with Calorie Restriction," *Obesity Update* (1991): 7.

A study was made of more than 4500 patients, including 652 with non-insulin-dependent diabetes, enrolled in a Pritikin Longevity Center lifestyle modification program. The patients underwent a 26-day dietary shift to low-fat, high-complex-carbohydrate, high-fiber, low-cholesterol, and low-salt foods. Aerobic walking was also a significant part of the program. Results showed a reduction in fasting glucose levels, and 71 percent of those patients on oral hypoglycemic medication, as well as 39 percent on insulin, were able to stop taking medication.

R. J. Barnard et al., "Diet and Exercise in the Treatment of Non-Insulin-Dependent Diabetes Mellitus," *Diabetes Care* 17, no. 12 (December 1994): 1469–72.

BREAST-FEEDING VERSUS COW'S MILK

Two studies found a significant link between the consumption of cow's milk during the early months and years of life and the risk of developing diabetes relative to children who were breast-fed only.

Dan Hurley, "Studies Confirm Diabetes Risk from Cow's Milk in Infants," *Medical Tribune* (February 5, 1995): 11.

Epidemiologic data show that an absence or short duration of breast-feeding, early introduction of cow's milk into the diet, and a high intake of nitrates and nitrosyl compounds can increase the risk of insulin-dependent diabetes. Obesity is also a serious non-insulin-dependent diabetes risk factor.

S. M. Virtanen and Antti Aro, "Dietary Factors and the Etiology of Diabetes," *Annals of Medicine* 26 (1994): 469–78.

A study of children recently diagnosed with diabetes found that the earlier the introduction of dairy products and the greater their consumption, the higher several of their antibody titers were, which was associated with an increased risk of insulin-dependent diabetes.

S. M. Virtanen et al., "Diet, Cow's Milk Protein Antibodies and the Risk of IDDM in Finnish Children," *Diabetologia* 37 (1994): 381–87.

A study found that insulin-dependent diabetics are immune to cow's milk albumin and that antibodies to albumin peptide can react with beta-cell-specific surface protein, which can lead to dysfunction in the islets.

Jukka Karjalainen et al., "A Bovine Albumin Peptide as a Possible Trigger of Insulin-Dependent Diabetes Mellitus," *New England Journal of Medicine* (July 30, 1992): 302–7.

HERBS/PLANT EXTRACTS

A study found that five non-insulin-dependent diabetics experienced a mean reduction in fasting blood sugar of 273 to 151 mg/dl following 14 weeks of taking a half teaspoon 4 times daily of aloes.

Nadia Gnhannam et al., "The Antidiabetic Activity of Aloes," *Hormone Research* 24 (1986): 288–94.

Results of a study showed that 54 diabetics taking 500–600 mg a day of bilberry (*Vaccinium myrtillus* extract) over a period of 8 to 33 months experienced a 30-percent decrease in structural glycoprotein and near-total normalization of polymeric collagen.

G. Lagrue et al., "Pathology of the Microcirculation in Diabetes and Alterations of the Biosynthesis of Intracellular Matrix Molecules," *Front Matrix Biol. S Karger* 7 (1979): 324–25.

The juice as well as the seeds or dried fruit of unripe bitter melon have been found to have oral hypoglycemic activity. Bitter melon contains numerous compounds with such effects, particularly the polypeptide p-insulin.

J. Cunnick and D. Takemoto, "Bitter Melon (*Momordica Charantia*)," *Journal of Naturopathic Medicine* 4, no. 1 (1993): 16–21.

A study administered 5 g of dried bitter melon powder 3 times a day or a single morning dose of 100 ml of an aqueous extract of bitter melon to type II diabetics. Results showed a significant drop in blood sugar of 54 percent in those taking the aqueous extract after 3 weeks and, after 7 weeks, a drop from 8.37 to 6.95 in glycosylated hemoglobin. Twenty-five percent of those who received the dried powder experienced a reduction in blood sugar.

Y. Srivastava et al., "Antidiabetic and Adaptogenic Properties of *Momordica Charantia* Extract: An Experiment and Clinical Evaluation," *Phytotherapy Research* 7 (1993): 285–89.

Researchers found that in type II diabetics, 50 ml/day of bitter melon juice significantly reduced concentrations of blood glucose, and that a smaller yet still significant effect resulted from daily consumption of fried bitter melon as well.

B. A. Leatherdale et al., "Improvements in Glucose Tolerance Due to *Momordica Charantia* (Karela)," *British Medical Journal* 282 (1981): 1823–24.

A topical 0.075-percent capsaicin cream was applied to areas of pain in patients with diabetic neuropathy four times a day for 8 weeks. The cream produced significant relief when these patients were compared to those receiving a nonactive cream.

The Capsaicin Study Group, "Treatment of Painful Diabetic Neuropathy with Topical Capsaicin: A Multicenter, Double-Blind, Vehicle-Controlled Study," *Archives of Internal Medicine* 151, no. 11 (1991): 2225–29.

Ten insulin-dependent type I diabetics took 100 mg of defatted fenugreek seed powder daily for two 10-day periods. Results: a significant reduction in cholesterol LDL, VLDL, triglycerides, and fasting blood sugar; improved glucose tolerance; and a 54 percent decrease in daily urinary glucose excretion.

R. D. Sharma et al., "Effect of Fenugreek Seed on Blood Glucose and Serum Lipids in Type I Diabetes," *European Journal of Clinical Nutrition* 44 (1990): 301–6.

Powdered fenugreek seed soaked in water administered to type II diabetics was found to significantly reduce glucose levels after meals.

Z. Madar et al., "Glucose-Lowering Effect of Fenugreek in Non-Insulin-Dependent Diabetics," *European Journal of Clinical Nutrition* 42, no. 1 (1988): 51–54.

Results of a study demonstrated reductions in serum cholesterol and 24-hour urinary glucose output, and significant improvements in blood sugar control and insulin responses of type II diabetics given 25 g a day of fenugreek seeds for 3 weeks.

R. S. Sharma, "Effect of Fenugreek Seeds and Leaves on Blood Glucose and Serum Insulin Responses in Human Subjects," *Nutrition Research* 6 (1986): 1353–64.

A study found that diabetic rats intravenously administered 50 mg per day of garlic oil showed a 64 percent reduction in blood and urine glucose levels after 29 days compared to controls. Reduction in the elevated serum total esterified fatty acids and serum cholesterol levels was also seen in the diabetic rats on garlic oil.

G. I. Adoga and M. B. Ibrahim, "Effect of Garlic Oil on Some Biochemical Parameters in Streptozotocin-Induced Diabetic Rats," *Medical Sciences Research* 18 (1990): 859–60.

In a study of diabetic rabbits, oral administration of an onion preparation for 7 days improved glucose tolerance and fasting blood levels.

P. T. Mathew and K. T. Augusti, "Hypoglycaemic Effects of Onion, Allium Cepa Linn. on Diabetes Mellitus—A Preliminary Report," *Indian Journal Physiol. Pharmacol.*, 19, no. 4 (October–December 1975): 213–17.

Ginseng root powder enhanced glucose-induced insulin release from an isolated pancreas in the rat.

Tao Zhang et al., "Ginseng Root: Evidence for Numerous Regulatory Peptides in Insulinotropic Activity," *Biomedical Research*, 11, no. 1 (1990): 49–54.

A double-blind study examined the effects of a *Coccinia indica* extract, a common Ayurvedic antidiabetic medicine, on uncontrolled maturity-onset diabetes. After 6 weeks, 10 of the 16 patients given the extract experienced significantly improved glucose tolerance, while none of the controls showed significant improvement.

A. K. Azad Khan et al., "*Coccinia Indica* in the Treatment of Patients with Diabetes Mellitus," *Bangladesh Medical Research Council Bulletin* 5, no. 2 (December 1979): 60–66.

Cotton seed proved to be effective in reducing the blood sugar levels and blood cholesterol of diabetic mice.

J. Sadique et al., "Hypoglycemic Effect of Cotton Seed Aqueous Extract in Alloxan-Induced Diabetes Mellitus in Rats," *Biochemical Med. Metab. Biol.* 38, no. 1 (August 1987): 104–10.

Fifteen diabetics treated with Artemisia herba-alba extract experienced a lowering of elevated blood sugar. All but one of the patients showed remission of diabetic symptoms.

N. S. Al-Waili, "Treatment of Diabetes Mellitus by Artemisia Herba-alba Extract: Preliminary Study," *Clinical Experiments in Pharmacology Physiology* 13, no. 7 (July 1986): 569–73.

Type II diabetics on conventional oral antihyperglycemic agents were supplemented with an extract of *Gymnema sylvestre* leaves (GS4). Results showed significant reductions in blood glucose, glycosylated hemoglobin, and glycosylated plasma proteins, and in the conventional drug dosage required. Of the 22 diabetic patients on conventional drugs, 5 were able to maintain blood glucose homeostasis solely with GS4, and were thus able to discontinue the medication.

K. Baskaran et al., "Antidiabetic Effect of a Leaf Extract from Gymnema Sylvestre in Non-Insulin-Dependent Diabetes Mellitus Patients," *Journal of Ethnopharmacology* 30, no. 3 (October 1990): 295–300.

Insulin-dependent diabetics in a study were given 400 mg/day of GS4. Results found reductions in fasting blood glucose and glycosylated hemoglobin, glyco-sylated plasma protein levels, and insulin require-ments.

E. R. Shanmugasundaram et al., "Use of Gymnema Sylvestre Leaf Extract in the Control of Blood Glucose in Insulin-Dependent Diabetes Mellitus," *Journal of Ethnophar-macology* 30, no. 3 (October 1990): 281–94.

An ethnobotanical survey was made of the medicinal plants of Israel. The species identified as hypo-glycemic treatments include *Achillea fragrantissima, Ammi visnaga, Atriplex halimus, Capparis spinosa, Ceratonia siliqua, Cleome droserifolia, Eryngium creticum, Inula viscosa, Matricaria aurea, Origanum syriaca, Paronychia argentea Lam, Prosopis farcta, Salvia fruticosa, Sarcopoterium spinosum,* and *Teu-crium polium.*

Z. Davini et al., "Plants Used for the Treatment of Diabetes in Israel," *Journal of Ethnopharmacology* 19, no. 2 (March–April 1987): 145–51.

A study examined the effects of the Soviet antidiabetic medicinal plant arfazetin on type I and type II diabet-ics. Type I patients received the arfazetin combined with insulin. Type II patients received it via infusion in addition to hypoglycemic drugs. Results showed the arfazetin to have hypoglycemic activity.

V. D. Korotkova et al., "Arfezetin v lechenii Sakhamogo Dia-beta," [Arfezetin in the Treatment of Diabetes Mellitus], *Probl. Endokrinol. (Mosk.)* 34, no. 4 (July–August 1988): 25–28.

A study examining the effects of an extract contain-ing *Phaseolus vulgaris* (pod), *Morus alba* (leaf), and *Vaccinum myrtillus* (leaves) in diabetics showed that the extract significantly lowered glycemia values.

C. Ionescu-Tirgoviste et al., "Efectul Unui Amestec pe Plante Asupra Echilibrului Metabolic la Bolnavii cu Diabet Zaharat de Tip 2" [The Effect of a Plant Mixture on the Metabolic Equi-librium in Patients with Type-2 Diabetes Mellitus], *Rev. Med. Interna. Neurol. Psikhiatr. Neurochir. Dermatovenerol. Med. Intern.* 41, no. 2 (March–April 1989): 185–92.

A herbal product containing guar gum, methi, tandika, and mesha shringi was tested on diabetic patients and found to be an effective blood-sugar-low-ering agent.

B. Sadhukhan et al., "Clinical Evaluation of a Herbal Antidi-abetic Product," *Journal of the Indian Medical Association* 92, no. 4 (1994): 115–17.

Powdered burdock root was shown effective in inhibiting hyperglycemia after a starch meal in dia-betics.

A. A. Silver et al., "The Effect of the Ingestion of Burdock Root on Normal and Diabetic Individuals: A Preliminary Report," *Annals of Internal Medicine* 5 (1931): 274–84.

A contolled study showed that broiled nopal stems taken in 500 g doses yielded mean reductions of 17 percent for glucose levels and 50 percent for insulin levels in type II diabetics.

A. C. Frati-Munari et al., "Hypoclycemic Effect of Opuntia Streptacantha Lemaire in NIDDM," *Diabetes Care* 11 (1988): 63–66.

Dandelion root has been shown to cause hypo-glycemic effects in animal studies. A likely explana-tion for this is that the root improves kidney function, particularly with respect to the kidney's ability to cleanse blood and resorb nutrients.

D. B. Mowrey, *The Scientific Validation of Herbal Medicine* (New Canaan, Conn.: Keats Publishing, 1986): 67.

Huckleberry is related to uva-ursi, and its leaf is a com-mon naturopathic treatment for diabetes. Neomyri-licine is the active ingredient.

Mowrey, *Scientific Validation of Herbal Medicine* (New Canaan, Conn.: Keats Publishing, 1986): 67.

A study found that pulp juice of Momordica charan-tia significantly lowered fasting blood glucose levels in rats.

J. Wellhide et al., "Effect of *Momordica Charantia* on the Glu-cose Tolerance in Maturity Onset Diabetes," *Journal of Ethnopharmacology* 17 (1986): 277–82.

The fruit juice of *Momordica charantia* significantly improved the glucose tolerance of 73 percent of maturity-onset diabetics examined.

A. Liaquat et al., "Studies on Hypoglycemic Effects of Fruit Pulp, Seed, and Whole Plant of *Momordica Charantia* on Normal and Diabetic Model Rats," *Planta Medica* 59 (1993): 408–12.

A placebo-controlled study examined the effects of ginseng taken for 8 weeks by newly diagnosed non-insulin-dependent diabetics. Results showed that ginseng elevated mood, improved psychophysical performance, and reduced fasting glucose and body weight.

E. A. Sotaniemi et al., "Ginseng Therapy in Non-Insulin-Dependent Diabetic Patients," *Diabetes Care* 18, no. 10 (October 1995): 1373–75.

EXERCISE

A study compared two groups of non-insulin-dependent diabetics. One group was managed by diet alone, and the other was put on the same diet combined with exercise (10,000 steps per day). Results: Both groups lost significant amounts of weight, although the exercise group lost more. Also, the exercise group experienced significant increases in their glucose infusion rates and metabolic clearance rates.

K. Yamanouchi, "Daily Walking Combined with Diet Therapy as a Useful Means for Obese, Non-Insulin-Dependent Diabetes Mellitus Patients Not Only to Reduce Body Weight but Also to Improve Insulin Sensitivity," *Diabetes Care* 18, no. 6: 775–78.

Experimental findings suggest that upper arm exercise might be a useful alternative to insulin in cases of gestational diabetes.

L. Jovanovic-Peterson and C. M. Peterson, "Is Exercise Safe or Useful for Gestational Diabetic Women?" *Diabetes* 40, no. 2 (December 1991): 179-81.

Researchers looked at the link between physical activity and glucose tolerance. They found that diabetes was inversely associated with physical activity levels and that the strongest indicators of the 2-hour blood glucose level at baseline were age, family history of diabetes, and physical activity. Subjects ranking among the lowest with respect to physical activity levels had a 2.7 times greater risk of diabetes than high-activity subjects.

A. Schranz et al., "Low Physical Activity and Worsening of Glucose Tolerance: Results from a Two-Year Follow-up of a Popular Sample in Malta," *Diabetes Research and Clinical Practice* 11 (1991): 127–36.

A large study of over 87,000 middle-aged American women free of major disease found that women engaging in vigorous exercise once a week or more had a significantly lower risk of non-insulin-dependent diabetes compared with women who did not exercise each week.

J. E. Manson et al., "Physical Activity and Incidence of Non-Insulin-Dependent Diabetes Mellitus in Women," *Lancet* 338 (September 28, 1991): 774–78.

Numerous studies link physical activity with the prevention of non-insulin-dependent diabetes, according to a review.

S. P. Helmrich et al., "Prevention of Non-Insulin-Dependent Diabetes Mellitus with Physical Activity," *Med. Sci. Sports Exerc.* 26, no. 7 (July 1984): 824–30.

YOGA

A study found that 104 out of 149 non-insulin-dependent diabetics experienced a fair to good response following yoga therapy, with decreases in requirements of oral hypoglycemic medication observed.

S. C. Jain et al., "A Study of Response Pattern of Non-Insulin Dependent Diabetes to Yoga Therapy," *Diabetic Research and Clinical Practice* 19 (1993): 69–74.

Yoga has been shown to increase body sensitivity to insulin injections, thus decreasing levels of anti-insulin hormones, such as adrenaline, in the body.

L. Rogers, "Yoga May Help Fight Diabetes," *London Evening Standard* (December11, 1989).

TRADITIONAL CHINESE MEDICINE

Chinese medical folklore identifies guava as an effective treatment of diabetes. Guava has been shown to have blood-glucose-lowering effects when administered orally to maturity-onset diabetics, as well as to healthy subjects.

J. T. Cheng and R. S. Yang, "Hypoglycemic Effect of Guava Juice in Mice and Human Subjects," *American Journal of Chinese Medicine* 11 (1983): 74–76.

Significant correlations were found between intake of broiled stems of *Opuntia streptacantha* and a decrease in serum glucose levels in type II diabetics.

A. C. Frati-Munari et al., [Hypoglycemic Action of Different Doses of Nopal (*Opuntia Streptacantha* Lemaire) in Patients with Type II Diabetes Mellitus], *Arch. Invest. Med.* (Mexico) 20, no. 2 (April–June 1989): 197–201.

It was found that the traditional Chinese medication *tian-shou* liquor (TSL) significantly decreased cholesterol and blood sugar concentrations in diabetics.

L. L. Zha, [Tian-shou Liquor on Activity of Cell Membrane and Energy Metabolism in Diabetes Mellitus], *Chung Hsi I Chieh Ho Tsa Chih* 10, no. 8 (August 1990): 455–57, 451.

The administration of *ke-tang-ling* to non-insulin-dependent diabetics produced significant decreases in blood glucose levels, particularly in non-obese subjects.

Z. Wang and Z. Yin, [Effect of *Ke-Tang-Ling* Administration on the Function of Pancreatic Islets Cells in Non-Insulin-Dependent Diabetes Mellitus], *Chung Hsi I Chieh Ho Tsa Chih* 10, no. 3 (March 1990): 137–40, 130.

Jiang tan san (JTS) significantly lowered the levels of blood glucose, blood lipids, and blood pressure in non-insulin-dependent diabetics.

Y.X. Ni et al., [Clinical Study on *Jiang Tang San* in Treating Non-Insulin Dependent Diabetes Mellitus Patients], *Chung Kuo Chung Hsi I Chieh Ho Tsa Chih,* 14, no. 11 (November 1994): 650–52.

A study compared type II diabetics who received treatment with Western medicine plus foot reflexotherapy with those who received western medicine alone. Results indicated that the patients receiving both treatments performed much better after 30 days, with significant reductions in fasting blood glucose levels.

X. M. Wang, [Treating Type II Diabetes Mellitus with Foot Reflexotherapy], *Chung Kuo Chung Hsi I Chieh Ho Tsa Chih* 13, no. 9 (September 1993): 517, 536–38.

A study found *jin-qi-jiang-tang-pian* (JQJTP) to be effective in treating diabetics.

X.C. Liang et al., [Clinical and Experimental Study on Effect of *Jin-qi-jiang-Tang-pian* on Qi-yin Deficiency and Hyperactivity of Diabetes Mellitus], *Chung Kuo Chung Hsi I Chieh Ho Tsa Chih* 13, no. 10 (October 1993): 579, 587–90.

BIOFEEDBACK

A study showed that, of six diabetics taking insulin, a biofeedback-assisted stress management program led to a reduction of insulin requirements in four.

L. Rosenbaum, "Biofeedback-Assisted Stress Management for Insulin-Treated Diabetes Mellitus," *Biofeedback Self-Regulation* 8, no. 4 (December 1983): 519–32.

Biofeedback and relaxation training were shown to produce significant increases in peripheral blood circulation in diabetic patients.

B. I. Rice and J. V. Schindler, "Effect of Thermal Biofeedback-Assisted Relaxation Training on Blood Circulation in the Lower Extremities of a Population with Diabetes," *Diabetes Care* 15, no. 7 (July 1992): 853–58.

A study examined the effects of biofeedback-assisted relaxation in 18 type I diabetics. Results showed that blood glucose levels were improved significantly in those diabetics receiving the treatment compared to controls.

A. McGrady et al., "Controlled Study of Biofeedback-Assisted Relaxation in Type I Diabetes," *Diabetes Care* 14, no. 5 (1991): 360–65.

ELECTRICAL NERVE STIMULATION

Electrical nerve stimulation produced significant positive results in the treatment of chronic diabetic ulcers after 12 weeks, a controlled study showed.

T. C. Lundeberg et al., "Electrical Nerve Stimulation Improves Healing of Diabetic Ulcers," *Annals of Plastic Surgery* 29, no. 4 (October 1992): 328–31.

CHELATION THERAPY

Twenty-four of 32 diabetics receiving chelation therapy with deferoxamine were able to come off all medication within 8–13 weeks.

P. Cutler, "Deferoxamine Therapy in High-Ferritin Diabetes," *Diabetes* 38 (October 1989): 1207–10.

OZONE THERAPY

A study of 120 diabetics found that a combination of insulin therapy, diet, and hyperbaric oxygenation resulted in significant improvement of tissue metabolism.

I. M. Kakhnovskii et al., [Effect of Insulin Therapy and Hyperbaric Oxygenation on the Enzyme Activity of Tissue Metabolism in Diabetes Mellitus], *Probl. Endokrinol.* (Moscow) 28, no. 6 (November–December 1982): 11–17.

RELAXATION

In a study of hospitalized non-insulin-dependent diabetics, five days of training in progressive relaxation resulted in an improved glucose tolerance that didn't affect insulin sensitivity or glucose-stimulated insulin secretory activity.

R. S. Surwit and M. N. Feinglos, "The Effects of Relaxation on Glucose Tolerance in Non-Insulin-Dependent Diabetes," *Diabetes Care* 6, no. 2 (1983): 176–79.

8. EATING DISORDERS

Eating disorders have plagued women in Western societies as a byproduct of the objectification of women found in advertising, the underlying message being that if you are not thin and beautiful you have no value. Today in America this message is getting out to women at a younger and younger age. But when it comes to which individual women will suffer from anorexia, bulimia, or obesity and, perhaps most importantly, which women who suffer from one of these conditions will respond well to proper treatment, strict physiological factors come into play separate from the psychological and societal issues.

Causes

Research shows that the eating disorders anorexia nervosa, bulimia, and obesity may be the result of a zinc deficiency. Dr. Alexander Schauss, Ph.D., C.E.D.S., a clinical psychologist and eating disorders specialist from Tacoma, Washington, reports that science has long been aware of this connection. "We've known, from at least the 1930s, that when animals were experimentally placed on diets deficient in zinc, those animals would develop anorexia. Our interest in eating disorders in relationship to zinc has to do with the observation that when humans are placed on zinc-deficient diets, they too develop eating disorders.

"By characterizing three of the most common eating disorders," Dr. Schauss continues, "you can see how vital zinc is. In morbid obesity, when people are significantly overweight in such a way that it could shorten their life span or increase their risk of disease, we know that there is an inverse relationship between the level of obesity and the level of zinc, meaning that the more obese they are, the less zinc they have in the body. We don't know yet whether this is cause or effect, but it is a very important observation because at the other end of the continuum, with anorexia nervosa, self-induced starvation, we also have individuals who are generally always zinc-deficient. We believe there is strong evidence today, from studies done at the University of Kentucky School of Medicine, at Stanford University, and the University of California at Davis, in addition to our research institute's work, that the lower the zinc status, the more likely it is that the patient will not recover from any treatment plan to resolve their anorexia."

Stress is commonly associated with the onset and continuation of eating disorders, and can also be understood in terms of zinc loss, since constant mental stress results in the depletion of this mineral. In 1975 it was reported that between ages fifteen and twenty, zinc loss due to stress is at its lifetime peak. Women are more prone to stress-related zinc loss than males, and therefore more likely to have eating disorders. Dr. Schauss explains, "The answer may lie in the fact that males have prostate glands and women do not. Zinc is highly concentrated in the prostate in males; it provides a mineral that is essential for the development, motility, viability and quantity of sperm. If a male is under psychological stress, it can catabolize or seek out storages of zinc in the prostate. Since women don't have a prostate, they will catabolize the zinc from other tissue.

"In women, the richest source of zinc is found in muscle tissue and bone. A common feature of anorexia is muscle wasting and an increased risk of osteoporosis. Anorexics actually catabolize or eat their own tissue as a way of releasing nutrients that they are not getting in the diet. The last muscle, and one that only contains about 1 percent zinc, is the heart muscle. When the body starts to scavenge zinc out of heart muscle tissue, it can interfere with the heart's function, which contributes to bradycardia, tachycardia, arrhythmia, and eventual heart failure. It is particularly dangerous when patients with damaged hearts are in recovery. As they put on weight, they add extra pressure to the heart. That is what killed the singer Karen Carpenter, for example."

Symptoms

Anorexia is signaled by muscle wasting, loss of menstrual periods, body image problems, and an exaggerated fear of becoming fat. Bulimia is characterized by compulsive eating and forced vomiting or the use of laxatives or diuretics to eliminate much of the calories that are consumed during binge episodes. Obesity is seen as an enormous increase in the ratio of fat to muscle. A common dual diagnosis is depression, which can be treated with numerous safe, non-habit-forming, and natural alternatives to drugs.

Clinical Experience

LIQUID ZINC. Liquid zinc has a positive effect in the treatment of eating disorders, as it is directly absorbed into the blood. Powders, tablets, and capsules, which must first be broken down by the stomach and absorbed by the small intestine, do not work as well because many eating disorder patients are unable to digest nutrients properly. Dr. Schauss has found only one brand available in the

United States, Zinc Status (supplied by Ethical Nutrients, San Clemente, California), to be effective in clinical trials. Other liquid zincs are not autoclaved (sterile); although they are cheaper, they have not proved effective. Once the patient shows marked improvement, a good zinc supplement will do unless deterioration occurs, when the more expensive Zinc Status is needed again.

While results are not usually immediate, taking from several days to weeks, once liquid zinc takes effect, its benefits are long-lasting. According to Dr. Schauss, "In fifteen years, I worked with hundreds of eating disorder patients. Until I saw this treatment, my colleagues and I felt that the best we could expect in long-term outcome, in treating patients with either bulimia or anorexia, was maybe a 20–30 percent recovery. In our five-year study, we found that bulemics had a 64.1 percent success rate after recovery on the liquid zinc treatment. In anorexic patients, our five-year follow-up study found an 85 percent recovery rate. These are extraordinarily high recovery rates for a condition that is considered difficult to treat and insidious."

Besides being highly effective, liquid zinc is inexpensive, costing between $12 and $15 a day. This makes it a first-choice treatment for eating disorders, especially when you consider the options. "Within twenty years of initial diagnosis, a British study found, 38 percent of patients with severe eating disorders are dead," says Dr. Schauss. "Many times the families have spent enormous amounts of money keeping their children alive, as the average institutional cost is about $650 a day."

Another favorable finding is that liquid zinc can lift the depression that is usually associated with eating disorders. Dr. Schauss reports, "In our eating disorder studies, we used a multi-dimensional design and evaluated the mood state of our patients. One of the first things to improve in patients was the degree of depression that they were experiencing based on psychometric instruments such as the Beck Depression Scale, the Profile of Mood Scales, and other depressive indices. The fact that we have discovered this antidepressive effect and could document it in patients under blind conditions is of great value."

Patient Story

DR. SCHAUSS GIVES THE FOLLOWING ACCOUNT OF ONE PATIENT'S RECOVERY:
We were doing blind studies, which means that neither I nor the patient were aware of whether they were receiving a placebo or liquid zinc. One of the women in the study was forty-seven years old. She was a psychotherapist who had been treating patients with eating disorders for the last fifteen years, and who herself had bulimia, involving about five binge/purge episodes per day for the last thirty-four years. She could hardly recount a single day in the last thirty-four years when she did not

engage in bulemic activity. We have a protocol in which we give a small amount of liquid zinc, about 5 or 10 ml, which is less than a tablespoon. We ask a person to swirl it around in his or her mouth for a few seconds and to tell us what he or she tastes. Zinc has a strong metallic taste. If the person can't taste the solution, it's evidence of a systemic zinc deficiency. This has to do with a zinc-dependent polypeptide known as gustin, which helps us to distinguish metallic tastes.

The zinc tasted like water to this woman. Since she couldn't taste anything, she thought that she was receiving a placebo. She followed the protocol, taking about 120 ml of the zinc solution spaced out through the day, about 30 or 40 ml each time on an empty stomach.

Four days later, she called back saying that she couldn't explain why, but she had no desire to binge or purge that day. That was the first day she could recall feeling that way in thirty-four years. This is very similar to the experience that we have had with hundreds of bulemics that we've studied.

We were intrigued as to how a simple nutrient, like zinc, could cause a major change in the way the brain functions and in the perceptions of the individual. When you've done something for thirty-four years, whether it's cigarette smoking, nail biting, or engaging in bulimia, you have to wonder how it is possible for that obsessive/compulsive type of behavior to disappear in just four or five days.

It has now been five years since that day, and she has never gone back to bingeing/purging. More importantly in terms of the study, she received no psychotherapy, nor did she have any contact with me personally. The protocol was given to her by a staff member. So we're quite convinced, in this case and in hundreds of others, that it was the liquid zinc that was effective, rather than some tangential treatment.

Hot News

Studies have found that dieting may produce alterations in the brain in women (and not in men), which in turn may produce brain deficiencies of, for example, L-tryptophan. This may partially explain the higher prevalence of eating disorders in women. Supplementation with tryptophan with pyridoxine has been shown to improve both eating behavior and feelings about eating. In women whose bulimia worsens in winter, light therapy has proven helpful. In the treatment of bulimia, zinc has proven helpful through its action on thyroid hormone conversion.

Obesity has been associated with low thyroid function in a substantial number of cases. Chromium supplementation, which can help speed up metabolism and stabilize blood sugar levels (reducing the desire to eat) has also proven helpful. Evening primrose oil has been shown to reduce appetite and contribute to weight loss in obese patients, as has ascorbic acid supplementation. Green tea has proven to be a much better weight-loss aid than amphetamines. *(See below.)*

NUTRIENTS/DIET

A study of 20 bulimic women proved that a nutrient-dense diet can end the urge to binge. For the first 3 weeks of the study, half of the subjects were placed on a 1400-calorie nutrient-dense diet and ceased to binge. The control group kept on binging until, at the end of the third week, they too were placed on the nutrient-dense diet, which proved to be a success for all the subjects. Even some 2.5 years after the initial treatment, all of the subjects had lost weight or maintained weight by choice without binging. The diet was free of suspected blood-sugar insulin-level destabilizers. It eliminated alcohol, caffeine, refined sugar, white flour, flavor enhancers, most salt, cigarettes, and medications. Supplements of vitamin C (1 g) and B complex vitamins were given, along with a multivitamin/multimineral supplement, daily.

S. Dalvit-McPhillips, "A Dietary Approach to Bulimia Treatment," *Physiol. Behav.* 33, no. 5 (1984): 769–75.

Eating disorders may easily lead to zinc deficiencies, and once this occurs it perpetuates abnormal eating patterns, since low zinc levels are associated with reduced taste and smell sensitivity. Zinc deficiency may result from poor diet, excess fiber consumption, vomiting, diarrhea, the zinc demands of rapid growth (i.e., in teenagers), or sweating.

C. J. McClain et al., "Zinc Status Before and After Zinc Supplementation of Eating Disorder Patients," *Journal of the American College of Nutrition* 11, no. 6 (December 1992): 694–700.

A study of 62 patients found a 54 percent rate of zinc deficiency in anorexics, and a 40 percent rate in bulimics.

L. Humphries et al., "Zinc Deficiency and Eating Disorders," *Journal of Clinical Psychiatry* 50, no.12 (December 1989): 456–59.

Studies demonstrate that zinc supplementation can curb eating abnormalities and promote weight gain. Zinc sulfate supplements of 45–90 mg daily given to 20 anorexia nervosa patients produced significant weight increases for most of them. Menstruation returned in 13 of the patients within 1 to 17 months.

S. Safai-Kutti, "Oral Zinc Supplementation in Anorexia Nervosa," *ACTA Pyschiatr. Scand.* 361, no. 82 suppl. (1990): 14–17.

In a placebo-controlled experiment, zinc gluconate supplements of 100 mg daily given to 35 female anorexics doubled the rate of increase in body mass in comparison to the placebo group.

C. L. Birmingham et al., "Controlled Trial of Zinc Supplementation in Anorexia Nervosa," *International Journal of Eating Disorders* 15, no. 3 (April 1994): 251–55.

Zinc supplementation has been shown not only to enhance appetite, taste sensitivity, and smell but also to enhance mental state. Zinc alleviates depression and anxiety.

D. Bryce-Smith and R. Simpson, "Case of anorexia nervosa responding to zinc sulphate," letter, *Lancet* 2 (1984): 350.

Tryptophan with pyridoxine improves both eating behavior and feelings about eating.

M. Mira and S. Abraham, "L-tryptophan as an adjunct to treatment of bulimia nervosa," letter, *Lancet* 2 (1989): 1162–63.

In women (and not men), dieting may create an increased need for L-tryptophan by altering brain serotonin function. This difference may explain the higher prevalence of eating disorders among women.

G. M. Goodwin et al., "Dieting changes serotonergic function in women, not men: implications for the aetiology of anorexia nervosa," *Psychol. Med.* 17, no. 4 (1987): 839–42.

Carnitine and cobalamin speed body weight gain and normalization of gastrointestinal functions, increase mental performance, and eliminate latent fatigue. This treatment promoted cerebral mass growth and led to full restoration of the normal structure of the neocortex after starvation.

M. B. Korkina et al., [Clinico-Experimental Substantiation of the Use of Carnitine and Cobalamin in the Treatment of Anorexia Nervosa], *Zh. Nevropatol. Psikhiatr.* (1986): 205.

Animal research shows that sugar acts like an opiate on feeding behavior. This may explain why sugar often triggers binges in humans—and why binge eaters prefer sweets.

Brain Res. Bull. 14, no. 6 (1985): 673–78.

LIGHT THERAPY

Like those with seasonal affective mood disorders, bulimics benefit from light therapy. When 17 female bulimics were treated daily for two weeks with early morning bright-white exposures for 30 minutes a day, all showed improvement with the treatment. Those whose symptoms noticeably worsened in winter (7 of the 17) improved the most.

R. W. Lam, "A Controlled Study of Light Therapy for Bulimia Nervosa," *American Journal of Psychiatry* 151, no. 5 (1990): 744.

BODY IMAGE

Body image is considered by some to be an important issue in the treatment of all addictions. Those with a positive body image are less likely to pollute their body with harmful substances, such as drugs or alcohol. Advertisements are one way women get the idea that their bodies are "faulty." Techniques for healing "faulty" body image include cognitive and behavioral approaches. Guided imagery and visualization can help.

"Body Image Work Leads to Addiction Recovery," *Addiction Letter* 9, no. 4 (April 1993): 1S.

A study of 40 white and black elderly women showed that the African-American women had more positive attitudes about their bodies than did the white women. The black women were 2.5 times as likely to be satisfied with their weight and 2.7 times as likely to think of themselves as attractive.

J. Stevens et al., "Attitudes toward Body Size and Dieting: Differences between Elderly Black and White Women," *American Journal of Public Health* 84, no. 8 (August 1994): 1322.

A study of 100 female undergraduates showed that sexual abuse and unhealthy eating habits were linked to overestimation of body size.

V. Byram et al., "Sexual Abuse and Body Image Distortion," *Child Abuse and Neglect* 19, no. 4 (April 1995): 507.

FROM THE MEDICAL LITERATURE ON OBESITY

America is one of the most overweight nations in the world, and the percentage of overweight Americans continues to rise. According to preliminary data from the Third National Health and Nutrition Examination Survey, 26 percent of American adults were overweight in the late 1970s. By the late 1980s, the number rose to 34 percent.

"Heavy News," *University of California, Berkeley Wellness Letter* 10, no. 2 (February 1994): 2.

NUTRITION

Obesity is associated with high blood pressure and poor glucose metabolism. However, a reduction in blood pressure is always accompanied by improvements in glucose metabolism. A study found that a high-protein, low-carbohydrate, calorie-restricted diet eliminated hypertension, corrected deficiencies in glucose metabolism, and reduced weight.

F. Nobels et al., "Weight Reduction with a High Protein, Low Carbohydrate, Calorie-Restricted Diet: Effects on Blood Pressure, Glucose and Insulin Levels," *Netherlands Journal of Medicine* 35, nos. 5–6 (December 1989): 295–302.

Obesity has been associated with low thyroid function. Zinc may play an important role in energy metabolism through its action on thyroid hormone conversion and insulin. A study of obese mice treated with both zinc and thyroxine resulted in a significant decrease in both serum triacylglycerols and body fat composition–even when the mice were on high-fat diets.

W. H. Lin et al., "Effects of Zinc and Thyroxine Treatment on Dietary-Obese Mice," *Proceedings of the National Sci. Counc. Repub. China* 11, no. 4 (October 1987): 3412–46.

Chromium picolinate, hydroxycitric acid (HCA), spirulina, ma huang, yerba mate, and kola nut speed up metabolism, so that fat is burned while muscle tone remains intact. Chromium reduces insulin resistance, which in turn decreases the storage of adipose (fatty) tissue and increases its metabolism. In addition, chromium helps stabilize blood sugar levels, which diminishes the desire to eat.

"Chromium Picolinate, HCA Help for Weight Loss," *Better Nutrition for Today's Living* 57, no. 3 (March 1995): 36.

Patients taking niacin-bound chromium in combination with HCA lost almost three times as much weight as patients taking placebos. In another study, volunteers averaged a 27 percent better response by taking 400 mcg of chromium picolinate rather than 200 mcg per day.

"Mainstays of Weight Loss: Exercise," *Better Nutrition for Today's Living* 57, no. 10 (October 1995): 38–41.

Supplementing a normal diet with gel-forming fibers such as guar gum produces a feeling of fullness that makes sticking to a diet easier for most people. Fiber may also improve metabolism.

U. Smith, "Dietary Fiber, Diabetes and Obesity," *International Journal of Obesity* 11, suppl. (1987): 27–31.

High-fiber diets have been shown to reduce serum lipids and blood pressure in slightly overweight women.

T. T. Solum et al., "The Influence of a High-Fibre Diet on Body Weight, Serum Lipids and Blood Pressure in Slightly Overweight Persons: A Randomized, Double-Blind, Placebo-Controlled Investigation with Diet and Fibre Tablets," *International Journal of Obesity* 11, suppl. (1987): 67–71.

When an air-expanded whole-wheat protein product (SNW) was used for 12 weeks as a meal substitute by moderately obese women, the women lost nearly twice as much weight as subjects placed on a standard low-calorie diet. Reductions in serum cholesterol and triglyceride measures were also greater for the SNW-users.

M. K. Fordyce-Baum et al., "Use of an Expanded-Whole-Wheat Product in the Reduction of Body Weight and Serum Lipids in Obese Females," *American Journal of Clinical Nutrition* 50, no. 1 (July 1989): 30–36.

Overweight women who took bean husk powder capsules prior to meals lost twice as much weight after 15 days and three times as much weight after 30 days as women receiving placebos. Similarly, reductions in waist measurement were twice as great for the bean husk group after 15 days and 3.5 times as great after 30 days.

A. Leomte, "A Double Blind Study Confirms the Effects on Weight of Bean Husk Arkocpas," *Revenue de l'Association Mondiale de Phytotherapie* 1 (1985): 41–44.

Dieters taking 3 g of glucomannan daily lost nearly twice as much weight as dieters receiving a placebo.

G. C. Reffo et al., "Glucomannan in Hypertensive Outpatients," *Current Ther. Research* 44, no. 1 (1988): 22–27.

Xanthum gum can produce a feeling of fullness that lasts from 90 minutes up to 5 hours.

M. Cairella and R. Godi, "Clinical Observations on the Use of Xanthum Gum in Obesity," *Clinical Deitol.*, 13, no. 1 (1980): 37–40.

A diet of 62 percent raw food produced a mean weight loss of 3.8 kg over a mean duration of 6.7 months in a sample of 32 hypertensive patients, most of whom were obese.

J. Douglass et al., "Effects of a Raw Foods Diet on Hypertension and Obesity," *South. Med. Journal* 78, no. 7 (1985): 841.

Sugar and other carbohydrates may produce an effect similar to opiates by increasing beta-endorphin production.

D. T. Fullerton et al., "Carbohydrate Ingestion, Hypoglycemia and Obesity," *Appetite* 6 (1985): 53–59.

Coenzyme Q10 may help dieters lose weight.

L. van Gaal et al., "Exploratory Study of Coenzyme Q10 in Obesity," in K. Folkers and Y. Yamamura, eds., *Biomedical and Clinical Aspects of Coenzyme Q* (Amsterdam: Elsevier, 1984): 369–373.

Evening primrose oil reduces appetite, especially for those with higher starting weights. In one study, half of those subjects taking the oil who were more than 10 percent above their ideal weight lost weight without dieting. The higher the starting weight, the greater the weight lost.

K.S. Vadadai and D. F. Horrobin, "Weight Loss Produced by Evening Primrose Oil Administration in Normal and Schizophrenic Individuals," *IRCS Journal Med. Science* 7 (1979): 52.

Evening primrose oil has a favorable effect on brown fat activation and the amount of brown fat in reserve, and it lowers blood pressure.

R. H. Lowndes and R. E. Mansel, "The Effects of Evening Primrose Oil on Serum Lipid Levels of Normal and Obese Subjects," in D. F. Horrobin, ed., *Clinical Uses of Essential Fatty Acids* (Montreal: Eden Press, 1982): 37–52.

One gram of ascorbic acid taken three times daily produced measurable weight loss after 1 week, with continued loss still noted after six weeks, a double-blind, placebo-controlled study found.

G. J. Naylor et al., "A Double-Blind Placebo Controlled Trial of Ascorbic Acid in Obesity," *Nutrition Health* 4 (1985): 25–28.

Large doses of ascorbic acid aid weight loss in obese patients, particularly those who are more than 33 percent above their ideal body weight.

G. J. Naylor, "A Double Blind Placebo Controlled Trial of Ascorbic Acid in Obesity," *IRCS Journal Med. Science* 10 (1982): 848.

Animals given tryptophan consumed less food, especially carbohydrates.

P. Morris et al., "Food Intake and Selection After Peripheral Tryptophan," *Physiol. Behav.* 40 (1987): 155–63.

Making a substantial change in eating habits to comply with a dietary program may be key to getting good weight-loss results. A study of breakfast-eating habits showed that breakfast eaters—subjects who normally eat breakfast—lost more weight when placed on a diet that excluded breakfast, while breakfast skippers—those who normally skipped the meal—lost more weight when placed on a diet that included breakfast.

D. G. Schlundt et al., "The Role of Breakfast in the Treatment of Obesity: A Randomized Clinical Trial," *American Journal of Clinical Nutrition* 55, no. 3 (March 1992): 645–51.

A dietary fiber supplement was shown to be an effective weight-loss aid. For mildly obese women in a randomized, double-blind, placebo-controlled experiment of long duration the fiber—but not the placebo—decreased heart rate and blood pressure, in addition to reducing subjects' weight. Also, fiber recipients were more likely to adhere to the program because the supplements significantly reduced feelings of hunger.

K. R. Ryttig et al., "A Dietary Fibre Supplement and Weight Maintenance after Weight Reduction: A Randomized, Double Blind, Placebo Controlled Long-Term Trial," *International Journal of Obesity* 13 (1989): 165–71.

The effect of 10 g of granulated guar-gum preparation taken twice a day was tested in comparison to commercially available bran on obese subjects. For 10 weeks, daily hunger feelings were rated; subjects showed greater reductions in hunger ratings with the guar gum than with the bran. Guar gum also resulted in greater weight reduction.

M. Krotkiewski, "Effect of Guar Gum on Body-Weight, Hunger Ratings and Metabolism in Obese Subjects," *British Journal of Nutrition* 52 (1984): 97–105.

HERBS/PLANT EXTRACTS

Green tea produces a significant reduction of triglycerides, weight, and waist size. Compared to a placebo group, obese dieting women who received green tea capsules prior to meals lost twice as much weight after 15 days and three times as much weight after 30. Their waist measurements were reduced twice as much after 15 days, and four times as much after 30 days.

"Clinical Study of Weight Loss Using Arkogelules' Green Tea," *Revenue de l'Association Mondiale de Phytotherapie*, June 1985.

Herbs can work better than amphetamines as weight-loss aids. Green tea in combination with wall germander results in weight loss slightly greater than that resulting from treatment with the drug dexfenfluoramine, without the side effects, a study showed. While the drug group experienced a steady increase in blood pressure, the green tea/wall germander group showed a slight decrease in systolic blood pressure. Additionally, slightly more than half (20 out of 39) of those on the drug complained of insomnia, nausea, and dry mouth; a portion of those subjects (3) discontinued treatment.

"Appetite Suppressants: Herbs or Amphetamines?" *Arkpharma's Phyto-Facts* 2, no.1 (1989): 2.

Hydroxycitric acid (HCA) reduces food intake, body weight, and serum triglyceride levels; studies with higher-order animals show a 46-percent reduction of food intake after a 3-mg/kg oral dose of HCA, and no rebound eating after discontinuation.

R. N. Rao and K. K. Sakariah, "Lipid Lowering and Antiobesity Effect of Hydroxycitric Acid," *Nutrition Research* 8 (1988): 209–12.

Kelp and bladder wrack provide the iodine required for a healthy thyroid as well as the nutrients and oxygen that increase the body's ability to burn off fat through exercise. Plaintain produces a feeling of fullness and reduces intestinal absorption of fats. This puts a limit on caloric intake and results in weight loss.

D. B. Mowrey, *The Scientific Validation of Herbal Medicine* (New Canaan, Conn.: Keats Publishing, 1986): 280.

Malabar tamarind is a natural food containing hydroxycitric acid, which substance, in animal studies, reduced food consumption. The fruit has been used for centuries in Asian countries with no harmful effect; sprinkled on food it makes meals more filling and satisfying.

W. Sergio, "A Natural Food, the Malabar Tamarind, May Be Effective in the Treatment of Obesity," *Medical Hypotheses* 27 (1988): 39–40.

When practitioners of natural medicine use ephedra for weight loss, they often use herbs like licorice and Panax ginseng and/or vitamin C, magnesium, zinc, vitamin B6, and pantothenic acid supplementation in order to support the adrenal glands.

M. T. Murray, "The Rational Use of Thermogenic Formulas," *American Journal of Natural Medicine* 1, no. 4 (December 1994): 5–7.

EXERCISE

Obesity increases the risk of coronary heart disease. Exercise increases cardiorespiratory capacity, decreases cholesterol and triglyceride levels, and helps to slow the loss of lean muscle mass in addition to helping with weight loss. For the best weight-loss and fitness results, an exercise program should continue even after a weight-loss diet ends. In a study of overweight postmenopausal women, a six-month follow-up check on exercise habits was added to a short-term diet. Subjects who were still exercising six months after the diet had significantly greater reductions in weight, fat tissue mass, and abdominal-to-total-body fat mass, as well as a significantly improved resting metabolic rates.

O. L. Svendsen et al., "Six Months' Follow-up on Exercise Added to a Short-term Diet in Overweight Postmenopausal Women—Effects on Body Composition, Resting Metabolic Rate, Cardiovascular Risk Factors and Bone," *International Journal of Obesity Related Metabolic Disorders* 18, no. 10 (October 1994): 692–98.

A total-body strength-training program can produce significant reductions in intra-abdominal adipose tissue.

M. S. Treuth et al., "Reduction in Intra-Abdominal Adipose Tissue after Strength Training in Older Women," *Journal of Applied Physiology* 78, no. 4 (April 1995): 1425–31.

TRADITIONAL CHINESE MEDICINE

When obesity is complicated by hypertension or cardiovascular disease, acupuncture should be combined with moxibustion, some feel. Studies show effectiveness rates of nearly 90 percent for this combination of treatments. Together, acupuncture and moxibustion have been shown to have a benign regulatory effect on overeating, blood pressure, lipid levels, and energy metabolism.

Z. Lieu et al., "Prophylactic and Therapeutic Effects of Acupuncture on Simple Obesity Complicated by Cardiovascular Diseases," *Journal of Traditional Chinese Medicine*, 12, no. 1 (March 1992): 21–29.

The active principle in refined rhubarb is an obesity-reducing drug known as Jiang-Thi Jian-Fei Yao (JZJFY). Research on rats shows that JZJFY reduces food intake, prolongs stomach evacuation, and accelerates intestinal movement.

H. M. Jin and D. H. Jiao, [Effect of Jiang-Zhi Jian-Fei Yao on Gastro-Intestinal Movement and Adipose Cell of Abdominal Wall], *Chung Kuo Chung Hsi I Chieh Ho Tsa Chih,* 14, no. 4 (April 1994): 230–31, 198.

Rats fed *Xiapangmei* all showed significant decreases in body weight and fat, food intake, and the intestinal absorption of glucose.

Z. Y. and Xu, "An Experimental Study by Single Blind Method on the Anti-Obesity Effect of *Xiaopangmei*," *Journal of Traditional Chinese Medicine* 9, no. 1 (March 1989): 5–8.

SUBLIMINAL SELF-HELP TAPES

Subliminal messages may not be responsible for the success attributed to subliminal self-help audiotapes designed for weight reduction, a study showed. Subjects who listened to such tapes lost no more weight than those in the placebo and control groups. All of the subjects believed in the possible effectiveness of subliminal audiotapes and were weighed once each week for five weeks. Researchers concluded that the apparent effectiveness of subliminal tapes may result simply from the fact that regular use makes subjects more conscious of their weight.

P. M. Merikle and H. E. Skanes, "Subliminal Self-Help Audiotapes: A Search for Placebo Effects," *Journal of Applied Psychology* 77, no. 5 (October 1992): 772–76.

OBESITY AND AYURVEDIC MEDICINE

Seventy obese patients participated in a double-blind, placebo-controlled clinical trial of Ayurvedic treatment. The treatment was seen to significantly decrease body measurements, including skin fold thickness and hip and waist measurements; it reduced serum cholesterol and triglyceride levels as well. Treatment was given for 3 months, and dietary intake was not controlled.

P. Prakash et al., "Ayurvedic Treatment of Obesity: A Randomised Double-Blind, Placebo-Controlled Clinical Trial," *Journal of Ethnopharmacology* 29 (1990): 1–11.

9. ENDOMETRIOSIS

Endometriosis is a condition in which the glands and tissues that line the inside of the uterus (the endometrium) grow outside the uterine cavity. Normally, cells build up in the uterus each month in preparation for pregnancy. They serve as a nest for an incoming embryo. When pregnancy does not occur, the lining sheds and appears as menstrual flow. With endometriosis, cells may attach themselves to the fallopian tubes, ovaries, urinary bladder, intestinal surfaces, rectum, part of the colon, and other structures in the area.

Causes

The exact cause of the condition remains a mystery, though several theories exist as to why it happens. These are some possible explanations:

Retrograde menstruation. Blood flows backward, instead of outwardly. It is thought to go out the fallopian tubes and into the pelvic and abdominal cavity. Once there, cells from the exiting blood implant themselves outside the uterus onto other tissues.

Lymphatic channels. Cells of the endometrium lining go through lymphatic channels, or migrate via blood, and then implant themselves outside the uterine cavity.

Genetic predisposition. Certain families are predisposed to the condition.

Immunologic failure. The immune system is deficient in some way, causing tissue to proliferate in abnormal areas. The thought is that through some type of immune deficiency, endometrial tissue gets activated at different times in the cycle through hormonal and chemical influences.

Childbearing. Childbearing in combination with methods of contraception may be responsible.

Symptoms

Endometriosis can produce slight or severe pain, ranging from mild cramps to agony and dysfunction. Pain results from swelling, inflammation, and scarring of affected tissues. It is usually cyclical, and most commonly occurs just before menstruation. Some women have pain during sexual intercourse any time in the month.

Where and to what degree pain is felt depends on the location of the endometrial tissue and the degree it has spread outside the uterus. Some women have pain during urination due to implants on the bladder. Some have pain during bowel movements due to colon and rectal implants. There can be ovarian pain or pain radiating to the back, buttocks, or down the legs. Upon a manual gynecological examination, there may be pelvic pain due to inflammation and scarring.

Internal bleeding may occur as well as nose bleeding or bleeding from another orifice, at certain times of the month. Any cyclic bleeding is suspect for endometriosis. Other symptoms that sometimes appear include bladder infections, fatigue, and lower back pain. Endometriosis may result in infertility when it interferes with ovarian function.

Clinical Experience

DIAGNOSIS

Endometriosis can be suspected in the presence of one or more of the symptoms listed above, but the only real way to confirm a diagnosis is with a surgical procedure, known as a laparoscopy, which allows the doctor to actually see and biopsy tissue. Sonograms and MRI scans may be helpful, but they are not definitive in making the diagnosis.

Proper diagnosis is important, notes Dr. Anthony Aurigemma, because while endometriosis is considered benign, it can become malignant.

CONVENTIONAL THERAPY

Treatment usually consists of medical prescriptions for pain control and reduction of endometrial growth. Antiprostaglandin medicines, such as Indomethacin, Ibuprofen, and Naprosyn, are often given to reduce pain.

Another popular pharmaceutical, Danazol, is also used for this purpose, but in some women it does not provide total or lasting relief. Studies show Danazol to have a good effect after surgery to remove adhesions. After some of the adhesions have been removed, it may help an infertile woman become pregnant. A side effect of the drug is that it may increase cholesterol, especially the LDL variety, which is implicated in accelerated arteriosclerosis. Adverse effects of all the above drugs can include weight gain, edema, decreased or increased breast size, acne, excess hair growth on the face and perhaps even in the developing fetus, and deepening of the voice.

Hormones are sometimes given to fool the body into believing it is pregnant, since pregnancy seems to retard or prevent the development of endometriosis. This method appears to have some benefit, but side effects include depression, painful breasts, nausea, weight gain, bloating, swelling, and migraine headaches. Since side effects can be fairly severe, this is not a popular method.

Newer compounds, called gonadotropin-releasing hormone compounds, are sometimes given by injection. These suppress the pituitary gland from releasing the female hormones FSH and LH, causing what is called a clinical pseudomenopause. They help to reduce pain in many women, and to decrease the size and volume of endometrial tissue after surgery.

Through the advanced surgical technique of Female Reconstructive Surgery (FRS), developed by Dr. Vicki Hufnagel, the uterus and ovaries can be repositioned, thus reducing the deep pelvic pain that is associated with endometriosis.

NATUROPATHY

Dr. Tori Hudson believes there is most support for the immunological weakness theory of endometriosis because women with the condition have altered immune cells, and fewer T-lymphocytes. By improving immune function with supplements, diet, and botanicals, she claims to help many patients: "I've seen women with severe pelvic pain, who were scheduled for surgery one month from the date that I saw them. My treatment helped them to recover completely without the surgery." She adds that most, but not all, women respond to her protocol, which is designed to stimulate a maximal immune response. The basic program consists of the following:

ANTIOXIDANTS.
Vitamin C: to bowel tolerance, up to 10,000 mg
Beta carotene: 150,000–200,000 IU
Selenium: 400 mcg
Vitamin E: 800–1200 IU

DIET. Changes in the diet are made to further stimulate the immune system. This is accomplished by lowering fat, adding whole grains, vegetables and fruits, and eliminating immune system inhibitors such as coffee, sugar, alcohol, and high-fat foods. Foods such as cheese and meat have high amounts of estrogen and are omitted, as estrogen aggravates the disease. A mostly vegetarian diet is best for lowering estrogen and stimulating the immune system.

BOTANICALS. Two botanical formulas are included. One contains chaste tree berry, dandelion root, motherwort, and prickly ash in equal amounts. One-half teaspoon is taken three times daily. The other formula contains small doses of toxic herbs that must be carefully prescribed by a naturopathic physician.

In addition, Dr. Hudson sometimes prescribes natural progesterone made from wild yam. The wild yam extract is converted in the laboratory to natural progesterone.

In addition, Dr. Hudson sometimes prescribes natural progesterone made from wild yam. The wild yam extract is converted in the laboratory to natural progesterone.

ASIAN MEDICINE

Dr. Roger Hirsch, a naturopathic doctor in Santa Monica, California, specializing in Asian medicine, says that the Chinese approach to gynecological imbalance is a holistic one: "What do I mean by holistic? It treats the mind and body as an integral unit like a gloved hand. If you move the hand, what is moving, the glove or the hand? The body or the mind? They move in concert. If there is a psychological, emotional, or spiritual imbalance, it may show up on the physical plane, and cause a 'stuckness' or endometrial situation."

The Chinese diagnose endometriosis by looking at the way the blood flows in the body, specifically in the pelvic cavity. This is determined by the appearance of the root of the tongue, which represents the pelvic cavity. "If a woman has endometriosis, there will be raised bumps and papillae in the back of the tongue and perhaps a greasy yellow coating," he says. "If you look at the back of your tongue in the mirror and see raised bumps that are red and fiery, especially during the time of menstruation, you may well have endometriosis." *(For an explanation of how Asian medicine treats endometriosis as it relates to infertility, see chapter 14, Infertility.)*

HELLERWORK

Hellerwork is a bodywork technique derived from Rolfing. Both modalities are similar in that they work to improve body structure with deep tissue work, but Hellerwork is different in that it is not painful. Certified Hellerwork practitioner Sarah Suatoni, from Pelvic Floor Rehabilitation Laboratory for Women with Endometriosis at St. Luke's Hospital in New York City, gives an overview of the process: "There are three components to Hellerwork. There is a hands-on part, which feels much like a massage, a movement educational aspect, and a mind/body dialogue aspect. I will talk about each of these.

"In the hands-on process, we analyze the body much as a chiropractor would, looking at the posture, or the structure as we call it, to determine which parts of the body are out of balance. We look to see which myofascial tissue connections are creating this misalignment. Then we work with our hands to release it. That, in a sense, is also the beginning of movement education, because this isn't done to the client but with the client. In other words, I put my hands on a spot, and we work closely together with visual images or deep breathing to help the person identify the misalignment, feel it, and then release it.

"The second part of the work is movement education, in which we do very simple everyday movements. We look at how a person sits or stands. In the case of a computer programmer, we look at how they sit at their computer and use their arms. We look at whatever it is that may be contributing to the dysfunction in the body, and then we begin to look at how we can have the person move in a way that will not create the same problem.

"Last, but certainly not least, is mind/body dialogue. We work under the belief that our emotional patterns, memories, and attitudes are reflected in our bodies. In the same way one needs to look at a movement pattern in order to shift some sort of physical dysfunction, one needs to look at emotional patterns or beliefs in order to shift those as well. We dialogue with clients in order to identify underlying emotions or memories. Then we look at how clients might better facilitate emotions or memories, so that they are not manifesting them through physical dysfunctions.

"This work is a process where people come in for eleven sessions. Once a week for an hour-and-a-half is ideal although other time frames are possible. Each session touches upon a different part of the body and different aspects of the being."

Suatoni tells how she began using Hellerwork to treat endometriosis and similar chronic conditions: "I met Dr. David Kauffman, a urologist, who determined that women with interstitial cystitis had severe spasm of the pelvic muscles. He has since started working with patients with endometriosis, vulvodinia, vestibulitis, and a number of other conditions that show the same symptoms of severe spasm or contraction. Dr. Kauffman was using biofeedback and felt that he needed someone who did hands-on work to accompany the biofeedback treatments. That's how I began.

"I determined that he was indeed right. When I put my hands on the deep pelvic muscles, they were in severe contraction. We do not know why this is so. Whether it is a cause or effect of the disease is still a question. We do know, however, that teaching women to feel those muscles, and to learn to relax them, releases a great deal of pain.

"I do a normal series of Hellerwork on these patients because each part of the body is connected to every other part. It's the hip-bone-connected-to-the-knee-bone thing. If the pelvis is in contraction, it has been affected by all the other related areas. So I work on the whole body as well as the pelvis area.

"I find that most of my patients do not know how to relax. Education is extremely useful. I place my hands into the deep pelvic muscles and teach women how to feel them. The beginning of the process is just to help them locate the muscles, feel the muscles, and then learn that they have control over them. They can, in fact, relax and release the contractions.

"The second part of the process involves movement. We look at the way women walk, sit, and breathe. Slowly they begin to realize that they have been holding onto these muscles all their lives. This insight is the beginning of their awareness of what is happening.

"Then we look at different situations in their lives that tend to exacerbate their condition. Issues of control are often involved. For example, when they are having a big fight with somebody or having a difficult day at work, they tend to grip these muscles tighter. Once women make this connection, their awareness is further enhanced. They realize that on a really bad day they grip those muscles tightly. Hopefully, once they identify what is happening, they can begin to release. Then much of their pain is greatly alleviated.

"So the process is really an educational process about the whole body. Specifically, it is a process of learning about how not to grip and grab those muscles so that they do not spasm and create pain.

"The last part of this looks at emotional patterns that may be creating some of the physical problems. Endometriosis, in particular, has been called the working woman's disease. On an emotional level, the disease is speaking to masculine/feminine aspects being out of balance. Most of these women lead very ambitious, fast-paced lives. They are doers and achievers who are often magnificently bright, aggressive, and successful. But they are not really in touch with their feminine aspect. I am using feminine in the Jungian sense, which refers to receptivity and surrender, and which applies to men or women. These aspects of being are less present in their lives. In a sense, the disease is a voice saying, 'It is time to bring life into better balance.' Certainly, the disease forces them to do that because most women must slow down, receive help, and do things that they have never done before. Ideally, women begin to replace the receiving they get through medical care with receptivity in other aspects of their lives, and disease symptoms lessen.

"Although this process deals with mind/body relationships, this does not imply that these diseases are imaginary. Some women have been told for years that their disease is all in their head, when there are all kinds of physical evidence for the disease. Rather, the disease is the result of a set of relationships between the mind and body. Hellerwork and other forms of bodywork help because they are process-oriented and look at relationships. Once women start understanding these relationships, they find that they have a whole lot of power to overcome disease and regain health."

HOMEOPATHY

Homeopathy is another holistic therapy that addresses underlying emotional causes. Dr. Aurigemma has been treating his patients homeopathically for ten years and claims that the therapy is completely safe and highly effective. "There is no doubt in my mind that something actually happens and that it helps people," he says. "I utilize the remedies because I see them work. What spurs me on is the continuous improvements of most of the patients I see."

Patient Stories

DR. AURIGEMMA OUTLINES ONE PATIENT'S PROGRESS
WITH HOMEOPATHY: A thirty-five-year-old woman, who was diagnosed with endometriosis via laparoscopy in 1981, came to my office in February 1993. She had a history of migraine headaches, vaginal yeast infections, pain beginning in her hips and going down to her knees, as well as mid-month pain in the uterine area, shooting, throbbing ovarian pain, pain while running, and pain after overeating. Premenstrually, she experienced headaches, anger, bloating, crankiness, and sensitivity. She had headaches the last day of her menstrual cycle, and the day after the menstrual cycle ended.

In homeopathy, part of the diagnostic process includes an assessment of how people appear. These were some of her personality characteristics. She was bright, lively, and pleasant. Even though she seemed to be in pain, she was not irritable. She said she alternated between being warm and chilly and that she easily got overheated. In addition, she claimed to be spontaneous and very quick to act. Also, she was an animal rights activist who took in strays. She said that she did not harbor anger. Instead, she tried to get things out in the open. In terms of her eating habits, she was not a very thirsty person. She liked to drink cold water and herb teas, and she would occasionally have a glass of wine with a steak dinner. She said that she liked salads, spicy foods, and borscht, but that creamy foods were too rich. She smoked one to two cigarettes per day, two or three times per week.

Her fears included claustrophobia, not liking to be in tunnels, elevators, or crowds. Thunderstorms bothered her. She was somewhat weepy at sentimental movies.

I studied her symptoms, personality characteristics, foods, likes and dislikes, and fears. Based on this information, I came up with a particular homeopathic remedy which I asked her to take twice a day, four or five days a week.

Approximately three months later, she reported feeling 70–80 percent better. Her uterine pain and headaches had decreased, pre-menstrual symptoms were less severe, and there was an almost total disappearance of her yeast infection. At that point, she was given one single dose of the same remedy, but in a higher potency. I gave this to her in the office and it was not repeated.

A month later, she returned, and said that she was improving further. There were no headaches at all with her period and very little pain. The yeast flared up, but then got better. On that visit, I gave her no remedy at all and told her to come back in three months, or if symptoms started to return.

Three months later, in September, she came back with some return of headaches when the period was stopping. Even so, headaches were still about 50 percent better than they had been in the first place. The yeast infection was 90 percent improved, and the monthly pain was about 75 percent better overall. This is without any further remedy.

At this point, I gave her another dose of the same remedy to take daily, five days per week. That was three months ago. Since that time, I have not seen her. She reports being between 75 and 80 percent better overall, and 90 percent better with her yeast infection. These subjective estimates of health are given to me by the patient, since there is no physical way to measure improvement. She is more functional, better able to do things, happier, and pleased with the treatment. She plans to continue.

Her symptoms are fewer, and certainly less intense. In seven months, her periods became easier, and between periods she feels more comfortable. There were no side effects from the remedy other than an aggravation of her yeast infection for a few days which then subsided. That was due to a higher potency of the remedy. Homeopathic remedies can aggravate symptoms. Very often that aggravation is a sign that the remedy is correct and is bringing things to a head, getting the body to focus on the problem, and then getting rid of it.

She is functioning better, she is less uncomfortable, but we do not know whether or not the endometrial tissue has shrunken or gone away. The only way to really know that is by doing another laparoscopy, but a person is unlikely to undergo surgery when feeling better.

LINDA DESCRIBES HER EXPERIENCE TREATING ENDOMETRIOSIS WITH AYURVEDIC MEDICINE: I had constant abdominal pain from the endometriosis for twenty-one days out of every month. For many years, I took eight to ten aspirin a day and sometimes stronger painkillers. In four years, I had been to three gynecologists, two internists, and a gastroenterologist. I had laparascopic surgery and then was given Lupron injections. Lupron is a drug that blocks estrogen and causes the endometrial tissue to shrink. After three months on Lupron, the pain from the endometriosis was gone, but there were some terrific side effects. Hot flashes interfered with my sleeping. I also had a lot of trouble with joint pain. But by far the worst side effect was loss of bone density. This is the reason why you are not supposed to take drugs like Lupron for more than six months in your lifetime. After I stopped taking Lupron, the endometriosis came back within a month or two. At that point, my gynecologist said my best options were another drug that could also affect bone density or a complete hysterectomy. It seemed as if I didn't have any acceptable options left.

At that point, I found Dr. Lonsdorf, an Ayurvedic doctor, who recommended certain herbal mixtures for me. She also suggested other simple measures that are simple to follow and of benefit to everyone: sipping hot water throughout the day to aid digestion, eating the main meal in the middle of the day and eating less toward the end, cutting down on meat and working toward a more vegetarian diet, getting to bed by ten and up by six—that is, trying to get more in touch with the circadian rhythms—using massage to stimulate circulation, and practicing meditation to calm the mind.

I incorporated as many of these suggestions into my life as I comfortably could. Within a few weeks, the pain from the endometriosis was almost completely gone. I have been under Dr. Lonsdorf's care for almost a year and a half and almost never have any discomfort anymore. I have much more energy and am much calmer. Some other problems I had, like low blood sugar, have also cleared up. In fact, the Ayurvedic medicine helped me so much that my husband and both our daughters see Dr. Lonsdorf now.

DR. ANTHONY PENEPENT DESCRIBES ONE PATIENT'S SUCCESS TREATING HER ENDOMETRIOSIS WITH NATURAL HYGIENE: One woman came to see me who was on prescription narcotic medication for the pain. The medicine gave her no relief, and she was at the point of wanting a hysterectomy to get relief from the pain. I put this woman on a natural hygienic regimen for a couple of weeks. First, she fasted for five days. Then she followed up with a nutritional plan.

Let me briefly describe a typical hygienic regimen. The patient has a breakfast consisting of a vegetable juice or a vegetable/fruit juice combination, a blended salad, a piece of fruit, perhaps some hot cereal and a couple of soft boiled egg yolks. For lunch the patient has a vegetable juice or vegetable/fruit juice combination, a blended salad, a cup or a little more than that, a piece of fruit, and then some raw nuts or unsalted raw milk cheese. For the evening meal, the patient starts with juice again, blended salad, tossed salad, steamed vegetables such as string beans, broccoli, or escarole. Then she goes on with the main course, which includes a steamed potato or yam, natural brown rice or other whole grain, and a legume. I also might supplement the meal with egg or cheese, depending on the protein needs of the woman. Of course, there are variations for individual patients.

Following this general plan, this patient was pain-free at the end of one month. That was ten years ago. Right now she is pregnant with her second child, whereas before she was infertile. Natural hygiene has tremendous implications for endometriosis. There is absolutely no reason why a woman should have pain or be infertile because of such a simple condition.

What I can see from my perusal of the literature is that endometriosis is plainly a condition of liver toxicity, where the liver is failing to completely break down the estrogen hormones that the body is manufacturing. These breakdown products wreak havoc in the form of endometrial tissue in the pelvic cavity.

Hot News

Dioxin has been implicated as a possible cause of endometriosis in women, based on animal studies. A new technique, beta-3 analysis, offers a nonsurgical alternative to laparoscopy for diagnosis, and in the field of treatment, a natural progesterone extracted from wild yam shows promise. *(See below.)*

Diagnosis of endometriosis is usually made by laparoscopy, in which a "belly-button cut" is made so that a lighted instrument may be inserted through the navel. An alternative has been tested: beta-3 analysis. This nonsurgical method has a positive predictive value and was shown to be 86 percent effective in a study.

G. Marino, "Protein Missing in Endometriosis Cases," *Science News* 146, no. 8 (August 20, 1994): 18.

Although over 5 million U.S. women have endometriosis, the cause is uncertain. Speculations include: menstrual blood that flows backward, a developmental disorder, and the lastest theory, dioxin exposure. In humans, high dioxin exposure may cause cancer and birth defects. A study on female rhesus monkeys shows that 79 percent of the monkeys exposed to low levels of dioxin on a daily basis developed endometriosis; severity was dose-related. People are exposed to dioxin from pesticides and certain types of waste incineration.

A. Gibbons, "Dioxin Tied to Endometriosis," *Science* 262 (1993): 1373.

Natural progesterone from wild yam can be used to treat endometriosis.

Neal Barnard, "Natural Progesterone: Is Estrogen the Wrong Hormone?" *Good Medicine*, Spring 1994, 11–13.

A study on mice supports the use of the traditional Chinese medicine keishi-bukuryo-gan (KBG) to treat uterine adenomyosis in humans.

T. Mori et al., "Suppression of Spontaneous Development of Uterine Adenomyosis by a Chinese Herbal Medicine, Keishi-Bukuryo-Gan, in Mice," *Planta Med.* 59, no. 4 (August 1993): 308–11.

10. ENVIRONMENTAL ILLNESS

Technological advance in our society has been accompanied by an unprecedented quantity of challenges to our bodies and our health. The ability to change our looks and our bodily processes with a pill or an implant, along with a variety of other types of changes, and combined with a multitude of potentially carcinogenic types of microscopic pollution in our air, water, homes, and workplaces, together cause an overload on our immune systems that can produce a type of condition called environmental illness. Women tend to be more prone to environmental illness than men. This is in part because a number of chemical toxins actually mimic estrogen in the body, causing an insufficiency in the hormone. Also, both birth control pills and silicone breast implants can compromise women's immune systems.

Causes

Dr. Stephen M. Silverman of Port Washington, New York, says that thousands of poisons in our food, water, and surroundings are responsible for environmental illness: "The first thing you must realize is that what you eat can have a tremendous effect on your immune system. One of the most toxic foods that people expose themselves to unknowingly, for example, is hydrogenated oil. People don't realize how widespread that ingredient is. It's in crackers, all commercial breads, potato chips, pretzels, and cookies, and it has a very strong damaging effect on the immune system.

"Along with what you eat, you must consider what you drink. Most people are being exposed to tap water, whether directly from their sink or outside when they buy a cup of coffee or tea. Probably one of the highest exposures to carcinogens comes from this source. In 1989, Ralph Nader's group identified over 2,000 chemicals commonly found in people's drinking water. When water is tested over the course of the year, it is tested for approximately 120 chemicals. When you are told that the water is safe to drink, it means that it safe for what it was tested. You have no idea about the other 1,900 chemicals. Insecticides and pesticides in the water have been associated with Long Island's high rate of breast cancer. Certainly, if they can create cancer, they can cause immune system damage.

"Among the other factors that can set you up for illness are the things you put on your body. I am talking about cosmetics, moisturizers, hair sprays. We know through medical applications of the nicotine and estrogen patches that what you put on your skin will be absorbed into the bloodstream. If you were to take a look at the ingredients of your cosmetics, hair sprays, underarm deodorants, you would see that they are loaded with chemicals. You have to realize that when you use these chemicals every day, they eventually get into the bloodstream. When you think about it, is it possible that these chemicals have no effect on your immune system? It's almost impossible.

"In addition, there are environmental factors. One of the most important rooms to be safe in is the bedroom. If you happen to have a carpet that is outgassing, by which I mean releasing chemicals at a very low level, and some of these chemicals are suspected carcinogens, despite how well you may be eating, you are going to get sick from that carpet. When we sleep at night, we are supposed to detoxify. Your body attempts to purify itself at night of any additives or toxins in foods that you may have eaten. If you have a toxic bedroom, where either the carpet, the paint on the wall, or a mattress loaded with formaldehyde is releasing gas, and if you're reacting to these chemicals, then eight hours a night, instead of restoring your immune system, you may be causing it severe damage."

"Research shows that women are more prone to environmental illnesses," says Heather Millar, author of *The Toxic Labyrinth*. "The reason is that many chemicals, such as formaldehyde, benzene, phenol, and chlorine have estrogen-mimicking properties. These chemicals take the place of estrogen in the body. The body thinks that it has enough estrogen and doesn't make enough of its own. Estrogen is responsible for reproduction as well as many other vital functions in the body. Problems occur when the body calls upon the estrogen it thinks it has, but doesn't.

"Silicone breast implants are making women terribly ill. They have a tendency to grow fungus inside the implant, which adds a problem to an already existing one. Fungus is extremely hard to get rid of once it starts to grow. After breast implants are removed, women do not feel better. This indicates that their immune systems have been damaged. It will probably take a very long time for them to recover, and we do not know the long-term effects."

Symptoms

Symptoms vary, depending on a woman's constitution, and may include fatigue, aching muscles, flulike feeling, ringing in the ears, burning in the eyes, headaches, migraines, disturbed sleep, shortness of breath, food allergies, heightened sense of smell, loss of balance, inability to concentrate, memory loss, anxiety, panic attacks, depression, and irritable bowel syndrome. There is a marked progressive debilitating reaction to consumer products, such as perfumes, soap, tobacco smoke, and plastics.

Clinical Experience

CONVENTIONAL APPROACH

Environmental illness was first recognized in the 1980s, but mainstream medicine still generally disregards this syndrome. When patients come in with the symptoms of sensitivity to a toxic environment, doctors often do not know the correct protocol. Standardized blood tests appear normal, leading doctors to assume that no problem exists.

Another problem is that most doctors today are not trained to work with a disease that affects the whole body. Millar, who suffered from the condition, notes, "In the medical community, we have created a world of specialists. Physicians are now neurologists, cardiologists, rheumatologists, and so on. We have gotten away from the old-fashioned approach. We no longer have general practitioners. Before, you would go to a doctor's office and tell him your history from start to finish. He would look at you as a whole individual, checking the psychological as well as the physical aspect of the body. Only then would he make an assessment.

"Now technology has compartmentalized the body. The neurologist only looks at the symptoms of numbness, tingling, and headaches. The rheumatologist only looks at arthritis, joint pain, aches. The infectious disease doctor only looks for infection. What happened to me was, I would go in and give a detailed history of what was happening. The doctor, according to his specialty, would look only at one specific area. He or she did not want to hear about the other symptoms I had.

"What we are failing to realize with all this super-technology in medicine is that the body works in harmony. You do not have one body system that works separately from something else. They all work together. So if you are having symptoms in one system, you are probably having symptoms elsewhere."

DIAGNOSIS

In her book, Heather Millar has a checklist to help people determine whether or not they may be suffering from environmental illness. These are some questions she asks people to consider:

Do I have a toxic lifestyle?

Have I had breast implants?

Does my environment contain chemicals that could be making me sick?

Do I feel ill at work?

Do I feel ill at home?

Do I live in a new home?

Have I recently painted or installed new carpet?

How much plastic do I have in the home?

Does my neighborhood contain chemicals that could be making me sick?

"Discovering the cause of the problem is a detective process," Millar says. "It involves taking a close look at your home, workplace, and neighborhood.

"Start with your home. You may ask, 'Why didn't we have these problems before? We always painted our house and put new carpet in.' What I'd like to suggest is that technology has changed a lot of chemicals and manufacturing processes. Since the 1980s, we have added more synthetics and are now seeing their effects. A lot of these products let out gas. The newness smell is a gas that is coming off. Basically, it's a chemical soup, which is very hazardous to our health. Also, since we live in energy-efficient buildings, we do not have the ventilation needed to lessen the concentration or these gases.

"Plastics present further problems. They have a lot of these estrogen-mimicking properties. Softer plastics have more toxicity. We used to live with metal, wood, and glass. These are far safer alternatives. When replacing plastic with wood, consider the type of finish on it. Does it smell?

"Then look at the workplace. Ask yourself, what are you doing as an occupation? Are you working with chemicals on an ongoing basis? Or are you working in an energy-efficient office building that was recently renovated? Is currently being renovated? Has no open windows? Do other people in the office frequently get colds and flus or feel unwell?

"Finally, examine your neighborhood. Where do you live? Do you have chemical manufacturing in your backyard? Is there some kind of toxic incinerator nearby? What is in your water supply? What kinds of pesticide regulations do they have for your neighborhood?

"You may react differently to toxins in your environment than your coworkers do. For example, in my workplace, which was extremely toxic, my symptoms were mainly neurological. Other colleagues were diagnosed with chronic fatigue. Still others experienced asthma or fibromyalgia, which is an aching of the muscles. We react differently depending upon our genetic predisposition."

Fortunately, there are physicians who do recognize the illness, and there are tests available to pinpoint the condition. Occupational health doctors and environmental physicians prescribe tests that look at solvent levels in the blood. They look at pesticide levels in the blood, and check mineral levels, which are usually low in people who suffer from chemical exposures.

DETOXIFICATION

Without detoxifying the system, all other steps to repair the body will be of no avail, says Dr. Silverman. "When people are ill they're frequently thinking, 'What should I take to repair my system?' But usually half of the battle is to figure out what is hurting the immune system. And more often than not, it is figuring out what can be taken away. People are under the impression that they can take B vitamins, minerals, and immune stimulants, and continue to drink toxic water with insecticides, pesticides and metals, eat foods that they react to, and get better. They don't get better, because although they are taking good nutrients, they are still poisoning their body."

Dr. Zane Gard, an expert in toxicology, reports methods of detoxification that have impressive results in the reversal of environmental illness: "Heat stress detoxification includes wood saunas, hot sand packing, steam baths and sweat lodges. The history of these approaches goes back several thousand years. Careful supervision is required. Heat stress detoxification can be effective, but requires knowledge of toxins and their potential effects on the body. If it is not administered properly, there can be a lot of complications, and the patient can actually end up worse.

"The biotoxic reduction program was designed with the toxic-chemical-syndrome patient in mind. It is a comprehensive, medically managed program, addressing toxicology, psychology, neurology, pathology, and immunology. The program must be followed seven days a week, three to five hours a day, for a minimum of two weeks. It would be nice to have off on Saturday and Sunday, but patients actually regress one or two days every time they take a day off during the first two weeks. So it has to be every day during that initial period.

"The program consists of increasing niacin, aerobic exercise, sauna therapy, and other therapies, as necessary. With those who have neurological damage, other therapies will be needed. Part of that is a therapy that stimulates the myelin sheaths to regenerate. As a result, many peripheral neuropathies completely reverse. In over eighty peripheral neuropathies, including MS, we have only two that did not fully recover.

"In a study of patients in our program, the average blood toxin levels after twenty-one days of therapy are as follows: toluene drops from 19.3 to an average of 0.34; ethyl benzine drops from 14.7 to 0.1; xylene drops from 72.9 to 0.94; 1:1 trichloroethylene goes from 7.7 to 0.92; and DDE goes from 5.7 to 1.8. We know that DDT, which is the parent compound of DDE, will be 97 percent removed within four months. You continue to detoxify for a good four months."

Patient Stories

HEATHER MILLAR

I started becoming ill a year before I realized what was happening. At first, I just thought I was tired. I was having trouble getting out of bed. I was dragging myself to work. I would come home feeling exhausted. Sometimes I had asthmalike symptoms where I couldn't quite catch my breath. I wondered why this started all of a sudden when I was thirty years old, because my understanding was that most people develop asthma as children. I attributed these symptoms to working and living a fast-paced lifestyle, and I ignored them. One day my wrist started to ache for no apparent reason, which made me wonder if I was getting arthritis. But I ignored that as well and thought it would go away. I had these warning signs for a year before collapsing at work in September 1993.

I woke up feeling as if I had the flu, but thought I was well enough to go to work. I had gone shopping with my mom that morning and had difficulty walking up stairs. When I arrived at work, I realized that I was feeling quite unwell, and that I would only be able to work part of my nursing shift. At the end of the first hour, I needed to go home because I was too ill to walk down the corridor and deliver medications to my patients. It was then that I returned to the nursing station and collapsed. I could hear, but I couldn't move. I felt as if I was paralyzed. I couldn't communicate with the other nurses who came to attend to me.

They took me to the emergency room, but I started to feel better and went home. I decided that I had the flu and that I would be better in three days.

Three days of flu evolved into a year and a half. During this time, I experienced many difficulties. The problem with environmental illness or chemical sensitivity is that you have a wide array of symptoms that come and go. You don't really know where to start and what connections to make. These are some of the symptoms I experienced.

Flu symptoms plagued me every day and became worse with time. As time passed, I was having more difficulty getting out of bed and walking around the house. I was extremely tired. No matter how much I slept, I just could not seem to get enough sleep. Even small tasks that shouldn't take much energy overwhelmed me. Cooking a meal was too much to even think about.

I also started having disturbed sleep. Despite my fatigue, I would wake up between two and four each night with numb hands. Sometimes I would have an incredible thirst. And sometimes I would wake up shaking as if I had a very high fever.

At one point I lost sight in my right eye. This happened for a short time but was extremely frightening nonetheless. All of a sudden, the vision in my right eye became completely silver, as if I was trying to look through a piece of tin foil.

I had headaches with stabbing pains in my temples and a burning sensation in the back of my neck, which made it difficult to turn my head. If you try to drive a car or move to do something, you realize how important it is to have range of motion in your neck.

The next month, I started to experience food allergies. It started with a few things. First, I wasn't tolerating wheat very well, and stopped eating it. Then I noticed that I did not feel well after drinking coffee and milk, so I eliminated that also. As the months progressed, I was unable to tolerate more and more foods. By January, I was virtually down to two foods: lamb and yams. By February, I lost my tolerance for everything. I was caught in a vicious cycle. I knew I needed to get nutrition in order to turn my health around, but eating these foods would make me even sicker.

As I became increasingly ill, my sense of smell became more and more acute. All of a sudden perfumes were a problem. I absolutely hated going to the department store and passing the perfume counter. I couldn't stand the smell of car exhaust either. I even avoided the hardware store because of the strong smell in there. Going to public places became difficult, as many people wear scented products, such as clothes washed in scented laundry detergents, perfumes, and aftershaves. I would walk into a room and if someone had perfume on, I would suddenly feel like I had the worst flu. My shoulders and muscles would start to ache. I would feel short of breath. I would get a headache.

A heightened sense of smell is part of the illness. People who are not affected need to understand that when individuals with environmental illness ask, "Please do not wear that fragrance because it makes me feel sick."

I also started to have ringing in my ears. That would come and go so I never could associate it with any particular event. Sometimes it would affect one ear, sometimes both. It was bothersome trying to have a conversation with somebody and trying to hear them over the ringing in my ears.

Additionally, I felt dizzy. I had days when it was even difficult for me to stand up and navigate my way to the bathroom. Several times I would fall over.

One of the most disturbing symptoms that I had was difficulty concentrating. I could no longer read something from start to finish. It would take me three to four times to read material that should have been comprehended in the first reading.

I also noticed that I was forgetful. Previously, I had an exceptional memory. All of a sudden I noticed that I couldn't remember things that were extremely important. At thirty, I was wondering if I was getting the beginning stages of Alzheimer's, the loss of memory was so apparent. Some days my memory was better than others, and some days my ability to concentrate was better than others.

Then there were the panic attacks. My heart would race while I was driving my car on the interstate. I did not understand why I felt better on residential streets. Later, I realized that the reason I was having difficulty on the interstate was that the exhaust was so much more prevalent there than on residential streets. Every time I was exposed to exhaust, it would make my heart race; it would make me feel anxious; I would have difficulty concentrating.

The other place I felt extremely anxious was in shopping malls. I have since learned that there are extremely high levels of chemicals in shopping malls, such as formaldehyde, emitted by new building materials. These synthetics are highly toxic. What I couldn't understand was why I felt anxious at some times and not others. The reason was that some shopping malls are less toxic than others, and some stores, because of the types of merchandise they carry, are also better than others.

The day I collapsed at work was the last day I worked as a nurse. I kept assuming that within a month I would feel better and go back to my job. One month rolled into two, two months into three, and three months into a year and a half.

Being a nurse, I felt that I would receive the support I needed. After all, I was a medical person myself. What I experienced instead was how the patient feels when he or she is told that nothing is wrong. I had always been on the other side of things. I found this new perspective extremely alarming.

The medical community has become technologically based. Everything relies on a diagnostic test. I would go in and they would run a gamut of tests. Like most people with environmental illness, the standard tests would come back negative. The doctors would then tell me that there was nothing wrong. This was disturbing because I was extremely ill. I was so sick that I could hardly get up off the couch. Nor could I make myself a meal. Going to the bathroom was even an effort. How, on a diagnostic test, could I look perfectly normal?

When the doctors could not diagnose me, they said that I was suffering from stress. But this was not the case. Before I got sick, my life was wonderful. I had one of the least pressured jobs I had ever had, and I was enjoying what I was doing. At the end of a contract I would go to Europe for a month and take a vacation. I was about to get married. My life couldn't have been better.

Stress is becoming the catch-all diagnosis in the medical community. We must ask why so many people in our society are being told that they have stress, panic disorder, anxiety, and depression. That category is growing larger and larger. People have to ask, Why is this happening in our society? Is something chemical bringing this on? Do we need to make changes in the environment?

If you are feeling some symptoms of toxicity, it is time to take action now. Don't wait until you end up, as I did, in a wheelchair, bed-ridden, and completely without tolerance to food.

DR. GARD ON ONE PATIENT'S EXPERIENCE:

A fifty-six-year-old Caucasian female came to us with swollen, painful joints, especially in the right knee. She was scheduled for a knee replacement. History indicated that she worked in a closed building as a counselor to students. Nine of the twelve teachers in this building had similar problems. Most of the complaints started following new carpet installation.

A biotoxic reduction was started. Within the first hour of the program, she was able to bend her right knee. By the second day, she was able to move with less difficulty, and ride the stationary bike. Upon completion, she was pain-free and had full range of motion in all joints. This was over four years ago, and the patient is still well.

Her laboratory work revealed toluene, 24.9 before the program and 1.4 after; ethyl benzine, 12.3 before and none after; xylen, 83.2 before and none after; styrene, 123.6 before and none after; chloroform, 5.4 before and none after; 1:1 trichlor, 1.4 before and 0.5 after; tetrachloroethylene, 1.5 before and none after; dichlorobenzene, 11.1 before and 4.3 after.

11. FATIGUE

In 1988 a state of constant exhaustion was termed "chronic fatigue syndrome" by the Centers for Disease Control in Atlanta, Georgia. Dr. Nancy Lonsdorf, medical director of the Maharishi Ayurveda Health Center in Washington, D.C., and coauthor of *A Woman's Best Medicine,* defines fatigue as an imbalance in the body's rest/activity cycle: "According to Ayurvedic principles, the nature structures in rest cycles allow the body to recover from activity cycles. A state of chronic fatigue means that the body has not fully rejuvenated itself."

Causes

Michael Vesselago, M.D., former chief medical resident at the Virginia Mason Medical Center in Seattle, Washington, says that new research sees chronic fatigue syndrome as the end result of an immune disorder: "It is well known that chronic fatigue syndrome is linked to viral diseases, such as Epstein-Barr and herpes viruses. Other people have found that some people with this condition test very high for a yeast called candida. Then there are those who have musculoskeletal problems. They ache terribly and become disabled from a disorder called fibromyalgia, which simply means pain in the muscles related to a thickening and tightening of muscle fibers. My colleagues and I have all seen these people, some with viral diseases, some with candida, and some with musculoskeletal diseases. It all seems to point in the direction of the immune system. We are looking at the immune system somehow being damaged, the result being a chronic viral infection, a chronic overgrowth of what is normally a friendly organism, or a chronic dysfunction of the muscles, which forms a prominent symptom."

Often immune system dysfunction is preceded by adrenal exhaustion brought on by chronic stress and overactivity: "It is very clear to me that the pace of life is enormous these days," says Dr. Vesselago. "We all experience that. People are trying to fit everything into the day without there being enough time. They are working under demands that are too great, trying to please too many people who are asking them to do too many things, not having enough time for their family, and on and on. This drains the adrenal system."

Symptoms

Chronic fatigue syndrome is characterized by extreme tiredness, which can last for years. Usually it begins after the onset of flulike symptoms. Many people have difficulty getting out of bed and may become weakened to the point of needing to lie down all the time. It may be accompanied by depression, irritability, headaches, low grade fever, infection, confusion, focusing difficulties, spaciness, diarrhea, sharp muscle pain and weakness, swollen glands, and sleep disorders.

Clinical Experience

AYURVEDA

Dr. Lonsdorf reports that many of her clients overcome fatigue by adhering to the basic rules of Maharishi Ayurveda, which address rest, activity, digestion, cleansing and meditation:

Rest. "One of the simplest things we can do is pay attention to our sleep cycles. Many Americans just don't get enough sleep. They think they should be able to get by with five, six or seven hours when most of them need eight or more.

"When we sleep and awaken is also important. This has to do with an understanding of the three *doshas*, or fundamental principles, that operate in nature. *Doshas* are expressions of nature's intelligence that guide all activity in our bodies and in nature. These three fundamental principles are called *vata, pitta,* and *kapha. Vata* governs movement, everything that flows in the body, all digestive action down to elimination, and all circulation. *Pitta* is the energy cycle, the fire and transformation. Last is *kapha,* the structural *dosha,* the muscles, bones, and connective tissue that give substance to the body. It includes everything that holds the body together as one piece of matter.

"*Vata, pitta, kapha* govern our rest/activity cycles. For best sleep, Ayurveda tells us that we should start our rest during the cycle that is organized for calming down. This is the *kapha* time, between six and ten in the evening. Most people naturally start to feel sleepy then. If we go to sleep at this time, we will fall asleep quickly and our sleep will be the most rejuvenating.

"The other side of the coin is getting up. Benjamin Franklin had the right idea when he said, 'Early to bed, early to rise makes a woman healthy, wealthy and wise.' Ayurveda agrees with this and says that getting up early gives us more energy throughout the day. If we get up during *vata* time, between two and six in the morning, we will be the most active and energetic.

"It is very important for a woman to rest more during menstruation. This is a time for the body to rejuvenate, clear out, and purify. Limiting activity and resting more at this time gives women more energy for the entire month."

ACTIVITY. "We also need more physical activity to rejuvenate the body. Ayurveda teaches that different body types are suited for different types of exercise, and that we should exercise according to the dominant *dosha* in our system.

"Let's start with the *vata* type. The *vata*-dominant person is light in build with a small bone structure. The person tends to be high strung and energetic. These people should exercise, but not overexercise. Walking or bicycling thirty to sixty minutes at a comfortable, easy pace, or a light exercise like yoga, is best for this body type. Too much exercise causes this type of individual to become overly anxious, to not sleep well, and to become weak.

"The *kapha* body type is the opposite. This person has a heavy bone structure, and tends to put on weight and keep it on. Too little exercise results in lethargy, and a sluggish type of fatigue. The best type of exercise for overcoming this type of fatigue is a vigorous workout. Joining an aerobics class, or scheduling time regularly to walk with a friend helps to keep this person motivated as *kapha*-dominant people tend to procrastinate.

"*Pitta*, the middle body type, has a medium bone structure, and lots of natural energy. The person tends to be athletic and to enjoy sports. The only problem is that they are workaholics who can forget to take the time to exercise. The *pitta* type is dominated by heat, so cooling types of activities, such as skiing in the winter or hiking on a mountain trail in the summertime is more balancing, and tends to make them feel better.

"A couple of other points on exercise. It is very good to exercise in the morning, during that sluggish *kafa* time, 6 to 10 A.M. That will keep us going the whole day. It will improve metabolism, increase appetite and help our digestion. Altogether, that will give us more energy."

DIGESTION. "The third area of treatment for fatigue is digestion- and diet-related. According to the Ayurvedic system, how we digest food and how the cells of the body get nourished by that food is related to how energetic or how fatigued we feel. In fact, Ayurveda has a precise word for lack of good digestion, *ama*. *Ama* refers to residues, or improperly digested food molecules, that get deposited in the arteries, bones, or joints. *Ama* can be as simple as excess cholesterol, gallstones, or uric acid which can create gout, or to glucose-related end products that get stuck in the tissues and cause stiffness and aging. Good nutrition creates less *ama* and gives us more energy.

"I would like to add that it is best not to eat late at night as this can interfere with good sleep. Eating after eight o'clock is to be avoided. Less food in the evening gives us better, more rejuvenating sleep."

CLEANSING. "One other Ayurvedic treatment for fatigue cleanses the body of accumulated impurities or *ama*. It is known as *pancha karma*. *Pancha* means five, and *karma* means action; this therapy consists of five actions or treatments. It is basically a physical treatment involving several days' work with a trained technician. During this time, special herbal oils are applied to the body to soften impurities. Then some mild cleansing therapies, like herbalized steam, are used to open the channels of circulation. A mild herbal enema follows, which helps to eliminate contaminants. A study published in the *Journal of Social Behavior and Personality* reported that this therapy resulted in 40 percent less fatigue."

MEDITATION. "The imbalance between rest and activity also includes our perceptions about life. Basically, it says that every waking moment, we have our attention in the field of activity. We experience through the senses, we think, we emote, and we relate to other people. We are always active. When we take that awareness to the field of silence, we greatly energize our mind and nervous system. This has a tremendously rejuvenating effect. We do this through meditation. In Maharishi Ayurveda, we use TM, the transcendental meditation technique, because that has been scientifically shown to give excellent results in terms of improving health and reducing anxiety and other stress-related conditions."

NATUROPATHY

Gracia Perlstein, an alternative health care practitioner with a private practice in Belle Terre, New York, says that for chronic fatigue, food is the best medicine: "We really don't have any existing drugs on the market to help this condition. In fact, most drugs will weaken immunity and delay recovery further. Best to approach this with natural supports to inherent, healing processes." While there are no quick cure-alls, Perlstein makes the following recommendations to speed up recovery:

DIET. A diet of pure, dense, nutrient-rich, whole foods is imperative in this condition. You want to include plenty of fresh organic vegetables. Cruciferous vegetables, such as broccoli, cauliflower, and Brussels sprouts, are very important for their immune-enhancing properties. You want onions and garlic, the poor man's cure-all.

"Choose from a wide assortment of whole foods. Don't eat the same few over and over again. In this weakened state you can develop allergic responses to the same foods consumed in large amounts. Eating different foods will insure that you get a variety of nutrients, and that will keep you from developing allergic responses. Amaranth, quinoa, and other grains not commonly eaten by Americans are good to include.

"Really emphasize the green foods. Have a dark, green salad daily. Super green powders are very helpful as well. Add them to juices, but do not emphasize sweet fruit and carrot juice.

"Eat an adequate amount of high quality proteins. Best sources are vegetarian because of the low toxicity and ease of digestion. Good vegetarian proteins are tofu, tempeh, fortified soy milk, and legumes. You can benefit from small amounts of fresh fish because fish is high in omega-3 fatty acids. But there are some precautions you must take. Be sure to find a market that gets fish from clean, unpolluted waters, and make sure they do not dip it in chlorine, which is common practice. If you eat farm raised fish, it should be organically raised. If you eat poultry, it should be naturally raised as well, free of hormones and pesticide residues. Consume only small amounts of animal protein, no more than three to four ounces a day.

"The best way to have protein is in a soup. An excellent old Chinese recipe for an immune-enhancing soup combines a whole astragalus root with onions, garlic, ginger, and either free-range chicken, fish, tofu or tempeh. Some fresh green vegetables and a handful of brown rice are added to that. The soup is brought to a boil and then simmered. Some miso is added for flavor. This is highly nourishing, easy to digest, and excellent for helping a weakened individual regain strength.

"Drink plenty of pure water daily. In colder seasons, unsweetened herb tea, such as immune-supportive echinacea tea, is a very good source of liquids. Cold water is a little shocking to the digestive system for people with chronic fatigue syndrome so you want warm liquids, and plenty of them."

SUPPLEMENTS. To enhance energy further, try adding the following immune-enhancing supplements:

Multivitamin and mineral complex. This should be a good quality, hypoallergenic supplement. Be sure to get magnesium, chromium, and zinc. Many people with chronic fatigue are low in these.

Vitamin C. 5,000–10,000 mg Vitamin C should be taken throughout the day. Every two hours take 1,000–2,000 mg. Much higher doses can be taken with an intravenous vitamin C drip. This method has proven highly beneficial for overcoming chronic fatigue.

Coenzyme Q10. At least 75 mg

Acidophilus and bifidus. Take as directed by label.

Vitamin E. 400–800 units

Garlic capsules. 2 or more with meals

B complex. 100 mg 3 times per day

Vitamin B12. 100 mcg

Essential fatty acid supplement. 1–2 tbsp.

Geranium. 100 mg

HERBS. Herbs are nature's medicines. The ones listed here concentrate on building and strengthening the immune system:

> Echinacea
> Pau d'arco
> Cat's claw

Siberian ginseng
Astragalus

In addition, Perlstein reports excellent results with lomatium complex: "It is one of the best things I have found for overcoming chronic fatigue syndrome. If you were to use one herbal complex, that would be it."

EXERCISE. The little strength a person has can be improved through gentle exercise. Perlstein says, "Being outdoors is best. Try walking, even in cold weather. If you bundle up, you can do it. Getting fresh air is very, very important.

"In terms of physical disciplines, yoga and tai chi have wonderful balancing effects on the endocrine and immune systems. Some kind of physical discipline is imperative for regaining health."

MINDSET. Perlstein concludes by pointing out the strong mind/body connection for getting and overcoming chronic fatigue syndrome: "Studies show that chronic fatigue syndrome generally manifests itself in people who feel they have overwhelming life circumstances. They do not feel empowered to make positive changes in their lives. This has a damaging effect on their immune system.

"When you have chronic fatigue, you want to do your best to be optimistic. You want to be grateful for your life experiences. Try to focus on the positive. That will help to keep the body more balanced. When you do have emotional issues, try to resolve them completely. Do not repress negative emotions. Do not tell yourself that they are unimportant or inconsequential. It is very important to resolve your emotional conflicts completely.

"Creative movement is very helpful for that, dance, in particular, with beautiful music. If you feel you cannot confront an individual or a situation, at least put on music, and somehow work out the emotions with your body. Creative dance can help with this."

GETTING TO THE ROOT OF THE PROBLEM. Dr. Vesselago uses laboratory tests to diagnose his patients, and then treats them accordingly. He looks for viruses, and for excess candida, as well as for allergies, and stress: "I test the person for allergies with an IgE rast test and get back a report showing how the body responds to over 100 tested foods. We adjust the diet so that the person is no longer eating allergy-causing foods, and that alone brings about a significant improvement in over 70 percent of individuals.

"If someone collapses unduly fast, or wakes up tired, and requires several cups of coffee to get going, then I will focus on the adrenals first. I do a test for adrenal function that involves checking cortisol, which is one of the main adrenal hormones. From that, I get a picture of how well the adrenal glands are coping with stress during the day. Problems here are treated specifically with glandulars, vitamins, magnesium, and calcium. Sometimes I also have people take vitamin B12 injections to support adrenal function as well. Again, sometimes, just with adrenal treatment, people get 30 percent, 40 percent, 50 percent better inside a few weeks."

Dr. Vesselago looks at medical treatments as short-term help for making patients more comfortable and better able to function, but adds that changes must be made on a deeper level if they are to be lasting: "When we talk about wishing for the good old days, part of that wish is for a slower pace and a more humane way of life. So part of what I do is talk to people about their lives. I make them aware of how their motors are racing all the time. I encourage them to start an aerobic exercise program because rhythmic, sustained, repetitive, total body activity, supports the adrenals and dissipates much stress. Look at how you feel after you have been out for even a half hour's walk.

"I also recommend meditation. People are always racing around in heavy traffic or surrounded by phones that ring all day long. Even television has their minds racing a mile a minute. Turning inward for twenty minutes, once or twice a day with the eyes closed, allows the system to take time out.

"One technique for decreasing one's stress response is called breath awareness. A person can be aware of his or her breathing any time of day, during any activity. It really grounds one in the here and now. It brings the person's focus back to the body, and decreases stress. So there are little things that one can do just in the course of the day that make a difference."

Herbal Pharmacy

Plants containing phytochemicals with antifatigue activity, in order of potency:

Lactuca sativa (lettuce)
Cichorium endivia (endive)
Vitna mungo (black gram)
Chenopodium album (lamb's-quarters)
Raphanus sativus (radish)
Brassica pekinesis (Chinese cabbage)
Portulaca oleracea (purslane)
Avena sativa (oats)
Chrysanthemum coronarium (garland chrysanthemum)
Anethum graveolens (dill)
Taraxacum officinale (dandelion)
Amaranthus sp. (pigweed)
Cucumis sativus (cucumber)
Brassica chinensis (Chinese cabbage)
Spinacia oleracea (spinach)
Borago officinalis (borage)
Rheum rhaponticum (rhubarb)

Nasturtium officinale (berro)
Aralia cordata (udo)
Beta vulgaris (beet)

Patient Stories

JANET

After giving birth to my daughter by cesarean section, two-and-a-half years ago, I developed very bad chronic fatigue. I guess a number of factors contributed to this. I had a very long labor, I was given medication for pain, such as Demerol and morphine, and I had an epidural. I took a lot of antibiotics and, as every mother knows, I had major sleep deprivation.

When I was breast-feeding, my body was so fatigued that I didn't have enough milk to feed her. Because of that, she would wake up every hour to be fed. After a few weeks, I was so weak that I hardly had the strength to hold her to my breast. My lab work showed that I had elevated viral titres. I don't know how I got through many months of this.

Finally, I started on the vitamin C drips. I noticed a gradual change in a period of about nine months. At first, I noticed that I no longer needed to take frequent naps. Then, I noticed that I was no longer fatigued. I was able to clean the house without getting tired.

Today, my blood work shows that I have normal viral titres. I not only run after my two-and-a-half year old, but I also work. I take care of a vegetable garden, two dogs, a parrot, five chickens, and two turkeys. I feel great.

SHARON

I came down with an extraordinary flulike illness that left me completely incapacitated. Before this took place, I had been leading a very busy career life as an owner of a public relations firm and a producer of large theatrical events. Now I was lying in bed as sick as I could imagine being.

I tried everything. I went to Western clinics and had interns and infectious disease people working. I would get a little bit better and then it would reassert itself.

I was really desperate for a place to go and something to try. I finally went to the Maharishi Ayurveda Health Center in Lancaster. Within one week of treatment, I had received more help than I did from everything else that I had done up until that point.

I felt that they gave me a handle on what was happening to my body, why I was having this illness, and what I could do about it. Basically, the management of the illness was the treatment. They did not believe, nor did I, that anything exterior was going to heal my condition. It was going to involve changing my lifestyle, particularly the way my physical activity was manifesting in the world.

I live very close to the routine that they established for me during that initial week. It is why I think I am going to get over chronic fatigue syndrome. I am not entirely out of it, but I am extraordinarily better. And my ability to function as a normal human being keeps increasing all the time.

One of the primary changes I made has to do with diet. Specifically, I am eating foods that are consistent with my own body type, and cooking them in a way that makes them easy to digest. I went from a stir-fry mentality to a balance between grains and vegetables that are over-cooked. I eat in a very Indian style, I would say. I am enormously careful not to have meat, fat, milk products, without considering what time of day I am having them. In Ayurvedic fashion, I eat my main nutrients at noon. I drink a lot of water; I am careful to make sure I get at least eight glasses a day. Those, I think, are the biggest things. I try to have an evenness of routine regarding food, exercise, activity of all kind, that makes one day to the next very, very similar. Before I led a life that was extraordinarily up and down. It was deadline-oriented and involved many, many hours of work a day. Now I do not live like that. I do three or four hours of work in the morning. I slow down and take another walk and eat lunch. Then I work in the afternoon and then do the same.

All of that came from Ayurvedic medicine. I could have probably died of toxic shock from all the things that were suggested to me by combinations of internists and other American specialists. This is an all natural way of returning to health. I sent many people there. I don't believe that I would be where I am now if I had not done this.

Hot News

Recent research has thrown some light on possible underlying causes of chronic fatigue syndrome. One study found a link between acylcarnitine deficiencies and the symptoms of chronic fatigue syndrome. In another, CFS patients seemed to have a reduced antioxidant status. The parasite giardia may be an important cause of chronic fatigue, causing dysfunctional immune activation or transport of RNA viruses; therapies for giardia include grapefruit-seed extract, the herb *Artemisia annua*, and the medications quinacrine and metronidazole.

Substances that have shown promise in combating CFS include malic acid (extracted from apples); magnesium sulfate and magnesium chloride; broad-spectrum amino acid preparations; vitamins B6 and B1; high-dose immunoglobulin therapy; essential fatty acid supplementation; potassium and magnesium aspartates; evening primrose oil; licorice, which seems to increase the glucocorticol hormone activity that is deficient in patients with chronic fatigue syndrome; and an extract of the traditional Chinese medicinal herb *Astragalus membranous*, which enhances natural killer cell activity. *(See below.)*

NUTRITION AND DIET

A study evaluated 38 patients with chronic fatigue syndrome and 308 normal control patients for acylcarnitine levels in the serum found a possible link between acylcarnitine deficiencies and the symptoms of chronic fatigue syndrome. Patients with chronic fatigue syndrome who recovered from general fatigue also had an increase to normal in their acylcarnitine levels.

Hirohiko Kuratsune et al., "Acylcarnitine Deficiency in Chronic Fatigue Syndrome," *Clinical Infectious Diseases* 18, suppl. 1 (1994): S62–S67.

Leading health researchers are recommending a malic acid/magnesium hydroxide complex for the treatment of chronic fatigue syndrome. Malic acid (extracted from apples) is important in the Krebs cycle, where fats and sugar are converted to energy, and magnesium is important in the production of energy.

"A Follow-up on Malic Acid: CFID Buyers Club," *Health Watch* 3, no.1 (Spring 1993): 1–3.

Patients with chronic fatigue syndrome appear to have a reduced antioxidant status. Vitamin B6 deficiency may increase valine excretion, while zinc deficiency may cause low absorption of the branch chain amino acids and subsequent reduced output. Many chronic fatigue patients report that broad-spectrum amino acid preparations help their conditions.

K. K. Eaton and A. Hunnisett, "Abnormalities in Essential Amino Acids in Patients with Chronic Fatigue Syndrome," *Journal of Nutritional Medicine* 2 (1991): 369–75.

The authors note deficiencies of magnesium, vitamin B1, and essential fatty acids in chronic fatigue patients, and correction of these deficiencies has resulted in clinical improvement. Changes in relaxation and resting indices with myothermography have been documented in patients with magnesium deficiency, and the authors have found a good correlation between myotherapy and magnesium status in chronic fatigue patients.

J. M. Howard et al., "Magnesium and Chronic Fatigue Syndrome," *Lancet* 340 (August 15, 1992): 426.

A general review article of chronic fatigue syndrome showed benefit from therapies using intravenous Acyclovir; B12-folic acid-liver extract injections; Efamol Marine; and magnesium sulfate, given intramuscularly.

S. D. Shafran et al., "Chronic Fatigue Syndrome," *American Journal of Medicine* 90 (June 1991): 730–40.

Twenty individuals with chronic fatigue syndrome had lower red cell magnesium concentrations than did 20 matched controls. Those patients treated with magnesium chloride claimed to have improved energy levels, better emotional states, and less pain. The authors conclude that chronic fatigue syndrome patients have slightly lower magnesium levels than controls, and that magnesium therapy appeared to be of benefit.

I. M. Cox et al., "Red Blood Cell Magnesium and Chronic Fatigue Syndrome," *Lancet* 337 (March 30, 1991): 757–60.

A study of students in a rural school district in upstate New York found that circumstances that increased the risk of chronic fatigue syndrome included CFS in other family members, ingestion of raw milk, and a history of allergy. The authors conclude that a combination of environmental and host factors, including the possibility of an infectious agent, may be involved in the etiology of chronic fatigue syndrome.

K. M. Bell et al., "Risk Factors Associated with Chronic Fatigue Syndrome in a Cluster of Pediatric Cases," *Review of Infectious Disease* 13, suppl. 1 (1991): S32–S38.

A study assessing the effectiveness of intravenous immunoglobulin G in treating chronic fatigue syndrome concluded that high-dose immunoglobulin therapy is effective in a significant number of patients, with improvement in both subjective and objective immunologic parameters.

Andrew Lloyd et al., "A Double-Blind, Placebo-Controlled Trial of Intravenous Immunoglobulin Therapy in Patients with Chronic Fatigue," *American Journal of Medicine* 89 (1990) 561–68.

Sixty-three patients with postviral fatigue syndrome received a combination of linoleic, gamma-linolenic, eicosapentaenoic, and docosahexaenoic acids or a placebo in a double-blind placebo-controlled trial. At one month 74% of the patients in the treatment group as compared to 23% in the placebo group reported improvement, and at three months it was 85% and 17% respectively. The authors conclude that essential fatty acid supplementation is safe and effective for the treatment of postviral fatigue syndrome.

P. O. Behan et al., "Effect of High Doses of Essential Fatty Acids on the Postviral Fatigue Syndrome," *ACTA Neurol. Scand.* 82 (1990): 209–16.

In a survey of vitamin C intake among 411 dentists and their wives, there was a significant inverse relationship between vitamin C intake and fatigue, with the mean number of fatigue symptoms among the low vitamin C users being double that among the relatively high users of vitamin C.

E. Cheraskin et al., "Daily Vitamin C Consumption and Fatigability," *Journal of the American Geriatric Society* 24, no. 3 (1976): 136–37.

During intellectual activity, iron-deficient women demonstrated reduction in efficiency, more noticeable fatigue in the course of a working day and week, and deterioration of body functions. Repletion with iron supplements raised the work volume and improved its quality. It also improved the state of health, activity and mood.

E. A. Kuleschova and N. V. Riabova, "Effect of Iron Deficiency of the Body on the Work of Capacity of Women Engaged in Mental Work," *Ter Arkh* 61, no. 1 (1989): 92–95.

Studies have found that 75–91% of treated patients experienced pronounced relief of fatigue during treatment with aspartates, compared to 5–25% of controls. Patients usually continued treatment for 4-6 weeks; afterward fatigue frequently did not return.

A. R. Gaby, "Aspartic Acid Salts and Fatigue," *Current Therapeutic Research* (November 1982).

Fifty-six out of 66 (85%) patients receiving aspartates reported an increase in strength or physical activity over 18 months, compared to only 9% of patients on placebo.

J. Hicks, "Treatment of Fatigue in General Practice: A Double Blind Study," *Clinical Medicine* (January 1964): 85–90.

Patients with persistent tiredness believed to be unrelated to depression, when placed on potassium and magnesium aspartates daily in divided doses, had a positive therapeutic response.

P. E. Formica, "The Housewife Syndrome: Treatment with the Potassium and Magnesium Salts of Aspartic Acid," *Current Therapeutic Research* (March 1962): 98–106.

HERBS/PLANT EXTRACTS

Some of the symptoms of chronic fatigue syndrome may reflect a mild glucocortic insufficiency. One author effected an almost complete recovery from chronic fatigue syndrome with licorice, which by increasing glucocorticol hormone activity can improve the hypocorticolism in patients with chronic fatigue syndrome.

Riccardo Basechetti, "Chronic Fatigue Syndrome and Licorice," *New Zealand Medical Journal* (April 26, 1995): 157.

The results of a study suggest that the parasite giardia may be an important cause of chronic fatigue, and dysfunctional immune activation or transport of RNA viruses by the parasite may account for systemic symptoms. Therapeutic treatments for giardia include grapefruit-seed extract, the herb *Artemisia annua*, and the medications quinacrine and metronidazole.

Leo Galland et al., "Giardia Lamblia Infection as a Cause of Chronic Fatigue," *Journal of Nutritional Medicine* 1 (1990): 27–31.

In clinical trials, evening primrose oil produced a marked clinical improvement in 85% of those with chronic fatigue syndrome. The researchers note that essential fatty acids such as are found in evening primrose oil are decreased in patients with severe Epstein-Barr virus infections.

"Evening Primrose Oil Benefits CFS patients," *Better Nutrition for Today's Living* 56, no. 5 (May 1994): 12.

TRADITIONAL CHINESE MEDICINE

F3, a form of carbohydrate derived from the traditional Chinese medicinal herb *Astragalus membranous,* was shown to have a beneficial effect on chronic fatigue syndrome patients by enhancing natural killer cell activity.

D.T. Chu et al., "The Effect of F3 on Natural Killer (NK) Cell Activity in the Patients with Chronic Fatigue Syndrome (CFS)," *Proc. Annu. Meet. Am. Assoc. Cancer Res.* 35 (1994): A3074.

HOMEOPATHY

Remedies for fatigue include *gelsemium* (yellow jasmine), *kali phosphoricum*, arsenicum album, pulsatilla (wind flower), and sulphur.

Frans Vermeulen, *Concordant Materia Medica* (Haarlem, The Netherlands: Merlijn, 1994).

12. HEART DISEASE

Heart disease among women is a much greater threat than many believe; twice as many women die from heart disease than from all forms of cancer combined. A major reason for this is the loss of estrogen that accompanies menopause, as estrogen protects the cardiovascular system.

Causes

Lowered estrogen is just one of many factors that contribute to heart disease in women. "Overall, there are 247 risk factors that can damage the heart," states Dr. David Steenblock, a complementary physician from California. "A risk factor is anything that injures the inner lining of the blood vessels that supply the heart with oxygen and nutrition. Any agent that injures the inner lining of the blood vessels, such as tobacco, air pollution, food additives, high blood pressure, and gasoline fumes, can initiate atherosclerosis, the so-called hardening of the arteries. The initial injury causes hardening of the arteries. Then the accumulation of such things as cholesterol, calcium, scar tissue, and fat causes atherosclerotic lesions, which gradually go on to occlude and block the arteries to the brain and to the heart. When the arteries to the brain are blocked you have a stroke, and when you have the blockage to the heart you have a heart attack."

Dr. Michael Janson, president of the American Preventive Medical Association and author of *Vitamin Revolution in Health Care*, describes other common heart ailments, some of which are precipitated by atherosclerosis:

Angina pectoris. "Clogged arteries leave the heart muscle with inadequate oxygen. As everyone knows, muscles hurt when exercised beyond their oxygen capacity. When not enough blood flows from the coronary arteries to the heart muscle, people experience pain in the chest. Sometimes they feel pain in the jaw, the shoulder, or even the wrist. Often, they do not realize that this is referred pain coming from the heart itself."

Congestive heart failure. "Hardening of the arteries to the heart can lead to a number of other problems. When heart muscle tissue functions inefficiently, more blood comes in than is pumped out. In other words, with each beat, the amount of blood being returned to the heart is more than the heart muscle can handle. Fluid backs up, and other tissues, such as the lungs and legs, can get congested. Congestive heart failure leads to shortness of breath, water in the lungs, and swelling of the ankles."

High blood pressure. "High blood pressure can be the result of dietary habits, lack of exercise, high stress, being overweight, too much caffeine, sugar, or alcohol in the diet, and particularly, too much salt in the diet. In the past few years, some reports have said that salt does not make much of a difference for most people. The fact is, that's not true. Even a slight elevation in blood pressure is enough to increase the risk of heart disease."

Symptoms

Heart disease is a gradual process that takes years to develop into a serious condition. At first there are no warning signs. If the coronary arteries become severely blocked, a person might experience shortness of breath or chest pains (angina pectoris) that are relieved by rest.

Clinical Experience

CONVENTIONAL TREATMENTS

HIGH-BLOOD-PRESSURE MEDICATIONS. Dr. Janson believes the general public is being misled into believing that high-blood-pressure medications are safe and always necessary: "We all hear advertisements on the radio telling us to stay on these medications for life. They say that no symptoms tell you whether or not your blood pressure is high. Therefore, if you are taking medication for your high blood pressure, you must stay on your medication and never, ever stop. That so-called public service announcement is really a sales pitch from the drug companies that make the medications. We know these medications actually cause more heart disease, and that they create side effects, in addition to the high blood pressure."

Dr. Steenblock warns, however, that patients who depend on medication to control high blood pressure should not self-discontinue: "Many people have this idea that since the doctor is not getting at the cause of their high blood pressure, it is somewhat illogical for them to take their blood pressure medicine. True, doctors often do not have the answer. Still, if you fail to take your medicine and your blood pressure gets out of control, you can develop heart disease and go on to have a stroke."

The solution here is to work with a complementary medical physician until heart health is restored. In some cases, medication may be needed long-term, even for a lifetime. But everyone can only better their situation by improving lifestyle and diet. The following sections can serve as guidelines:

RISK ASSESSMENT. Diagnosis is an important first step. Before beginning a program, a doctor should take the following factors into account: family history, blood pressure, cholesterol level, weight, and stress EKG tests. Following a risk assessment, a cardiovascular health program should be followed.

DIET. The power of the vegetarian diet in a cardiovascular health program was recognized in Dr. Dean Ornish's now-famous study, which placed heart patients on a protocol of healthy vegetarian foods, daily aerobic exercise, and relaxation. At the end of a year, his program showed that heart disease could be stopped and even reversed.

Dr. Paul Cutler, a complementary physician from Niagara Falls, New York, says, "Medicine in general owes Ornish a great deal of gratitude. He showed that a drastic reduction of fats was most important. I believe that the total dietary fats should be well below the typical average of 40 percent. Modern nutritionists are saying 30 percent. I try to get fat content down to 10 percent of the total calories. I see improvement in angina just by reducing the fats to that degree."

While the dangers of saturated fats to heart health are well known, Dr. Ray Peat, a distinguished scientific researcher residing in Eugene, Oregon, says unsaturated fats can be just as damaging: "Many people have been soaking their bodies in unsaturated vegetable oil diets for years. As a result, every time they get hungry or face stress, their blood sugar falls, their adrenaline rises, and these unsaturated fats are drawn out of storage. Once released, they immediately start poisoning the lining of the blood vessels and all the cell energy producing systems. In 1960, this effect was demonstrated by a group in England who saw that adrenaline, either natural or synthetic, caused damage to the circulatory system. It turns out that this occurs after unsaturated fats become mobilized. They hit the lining of the blood vessels, where they cause lipid peroxidative damage."

Dr. Janson adds that people should avoid foods such as sugar, salt, white flour, white rice, and particularly any shortening or hydrogenated vegetable oils found in products like margarine and Crisco: "Whenever you see vegetable shortening, hydrogenated vegetable oil, or partially hydrogenated vegetable oil on a label, it is important to avoid that product. These are not foods. In fact, I consider margarine to be an industrial waste product that is fashioned to resemble food."

He recommends a low-fat, whole foods diet that is mostly, if not completely, vegetarian: "Mostly, the diet should be high in complex carbohydrates, including whole grains, beans, vegetables, and fruits. Remember, flavonoids, which are plant pigments, are present in fruits and vegetables and in some beans and grains. These are very protective, and most of them are not available as supplements.

"I think the diet should be largely vegetarian, although a number of studies show that fish in the diet also reduces levels of heart disease and cancer. Fish may or may not be the reason for this. It may be that eating more fish means eating less chicken and meat. Cutting those foods out of the diet help cut down on heart disease."

EXERCISE. "Aerobic exercise and an improved diet should go hand-in-hand," notes Dr. Cutler. "Aerobics help the good cholesterol go up significantly, which in turn helps remove cholesterol from arterial walls after the cells are through with them so they are less likely to form plaque." Exercising aerobically means getting the heart rate up three or four times a week. A doctor can help determine how much exercise is needed.

Dr. Janson adds that people should stretch before and after an aerobic workout: "The stretching has another benefit in that it relaxes the body, and keeps people limber and more flexible. That makes it easier to continue an aerobic exercise program."

SUPPLEMENTS
Supplements provide wonderful support for the heart and sometimes help eliminate or reduce required dosages of medication. These are nutrients to know about:

ANTIOXIDANTS. These help prevent the heart from free radical damage, also known as oxidation. Antioxidant nutrients include vitamin E, beta carotene, vitamin C, and selenium. Free radicals damage the lining tissues of arteries, which leads to atherosclerosis and plaque deposits. Antioxidants, particularly vitamin C, can prevent this from happening by protecting the lining of the arteries. Vitamin E has several functions. Aside from being a protective antioxidant, it also reduces the stickiness of platelets, little blood fragments that initiate blood clots. This effect is helped by the addition of essential fatty acids and garlic. Minimizing free radical damage and keeping platelets from clogging up the arteries gives arteries a chance to heal and recover. There is more room for oxygen to flow through the arteries to reach tissues.

L-ARGININE. This amino acid has been receiving well-deserved attention in the medical literature for its ability to produce nitric oxide. Nitric oxide benefits the arterial walls in several ways. It helps the smooth muscles in the arterial walls to relax, thereby promoting an antiangina, antihypertensive, and antistress effect.

Additionally, research shows that L-arginine reduces the activation of platelets, the white cells that can initiate arterial spasm and plaque development. Other studies show L-arginine to slow down plaque development, and even reverse small amounts of plaque buildup. "I've seen it work," says Dr. Cutler. "Taking two to three grams of L-arginine per day has quite a marked antianginal effect. L-arginine now is a must in my protocol for nutrients. Usually I will start with about 1,000 mg per day, and raise the levels if that amount isn't helping."

L-CARNITINE. The heart muscle needs to burn fat for energy, and L-carnitine allows this to happen. Dr. Janson explains, "L-carnitine gets fat into the little engines inside the cells called mitochondria. These little mitochondrial engines are where fat is burned for energy. Your heart muscle needs to burn fat for energy, and the only way it can get the fat into that little engine is with the amino acid L-carnitine. At the same time, that inner mitochondrial membrane requires another nutrient to burn the fat, coenzyme Q10." Dr. Janson recommends people take 500 mg L-carnitine two to three times a day.

COENZYME Q10. This nutrient is for anyone with heart problems or who wants to prevent getting them. Along with L-carnitine, it helps prevent angina and protects the heart muscle by letting it burn fat for energy more easily. It also improves heart health by reducing blood pressure and arrhythmias of the heart. As an antioxidant, it prevents damage to the blood vessels that leads to hardening of the arteries. Therapeutic levels are between 50–150 mg for mild heart disease. More severe heart disease may respond to 200 mg.

MAGNESIUM. This mineral increases blood flow by allowing muscles in the arterial wall to relax. Usually 500–1,000 mg is needed.

NIACIN (VITAMIN B3). A fifteen-year study on the effects of niacin, published by the American Heart Association in the mid-1980s, connected use of niacin to a significant reduction in heart attacks and death from heart disease. Long-term niacin has also been associated with decreased rates in cancer. Niacin should be taken under medical supervision, as it can affect liver function. Dr. Janson adds, "Other B vitamins, such as folic acid and B12, can help to lower levels of homocystine in the blood, a risk factor for heart disease."

TAURINE. This amino acid is another important antioxidant that helps prevent atherosclerosis. Additionally, it can avert heart failure by improving strength of contraction. That improves the outflow of blood from the heart and reduces congestive heart failure. Generally, 500 mg are taken twice a day.

THYROID SUPPLEMENTS. Thyroid supplementation may normalize high cholesterol, according to Dr. Ray Peat, a scientific researcher from Eugene, Oregon: "High cholesterol indicates a thyroid hormone deficiency. A clear demonstration of this was seen in the 1930s in patients who had their thyroid glands surgically removed. After the operation, cholesterol levels became abnormally high, but they returned to normal with thyroid supplementation." He adds that thyroid extract is also linked to fewer heart attacks: "One of the foremost American researchers in the field, Brota Barnes, wrote *Solved: The Riddle of Heart Attacks* after finding that patients in one group had far fewer heart attacks than patients in another group. All the low-heart-attack group did differently was take thyroid when they needed it."

HERBS

Bugleweed. This is a remedy for heart palpitations and elevated blood pressure. It may also alleviate anxiety, since an elevated blood pressure is associated with a frequent fast pulse, anxiety, and agitation.

Cayenne. Capsicum, the active ingredient in cayenne, helps the heart in many ways. It stimulates circulatory function, lowers cholesterol, reduces blood pressure, and lessens the chance of heart attacks and strokes. By decreasing blood levels of fibrin, it also reduces the risk of blood clot formation that cause heart attacks and strokes.

Garlic. Among its many benefits, garlic helps lower blood pressure and decrease cholesterol and, when combined with vitamin E, lessens the frequency of blood clots in arterial walls. That helps to prevent heart attacks and strokes. Five hundred mg or more of deodorized garlic can be taken twice a day.

Biloba. Ginkgo helps improve small blood vessel circulation.

Hawthorn berry. Hawthorn is an overall heart tonic that works against arrhythmia, angina, blood pressure, and hardening of the arteries. It aids circulation, as well as ameliorating valvular insufficiency and an irregular pulse. Hawthorn berry can also correct acid conditions of the blood, and can be safely taken every day.

Mistletoe. Mistletoe is a cardiac tonic that stimulates circulation. Fifteen drops taken three times a day, or three cups of tea daily, help lower blood pressure and alleviate heart strain. Mistletoe should not be overused, nor should the berries be eaten.

Motherwort. Helps stabilize the electrical rhythm of the heart. The amount taken should be monitored by a doctor.

Wild yam. Stimulates production of DHEA. Low levels of this hormone have been related to higher incidences of heart disease. Wild yam can provide added protection and is completely safe.

Other herbs to consider include barberry, black cohosh, and butcher's broom.

CHELATION THERAPY

Dr. Steenblock describes the treatment: "Chelation is a therapy using an IV and a material called EDTA, which is basically a fancy vinegar molecule. It is put into a bottle that is hung up about two to three feet above the person's head. The person sits in an easy chair, and this material drips into a vein over a three-hour period. This modified vinegar molecule goes into the blood and circulates around the fluid spaces around all the cells of the body, cleaning all the tissue. Basically, it does a housecleaning, removing all the heavy metals, such as lead, uranium, and nickel. EDTA binds with calcium that has deposited in artery walls and is excreted from the body through the kidneys. In addition, it breaks down scar tissue and allows the arteries to become softer. In other words, it takes the *hard* out of hardening of the arteries."

When deciding whether or not to administer chelation therapy, Dr. Cutler tests patients for heavy metal buildup. "I look for elevated iron and copper levels in the blood. I also measure something called the serum ferritin, which reflects artery tissue levels of iron. If I start chelation, as the iron levels come down in the blood, there are also clinical improvements in angina and exercise tests. And there are angiogram and treadmill test improvements as well.

If I do not find any abnormality in these metals, I do what is called a challenge, which means I give one chelation treatment, collect urine for twenty-four hours afterward, and observe the metals that come out. Based on these results, I will make a decision as to whether I want to chelate the person."

Dr. Steenblock, who has administered chelation therapy for almost twenty years, uses the treatment more extensively. He explains why it so valuable to most individuals: "In their forties, most people develop some degree of atherosclerosis. This hardening of the arteries is due to cholesterol, scar tissue, fat, and calcium, which accumulate in the artery walls.

"You have to try to prevent all these risk factors by keeping your diet low in fat and cholesterol, by exercising, thinking properly, avoiding chemicals, and taking antioxidants to protect the inner lining of blood vessels. In addition, you can break down the scar tissue and remove calcium by the use of chelation.

"Studies show that if you start chelating in your forties you can actually reverse all the atherosclerosis as soon as it starts to develop. If you have done things that have not been perfect in your life–you haven't eaten right, you have been under too much stress, you smoked—by the time you are forty, you will have some degree of atherosclerosis. What I am saying is that chelation can reverse this process and keep those arteries more pristine.

"By the time you are sixty, the amount of calcium that has been deposited in your arteries is ten times more than what you had in your arteries at ten years of age. A man by the name of Al Fleckenstein, a leading doctor in cardiovascular drug research, stated in one of his books that the amount of calcium present in the walls of the arteries is the single most important risk factor for the development of atherosclerosis. In other words, as calcium accumulates in the walls of the arteries, it actually propagates the development of atherosclerosis. Atherosclerosis develops just because you are gradually accumulating this calcium. If you can remove the calcium somewhere between forty and sixty, you can change that ratio, reverse the whole process, and put off the development of atherosclerosis for a number of years. That's for prevention.

"Of course, if you have outright disease, you can be helped as well. I have been doing chelation since 1977, so I have treated thousands of patients, and most do not come for prevention. They come for treatment of disease. They come in with angina or claudication. With chelation, most of the time, these types of symptoms disappear. If they do not, it is usually because the person has got advanced disease and needs more than the standard thirty treatments. When people come in with advanced disease, who are seventy-five or eighty years old, I tell them that they need to start out with thirty treatments, that's one treatment twice or three times a week. They wait a month or two, and then come back and do another thirty. This process continues until we clean out these arteries because it takes time to reverse all of the terribly occluded blocked arteries that develop over many, many years of bad living." *(See also "Chelation Therapy" in chapter 1, Aging.)*

STRESS MANAGEMENT

Stress contributes to heart disease by increasing free radical damage to tissues and increasing spasms in the arterial walls. Some ways to overcome stress include exercise, deep breathing, visualization, tai chi, yoga, meditation, *qi gong*, mantras, massage, Reiki, biofeedback, and aromatherapy. An essential oil blend of ylang ylang, lavender or peppermint, and marjoram, added to oil and applied during massage, helps calm the system and may even lower blood pressure.

TREATMENT OF H. PYLORI

Dr. Paul Cutler says that recent research links the *H. pylori* bacteria to high incidences of heart attacks and strokes. Dr. Cutler explains the connection: "*H. pylori* causes ulcers and chronic gastritis. Most of us practitioners are well aware of the higher incidence of stomach complaints in our patients with heart disease. Apparently, this little bacteria, which comes in from contaminated foods, burrows its way into the stomach wall. In its attempt to fight off the body's defenses, it produces toxins that initiate plaque development and thickening of the blood. This points to a strong correlation between stomach ulcer disease and coronary artery disease."

Fortunately, this problem is simple to cure, says Dr. Cutler. "You can use one particular type of honey that is high in hydrogen peroxide, or cider vinegar, bismuth, and extracts from licorice. Or you can take a one-week course of three antibiotics to kill this bacteria, probably 97 percent of the time. It is very gratifying, as a physician, to see not only stomach symptoms but angina improve, and sometimes dramatically, with the treatment of this common bacterial parasite." *(See also chapter 20, Parasites.)*

PSYCHOLOGICAL, SOCIAL, AND SPIRITUAL FACTORS

Most healing programs focus on physical modalities. We look at diet, exercise, supplements, and substances to avoid. More and more, people are beginning to understand that more subtle factors have a powerful influence as well. Dr. Ron Scolastico, spiritual counselor and author of *Healing the Heart, Healing the Body,* believes that the process of remaining healthy involves four important elements: "The first element is our physical life, which most people know a great deal about. The second element looks at our mental life. It is becoming clearer and clearer that our thoughts promote or hinder health, and in some cases actually cause disease. The third element addresses our emotional lives. Feelings, particularly love, have a profound effect. The fourth element addresses spiritual factors. I believe those energies come from our soul, which is an incredible source of power, love, and wisdom, inside each of us."

Dr. Scolastico says that we need to draw upon each of these factors as needed. Sometimes we must take physical steps, such as seeing a doctor and taking medications or herbs, but sometimes that is not enough: "For example, one of my clients developed congestive heart failure after a painful divorce, along with pericarditis, which is an inflammation of the membrane surrounding the heart. She failed to respond to medical treatment, and her condition began to worsen. As I worked with her, she realized that she had lost touch with her soul. The divorce had wreaked such havoc in her emotional life that she could no longer feel love.

"Every day, for six months, she took an hour to connect with her soul. By doing this, she was able to regain a feeling of deep love for her body and herself. Today, she is symptom-free, and believes that without inner work, she might be dead. So many times, we need not only physical treatment but mental, emotional, or spiritual work to augment that process."

To promote health at every level, Dr. Scolastico advises the following:
Connect with your spiritual nature. Religious or not, we need to accept the existence of some benevolent, healing force larger than our personality and physical being. Once we realize we are never alone or abandoned, amazing changes can happen.

Be mindful of your thoughts. We all have negative thoughts, but this alone does
not cause illness. Swallowing them down and engaging them does. We must
learn to release negative ideas. This work takes time, and we should not be
hard on ourselves when our thoughts are less than perfect.

Follow physical principles of health. Living in a healthy way includes eating the
right foods, exercising, getting enough rest, play, and social activity. Giving
to others has a beneficial impact on health.

Create love in your life every day. This is perhaps most important of all. Research
shows that love impacts every aspect of our being, including the physical.
When we feel love, all body systems work better. The endocrine system produces beneficial hormones. Muscles relax, so that the flow of oxygen to the
cells increases. Immune system function is enhanced.

When we are filled with self-love, our health is strongest and our lives improve
all around. Recent studies show that teaching self-esteem improves academics,
as well as promoting emotional stability and greater health.

"A powerful way to enhance self-love," advises Dr. Scolastico, "is to notice
when you are creating negative thoughts and feelings about yourself. Then consciously create an experience of love for yourself right at that moment, using the
power of the word to augment the process. You can say, 'I just noticed I'm creating these negative thoughts and feelings about myself. I now choose to use my
imagination, my creativity, and my will to create an inner experience of love for
myself right now in this minute.'"

Another way to build love into our lives is to set aside time each day for building loving energy. Dr. Scolastico says, "For at least five minutes, use your mind,
open your heart, and create love in your feelings. You can do that by imagining
a person you love. Let your feelings for that person fill you as you bring that loved
one fully into your thoughts and feelings. Let the corners of your mouth lift up
in a smile. Just let your heart swell with love. You won't need a scientific test to
prove the benefits."

Equal in importance to self-love is the love we share with others. Connect-
ing with family, friends, and community gives us a sense of belonging that is
invaluable to our well-being. Recently, a link between social bonds and heart
health was reported in *Natural Health*. The magazine summarized thirty years
of research on the town of Rosetto, Pennsylvania, and concluded that the most
important risk factor for heart disease is a lack of community and intimate relationships. In this town, people lived in three-generation households, with grand-
parents, parents, and children. There was a lot of interaction among families and
much participation in community organizations. The incidence of heart disease
was virtually nil, even though residents ate high-fat diets and did not go out of
their way to exercise. In fact, there was less coronary heart disease in Rosetto
than in any other population in the United States.

Herbal Pharmacy

Plants containing phytochemicals with antihypertensive properties, in order of potency:

Viola tricolor hortensis (pansy)
Sophora japonica (Japanese pagoda tree), bud/flower
Oenothera biennis (evening primrose)
Lactuca sativa (lettuce)
Cichorium endivia (endive)
Vigna mungo (black gram)
Chenopodium album (lamb's-quarters)
Raphanus sativus (radish)
Portulaca oleracea (purslane)
Brassica pekinensis (Chinese cabbage)
Avena sativa (oats)
Amaranthus sp. (pigweed)
Chrysanthemum coronarium (garland chrysanthemum)
Anethum graveolens (dill)
Taraxacum officinale (dandelion)
Spinacia oleracea (spinach)
Cucumis sativus (cucumber)
Brassica chinensis (Chinese cabbage)
Allium cepa (onion)

Plants containing phytochemicals with antiarteriosclerotic properties, in order of potency:

Cucumis melo (cantaloupe), cotyledon
Juglans regia (English walnut)
Persea americana (avocado)
Cucumis sativus (cucumber)
Carthamus tinctorius (safflower)
Prunus armeniaca (apricot)
Papaver bracteatum (great scarlet poppy)
Helianthus annuus (sunflower)
Juglans cinerea (butternut)
Lagenaria siceraria (calabash gourd)
Bertholletia excelsa (Brazil nut)
Papaver somniferum (opium poppy)
Sesamum indicum (sesame)
Pinus edulis (pinyon pine)
Cannabis sativa (marijuana)
Cucumis melo (cantaloupe), seed

Cucurbita foetidissima (buffalo gourd)
Nigella sativa (black cumin)
Oenothera biennis (evening primrose)
Pinus gerardiana (chilgoza pine)

Plants containing phytochemicals with anticardiospasmic properties, in order of potency:

Theobroma bicolor (Nicaraguan cacao)
Cimicifuga racemosa (black cohosh)
Spirulina pratensis (spirulina)
Gentiana lutea (yellow gentian)
Ephedra sinica (ma huang)
Phaseolus vulgaris (black bean)
Vigna unguiculata (cowpea)
Aegle marmelos (bael de India)
Asparagus officinalis (asparagus)
Theombroma speciosum (macambo)
Helianthus annuus (sunflower)
Capsella bursa-pastoris (shepherd's purse)
Abelmoschus esculentus (okra)
Malva sylvestris (high mallow)
Agathosma betulina (buchu)
Sonchus oleraceus (cerraja)
Nasturtium officinale (berro)
Durio zibethinus (durian)
Arachis hypogaea (peanut)

Plants containing phytochemicals with antiarrhythmic properties, in order of potency:

Lactuca sativa (lettuce)
Portulaca oleracea (purslane)
Coptis chinensis (Chinese goldthread)
Cichorium endivia (endive)
Avena sativa (oats)
Vigna mungo (black gram)
Raphanus sativus (radish)
Chenopodium album (lamb's-quarters)
Brassica pekinensis (Chinese cabbage)
Anethum graveolens (dill)
Amaranthus sp. (pigweed)
Spinacia oleracea (spinach)
Cucumis sativus (cucumber)
Coptis japonica (huang lia)
Chrysanthemum coronarium (garland chrysanthemum)
Taraxacum officinale (dandelion)

Phaseolus vulgaris (black bean)
Strophathus gratus (quabain)
Brassica chinensis (Chinese cabbage)
Plants containing phytochemicals with antianginal properties, in order of potency:
Catharanthus lanceus (lanceleaf periwinkle)
Carya glabra (pignut hickory)
Carya ovata (shagbark hickory)
Chondrus crispus (Irish moss)
Portulaca oleracea (purslane)
Phaseolus vulgaris (black bean)
Papaver somniferum (opium poppy)
Avena sativa (oats)
Vigna unguiculata (cowpea)
Spinacia oleracea (spinach)
Tephrosia purpurea (purple tephrosia)
Ammi visnaga (visnaga)
Trichosanthus anguina (snakegourd)
Glycyrrhiza glabra (licorice)
Prunus serotina (black cherry)
Nyssa sylvatica (black gum)
Juniperus virginiana (red cedar)
Rhizophora mangle (red mangrove)
Symphoricarpos orbiculatus (buckbush)
Plants containing phytochemicals with anti-ischaemic properties, in order of potency:
Portulaca oleracea (purslane)
Ipomoea aquatica (swamp cabbage)
Panicum maximum (guinea grass)
Viola tricolor hortensis (pansy)
Moringa oleifera (ben nut)
Asparagus officinalis (asparagus)
Elaeagnus angustifolia (Russian olive)
Frangula alnus (buckthorn)
Ipomoea batatas (sweet potato leaf)
Bertholletia excelsa (Brazil nut)
Ribes uva-crispa (gooseberry)
Linum usitatissimum (flax)
Fagopyrum esculentum (buckwheat)
Ipomoea batatas (sweet potato root)
Capsicum annuum (bell pepper)
Capsicum frutescens (cayenne)
Pisum sativum (pea)
Lens culinaris (lentil)

Plant containing anti-infarctal phytochemicals:
   Jateorhiza palmata (calumba), root

Patient Stories

SYLVIA

An ultrasound test disclosed that my carotid arteries were 95 percent closed. I didn't want an operation, and while sitting in the doctor's waiting room, I discovered an alternative. While waiting to be examined, I overheard patients discussing chelation therapy.

After twenty-eight chelation treatments, my carotid arteries are only 70 percent closed. I plan to continue with this therapy. It has made a difference in my life. I also have osteoporosis. Since the chelation, I can walk more freely and without too much pain.

KAREN

I was looking for stress management because I have a pretty stressful job. When I was down in Port Jefferson, I saw a sign that read "Long Island Reflexology." I took the number and made an appointment to see Gerri Brill. That was three years ago. Since then, I've been diagnosed with moderate hypertension.

One evening, just out of the blue, I decided to take my pressure before I had a session, and then afterward. I found that whereas before the session, my pressure was 150/100, it fell afterward to 120/80, which is the ideal number. This convinced me that reflexology had some of the health benefits that I read about.

I find reflexology immensely energizing and relaxing, and go for a session every two weeks. It's an hour and a half of complete relaxation. You're away in a different place, and when you come back, you feel more energized and able to do your normal routine.

Hot News

Among the substances studies have shown to lower blood pressure are magnesium, fish oil, eicosapentaenoic acid (manufactured from sardine oil), beta carotene, vitamin C, and L-dopa. Rhubarb, garlic, cucumber vine, hawthorn, *Crataegus pinnatifida*, and ginkgo are heart-protective plants; berberine has proven to help regulate the heartbeat. Patients given gugulipid supplements showed a significant drop in total cholesterol. Ajoene, derived from garlic, and gingerol, derived from ginger root, inhibit clotting. Other, less concrete treatment modalities effective in fighting hypertension and heart disease include acupuncture, reflexology, and biofeedback. *(See below.)*

NUTRITION/DIET

Results of a placebo-controlled study found that mild to moderate hypertensive patients given daily doses of 365 mg of magnesium 3 times a day over an 8-week period experienced significant decreases in blood pressure.

M. P. Wirell et al., "Nutritional Dose of Magnesium in Hypertensive Patients on Beta Blockers Lowers Systolic Blood Pressure: A Double Blind Cross-Over Study," *Journal of Internal Medicine* 236, 1994): 189–195.

A review article notes that significant declines in systolic and diastolic blood pressure have been achieved through supplementation with 15 g of fish oil daily.

H. R. Knapp, "Fatty Acids and Hypertension," *World Review of Nutrition and Diet* 76 (1994): 9–14.

A study examined the effects of fish consumption on plasma fatty acid levels in coronary heart disease patients with a history of at least one acute myocardial infarction. Results showed that the fish diet significantly decreased stearic fatty acid after 4 weeks of fish consumption. Significant increases were seen in linoleic acid levels. Such findings lead the authors to conclude that the consumption of fish might provide benefits for coronary heart disease patients.

M. J. Santos et al., "Influence of Dietary Supplementation with Fish on Plasma Fatty Acid Composition in Coronary Heart Disease Patients," *Annals of Nutrit. Metab.* 39, no. 1 (1995): 52–62.

Thirty-one placebo-controlled studies on the role of fish oil in blood pressure were analyzed, and the oil was found to have a significant blood-pressure-lowering effect.

Martha Clare Morris et al., "Does Fish Oil Lower Blood Pressure? A Meta-Analysis of Controlled Trials," *Circulation* 88, no. 2 (August 1993): 523–33.

Results of a study showed that eicosapentaenoic acid, manufactured from sardine oil, has value in improving cardiovascular health.

Y. Tamura et al., "Clinical and Epidemiological Studies of Eicosapentaenoic Acid in Japan," *Prog. Lipid. Research.* 25 (1986): 461–66.

Daily oral doses of 6 g of L-carnitine given to ischemic heart disease patients in three divided doses had an antiarrhythmic effect.

V. Palalzzuoli et al., [The Evaluation of the Antiarrhythmic Activity of L-carnitine and Propafenone in Ischemic Cardiopathy], *Clin. Ther.* 142, no. 2 (February 1993): 155–59.

A review article notes that studies show carnitine has positive effects on various cardiovascular disorders. Carnitine supplementation can reverse cardiomyopathy in carnitine-deficient patients. Both animal and human studies suggest carnitine might have a role in the management of acute and chronic ischemic syndromes.

C. J. Pepine, "The Therapeutic Potential of Carnitine in Cardiovascular Disorders," *Clin. Ther.* 13, no. 1 (January–February): 2–21.

A study gave coenzyme Q10 to 6 untreated and 10 treated hypertensive patients. Results showed that 14 out of the 16 experienced significant reductions in systolic pressure, 11 out of 16 experienced significant reductions in diastolic pressure, and 9 out of the 10 treated patients experienced reductions of elevated pressures to a normal range.

K. Folkers et al., "Bioenergetics in Clinical Medicine, XVI: Reduction of Hypertension in Patients by Therapy with Coenzyme Q10," *Res. Commun. Chem. Pathol. Pharmacol.* 31, no. 1 (January 1981): 129–40.

Giving 100 mg of coenzyme Q10 daily to patients with advanced heart failure resulted in 67 percent of the patients experiencing improvement following the treatment.

S. A. Mortensen et al., "Long-term Coenzyme Q10 Therapy: A Major Advance in the Management of Resistant Myocardial Failure," *Drugs Exp. Clin. Res.* 11, no. 8 (1985): 581–93.

In a double-blind crossover study, chronic myocardial disease patients were given coenzyme Q10, which proved effective in treating their condition.

P. H. Langsjoen et al., "Effective Treatment with Coenzyme Q10 of Patients with Chronic Myocardial Disease," *Drugs Exp. Clin. Res.* 11, no. 8 (1985): 577–79.

In a placebo-controlled study, 100 mg/day of coenzyme Q10 were given to hypertension patients taken off all medications. Results showed that after a 2-week washout period and 10 weeks of supplementation with coenzyme Q10, there was an approximate 10-point drop in systolic blood pressure and a 7-point drop in diastolic pressure. Such findings were significant relative to controls, leading the authors to suggest that coenzyme Q10 may be a promising treatment for patients with hypertension.

V. Digiesi et al., "Effect of Coenzyme Q10 on Essential Arterial Hypertension," *Current Therapeutic Research* 47, no. 5 (May 1990): 841–45.

A study measured the levels of alpha-tocopherol and beta carotene concentration in adipose tissue samples taken from acute myocardial infarction patients, and compared them to controls. Results showed there to be no correlation between low alpha-tocopherol concentrations and myocardial infarction. However, results did suggest that myocardial infarction risk is reduced by high beta carotene concentrations.

A. F. Kardinaal et al., "Antioxidants in Adipose Tissue and Risk of Myocardial Infarction: The EURAMIC Study," *Lancet* 342 (December 4, 1993): 1379–84.

Results of a study support previous findings that deficiencies in plasma vitamin C, as well as cholesterol-standardized vitamin E, are associated with an increased risk of ischemic heart disease in Westernized countries.

K. F. Gey et al., "Relationship of Plasma Level of Vitamin C to Mortality from Ischemic Heart Disease," *Annals of the New York Academy of Sciences* 498 (1987): 110–23.

Vitamin C seems to help keep blood pressure down. A significant inverse relationship between systolic and diastolic blood pressure and plasma concentrations of vitamin C was found in healthy volunteers eating normal diets.

J. P. Moran et al., "Plasma Ascorbic Acid Concentrations Related Inversely to Blood Pressure in Human Subjects," *American Journal Clinical Nutrition* 57 (1993): 213–17.

A study examined the effects of vitamin B1 and nicotinamide on ischemic heart damage. Results showed that a single administration of thiamine and repeated nicotinamide administration produced cell-protective effects.

A. B. Shneider, [Anti-Ischemic Heart Protection Using Thiamine and Nicotinamide], *Patol. Fiziol. Eksp. Ter.* 1 (January–February 1991): 9–10.

Vitamin C levels were significantly lower in subjects with high blood pressure relative to controls.

W. Y. Tse et al., "Antioxidant Status in Controlled and Uncontrolled Hypertension and Its Relationship to Endothelial Damage," *Journal of Human Hypertension*, 8 (1994): 843–49.

Studies have shown that supplementation with 1 to 2 g of calcium is beneficial in lowering blood pressure.

Pavel Hamet et al., "The Evaluation of the Scientific Evidence for a Relationship between Calcium and Blood Pressure," *Journal of Nutrition* 125 (1995): 311S–400S.

A review article on blood pressure and dietary protein notes that data suggest the severity of hypertension and cerebrovascular disease can be reduced by adequate dietary protein intake coupled by a reduction in sodium intake, while patients suffering from renal vascular disease may benefit from a diet lower in protein.

W. M. Lovenberg and Yukio Yamori, "The Role of Dietary Protein in Hypertensive Disease," *Hypertension Pathophysiology, Diagnosis and Management*, 2nd ed. (New York, 1995).

Women between 18 and 28 years old were given 1,000 mg of calcium carbonate per day for 20 weeks. Results showed a significant inverse association between intake of dietary calcium and blood pressure.

K. B. Knight and R. E. Keith, "Calcium Supplementation on Normotensive and Hypertensive Pregnant Women," *American Journal of Clinical Nutrition* 55 (1992): 891–95.

In this study, 250 mg of L-dopa was orally administered to hypertension patients. Results: The L-dopa significantly reduced blood pressure relative to controls.

Ikuno Saito et al., "Effect of L-Dopa in Young Patients with Hypertension," *Angiology—The Journal of Vascular Disease* (September 1991): 691–95.

Results of a study showed that hypertensives were able to reduce their dependence on antihypertensive drugs through reductions of weight, dietary salt, and alcohol.

R. Stamier et al., "Nutritional Therapy for High Blood Pressure: Final Report of a Four-Year Randomized Controlled Trial—The Hypertension Control Program," *JAMA* 257, no. 11 (March 20, 1987): 1484–91.

A placebo-controlled study examined the effects of supplementation with 100 mcg/day of selenium for 6–8 weeks during late pregnancy in women at risk for pregnancy-induced hypertension. The treatment did prevent and decrease the incidence of gestational edema and pregnancy-induced hypertension relative to controls.

L. Han and S. M. Zhou, "Selenium Supplement in the Prevention of Pregnancy Induced Hypertension," *Chinese Medical Journal* 107, no. 11 (November 1994): 870–71.

An extensive review article on the link between diet and disease concludes that diet is a strong factor in the control of atheroscelorsis relating to general vascular disease, coronary heart disease, stroke, and hyperinsulinemia, hyperlipidemia, and hypertension as well.

R. W. Hubbar et al., "The Potential of Diet to Alter Disease Processes," *Nutrition Research* 14, no. 12 (1994): 1853–95.

HERBS/PLANT EXTRACTS

Analysis of eight trials on the effects of 600–900 mg per day of dried garlic powder administered for 12 weeks found that the garlic was of benefit to some patients with hypertension.

C. A. Silagy and A. W. Neil, "A Meta-Analysis of the Effect of Garlic on Blood Pressure," *Journal of Hypertension* 12 (1994): 463–68.

A garlic preparation was shown effective in lowering blood pressure.

F. G. McMahon and R. Vargas, "Can Garlic Lower Blood Pressure? A Pilot Study," *Pharmacotherapy* 13, no. 4 (July–August 1993): 406–7.

Ajoene, a garlic compound, may be useful in the acute prevention of thrombus formation induced by vascular damage.

R. Apitz-Castro et al., "Effect of Ajoene, the Major Antiplatelet Compound from Garlic, on Platelet Thrombus Formation," *Thrombosis Research* 68 (1992): 145–55.

Terminalia arjuna helps reduce risk factors for coronary heart disease.

S. Dwivedi et al., "Effect of *Terminalia Arjuna* on Ischaemic Heart Disease," *Alternative Medicine* 3, no. 2 (1989): 115–22.

A double-blind, placebo-controlled study gave 500 mg of *Terminalia arjuna* every 8 hours for 2 weeks to patients with refractory chronic congestive heart failure. Results showed patients benefited from the treatment relative to controls.

A. Bharani et al., "Salutary Effect of *Terminalia Arjuna* in Patients with Severe Refractory Heart Failure," *International Journal of Cardiology* 49, no. 3 (May 1995): 191–99.

Abana was shown effective in reducing both diastolic and systolic blood pressure in a double-blind study.

V. N. Dadkar et al., "Double Blind Comparative Trial of Abana and Methyldopa for Monotherapy of Hypertension in Indian Patients," *Japanese Heart Journal* 31, no. 2 (March 1990): 193–99.

A double-blind, placebo-controlled study examined the effects of 8 weeks of Abana supplementation on patients with ischemic heart disease and on ischemic heart disease patients with hypertension. Results showed that Abana causes a significant reduction in the severity and frequency of anginal episodes, significant improvements in ventricular function, and significant blood-pressure reduction.

J. A. Antani et al., "Effect of Abana on Ventricular Function in Ischemic Heart Disease," *Japanese Heart Journal* 31, no. 6 (November 1990): 829–35.

Cucumber vine may be a safe and effective treatment for hypertension.

G. L. Lu et al., [Clinical and Experimental Study of Tablet Cucumber Vine Compound in Treating Essential Hypertension], *Chung Hsi I Chieh Ho Tsa Chih* 11, no. 5 (May 1991): 274–76, 260–61.

A double-blind, placebo-controlled study gave 0.75 mg of processed rhubarb to pregnant women at risk for pregnancy-induced hypertension from the 28th week of gestation up through delivery. Only 5.7 percent of the women taking rhubarb developed hypertension, compared to 20.8 percent of the controls.

Z. J. Zhang et al., [Low Dose of Processed Rhubarb in Preventing Pregnancy Induced Hypertension], *Chung Hua Fu Chan Ko Tsa Chih* 29, no. 8 (August 1994): 463–64, 509.

Supplementation with *Ginkgo biloba* extract was heart-protective in a study.

N. Haramaki et al., "Effects of Natural Antioxidant *Ginkgo biloba* Extract (EGB 761) on Myocardial Ischemia-Reperfusion Injury," *Free Radic. Biol. Med.* 16, no. 6 (June 1994): 789–94.

Berberine was shown to help regulate heartbeat.

W. Huang, [Ventricular Tachyarrhythmias Treated with Berberine], *Chung Hua Hsin Hsueh Kuan Ping Tsa Chih* 18, no. 3 (1990): 155–56.

A controlled study found that patients taking 500 mg of cynarin per day for 50 days experienced significant reductions in their levels of total cholesterol, triglyceride, and pre-beta-lipoprotein.

M. Montini et al., "Controlled Trial of Cynarin in the Treatment of the Hyperlipidemic Syndrome: Observations in 60 Cases," *Arzneim Forsch.* 25, no. 8 (1975): 1311–14.

Bromelain (1,000–1,400 mg) was given to angina pectoris patients daily in this study, with results showing that symptoms disappeared in all of them within 4 to 90 days. Removal of the bromelain caused a recurrence of symptoms.

H. A. Nieper, "Effects of Bromelain on Coronary Heart Disease and Angina Pectoris," *Acta Med. Empirica* 5 (1978): 274–75.

Results of a controlled study showed a significant drop in total cholesterol in 70–80 percent of patients given 500 mg of gugulipid 3 times a day.

S. Nityanand, et al., "Clinical Trials with Gugulipid: A New Hypolipidemic Agent," *Journal Assoc. Phys. India* 37, no. 5 (1989): 323–28.

In a placebo-controlled study, 40-to-60-year-old patients with hyperlipidemia were given 2.25 g of purified gum guggal twice daily. It was shown effective in lowering cholesterol and triglycerides, and in raising HDL cholesterol levels.

S. K. Verma and A. Bordia, "Effect of *Commiphora Mukul* (Gum Guggal) in Patients with Hyperlipidemia with Special Reference to HDL-Cholesterol," *Indian Journal of Medical Research* 87 (1988): 356–60.

Crataegus pinnatifida leaves were used in a placebo-controlled study to treat angina, and were shown effective.

W. L. Weng et al., "Therapeutic Effect of *Crataegus Pinnatifida* on 46 Cases of Angina Pectoris—A Double Blind Study," *Journal of Traditional Chinese Medicine* 4, no. 4 (1984): 293–94.

Crataegus given to patients with decreasing cardiac performance produced significant improvements in exercise tolerance, heart rate, and overall well-being.

V. M. O'Conolly et al., [Treatment of Cardiac Performance (HYHA Stages I to II) in Advanced Age with Standardized *Crataegus* Extract], *Fortschr. Med.* 104 (1986): 805–8.

Glucomannan reduced total cholesterol and triglycerides in patients with high blood pressure.

G. C. Reffo et al., "Glucomannan in Hypertensive Outpatients: Pilot Clinical Trial," *Current Therapeutic Research* 44, no. 1 (July 1988): 22–27.

Crude leaf extracts of the plant *Rauwalfia* proved to be extremely effective in reducing blood pressure in hypertensive rats and dogs, a study found.

H. Piang-Nan et al., "The Hypotensive Effect of Leaf and Alkaloid of *Kwangtung Rauwalfia*," *Chinese Medical Journal* 81 (1962): 104–8.

Hawthorn extract helped heart patients experience significant decreases in systolic pressure and heart rate.

U. Schmidt et al., "Wirksamkeit des Extrak-tes LI 132 (600 mg/Tag) bei achitowchiger Therapie," *Munch. Med. Wschr.* 136, suppl. 1 (1994): S13–19.

Crataegus extract had a cardioprotective effect in a study with rats.

Y. Nasa et al., "Protective Effect of *Crataegus* Extract on the Cardiac Mechanical Dysfunction in Isolated Perfused Working Heart," *Arzneim Forsch/Drug Res.* 43, no. 9 (1993): 945–49.

EXERCISE

Close to 1.5 million people are diagnosed with coronary heart disease each year; approximately $47 billion is spent treating it. But studies suggest that exercise—even as moderate as gardening, dancing, and walking—may prevent much of the incidence of the disease.

"Public Health Focus: Physical Activity and the Prevention of Coronary Heart Disease," *JAMA* 270, no. 13 (October 6, 1993): 1529.

A study examined the effects of 40 minutes of brisk walking 3 times per week with or without reductions in salt consumption in sedentary patients receiving drug treatment for hypertension. Results: Lowering salt intake and increasing exercise levels could lower blood pressure for short periods of time.

Bruce Arrol et al., "Salt Restriction and Physical Activity in Treated Hypertensives," *New Zealand Medical Journal* (July 14, 1995): 266–68.

TRADITIONAL CHINESE MEDICINE

The effects of *Salvia miltiorrhizae* bge (SMB) and ligustrazine (L) on women with pregnancy-induced hypertension were studied. Both herbs demonstrated the ability to invigorate blood circulation by decreasing vasoconstriction.

S. Y. Liu et al., [The Effects of *Salvia Miltiorrhizae* Bge and Ligustrazine on Thromboxane A2 and Prostacyclin in Pregnancy Induced Hypertension], *Chung Hua Fu Chan Ko Tsa Chih* 29, no. 11 (November 1994): 648–50, 697.

Mailuoing was shown to lower blood pressure in pregnant women.

F. Luan et al., [Observation on Treatment of Mailuoing Injection for 46 Pregnancy Induced Hypertension Patients], *Chung Kuo Chung Hsi I Chieh Ho Tsa Chih* 15, no. 3 (March 1995): 153–55.

Feiyaning and ligustrazine were shown to be of benefit to heart disease patients.

S. M. Liu and T. Q. Tang, [Clinical and Experimental Studies of Feiyaning in Treating Pulmonary Arterial Hypertension in Cor Pulmonale], *Chung Kuo Chung Hsi I Chieh Ho Tsa Chih* 14, no. 8 (August 1994): 469–73.

Dasheng jiangya (DSJY) has a blood-pressure-lowering effect.

P.S. Shi, [Clinical and Experimental Study of No. 90–*Dasheng Jiangya* Oral Liquid in Treating Hypertension], *Chung Kuo Chung Hsi I Chieh Ho Tsa Chih* 14, no. 3 (March 1994): 145–47, 132.

Buyang huanwu decoction (BYHWD) was effective in treating coronary heart disease patients.

H. Zhang et al., [Clinical Study on Effects of *Buyang Huanwu* Decoction on Coronary Heart Disease], *Chung Kuo Chung Hsi I Chieh Ho Tsa Chih* 15, no. 4 (April 1995): 213–15.

Results of a study showed that *Astragalus membranaceus* was effective in significantly strengthening the left ventricular function in patients suffering from acute myocardial infarction and also produced an anti-free-radical effect relative to controls.

L. X. Chen et al., [Effects of *Astragalus Membranaceus* on Left Ventricular Function and Oxygen Free Radical in Acute Myocardial Infarction Patients and Mechanism of its Cardiotonic Action], *Chung Kuo Chung Hsi I Chieh Ho Tsa Chih* 15, no. 3 (March 1995): 141–43.

Astragulus membranaceus was shown to have a cardiotonic (heart-helping) effect.

S.Q. Li et al., [Clinical Observation on the Treatment of Ischemic Heart Disease with *Astragalus Membranaceus*], *Chung Kuo Chung Hsi I Chieh Ho Tsa Chih* 15, no. 3 (February 1995): 177–80.

ACUPUNCTURE

Results of a study showed that auricular acupuncture had a 100 percent short-term blood-pressure-lowering effect in 30 patients suffering from hypertension.

H. Q. Huang and S. Z. Liang, [Improvement of Blood Pressure and Left Cardiac Function in Patients with Hypertension by Auricular Acupuncture], *Chung Hsi I Chieh Ho Tsa Chih* 11, no. 11 (November 1991): 654–56, 643–44.

Acupuncture and electroacupuncture were shown effective as a substitute for drug therapy in patients with coronary heart disease, neurocirculatory dystonia, and essential hypertension.

S. A. Radzievskii et al., [The Effect of Acupuncture on the Hemodynamics and Tolerance for Physical Loads in Patients with Cardiovascular Diseases], *Vopr. Kurotol. Fizioter. Lech. Fiz. Kult.* 2 (March–April 1991): 30–33.

Researchers examined the effects of acupuncture on angina pectoris patients resistant to medical treatment. Patients receiving the acupuncture experienced a significant increase in cardiac work capacity compared to those receiving sham acupuncture.

S. Ballegaard et al., "Acupuncture in Severe, Stable Angina Pectoris: A Randomized Trial," *Acta. Med. Scand.* 220, no. 4 (1986): 307–13.

BIOFEEDBACK

Results of a study on the effects of biofeedback on hypertensive patients showed that the patients continued to experience benefits up to 3 years after their last treatment.

A. McGrady et al., "Sustained Effects of Biofeedback-Assisted Relaxation Therapy in Essential Hypertension," *Biofeedback and Self-Regulation* 16, no. 4 (1991): 399–410.

Biofeedback was used by high-blood-pressure patients, 77 percent of whom experienced significant drops in both systolic and diastolic pressures. A subsequent reduction in the use of antihypertensive drugs was achieved in 50 percent of the patients.

C. Patel and K. K. Datey, "Relaxation and Biofeedback Techniques in the Management of Hypertension," *Angiology* 27, no. 2 (February 1976): 106–13.

A study examined the effects of either relaxation training or relaxation training combined with biofeedback in pregnant women suffering from hypertension. Women in both groups experienced significant reductions in systolic and diastolic blood pressure compared to controls, and they required fewer trips to the hospital during their pregnancies.

B. C. Little et al., "Treatment of Hypertension in Pregnancy by Relaxation and Biofeedback," *Lancet* 1 (April 21, 1984): 865–67.

Researchers examined the effects of thermal biofeedback training combined with progressive muscle relaxation therapy on hypertensive patients. They found a significant drop in systolic and diastolic blood pressure in the treatment group compared to controls (progressive muscle relaxation therapy only).

Y. B. Hahn et al., "The Effect of Thermal Biofeedback and Progressive Muscle Relaxation Training in Reducing Blood Pressure of Patients with Essential Hypertension," *Image Journal of Nurs. Sch.* 25, no. 3 (Fall 1993): 204–7.

RELAXATION

A review article concluded that relaxation therapy is an effective means of reducing blood pressure.

R. G. Jacob et al., "Relaxation Therapy in the Treatment of Hypertension: A Review," *Archives in General Psychiatry* 34, no. 12 (December 1977): 1417–27.

BLOOD CLOTS

Greenland Eskimos and other groups who eat seafood have lower levels of cardiovascular disease than groups who do not. Fish oil is rich in eicosapentaenoic acid (EPA).

B. J. Holub, "Dietary Fish Oils Containing Eicosapentaenoic Acid and the Prevention of Atherosclerosis and Thrombosis," *Canadian Medical Association Journal* 139, no. 5 (September 1, 1988): 377–81.

Dietary saturated fats increase the risk of coronary heart disease. Diets low in long-chain saturated fatty acids and rich in linoleic acid prevent coronary heart disease; they reduce the platelet aggregation, decrease atherosclerosis, and inhibit arterial thrombosis.

G. Hornstra, "Dietary Prevention of Coronary Heart Disease: Effect of Dietary Fats on Arterial Thrombosis," *Postgraduate Med. Journal* (August 1980): 563–70.

A study compared a low-fat, high-fiber diet to the average Danish diet for 2 weeks with 21 healthy middle-aged subjects. The low-fat, high-fiber diet reduced atherogenic and thrombogenic tendencies.

P. Marckmann et al., "Low-fat, High-fiber Diet Favorably Affects Several Independent Risk Markers of Ischemic Heart Disease: Observations on Blood Lipids, Coagulation, and Fibrinolysis from a Trial of Middle-aged Danes," *American Journal of Clinical Nutrition* 59, no. 4 (April 1994): 935–39.

Nutritional antioxidants show antithrombotic effects, that is, they prevent the formation of clots in blood vessels.

M. F. McCarty et al., "An Antithrombotic Role for Nutritional Antioxidants; Implications for Tumor Metastasis and Other Pathologies," *Medical Hypotheses* 19, no. 4 (April 1986): 345–57.

Selenium was shown to be antithrombotic.

N. W. Stead et al., "Selenium (Se) Balance in the Dependent Elderly," *American Journal of Clinical Nutrition* 39 (1984): 677.

A study of chondroitin polysulfate showed that serum cholesterol was 10-20 percent lower and triglycerides were 27 percent lower for a treated group, as opposed to controls. Mean clotting time increased by 50 percent after 33 months of treatment.

K. Nakazawa and K. Murata, "The Therapeutic Effect of Chondroitin Polysulfate in Elderly Athersclerotic Patients," *Journal of International Medical Research* 6, no. 3 (1978): 217–25.

Chondroitin-4 sulfate prolonged thrombus formation and reduced serum cholesterol, a study of 120 coronary heart disease patients showed. Also, the treated group had fewer abnormal cardiac events over 6 years (10 percent versus 70 percent for the control group); and a lower death rate (7 percent versus 23 percent for the controls).

K. Izuka and K. Murata, *Experientia* 29 (1973): 255–57.

Reducing triglyceride levels with soy lecithin produces a similar reduction in platelet aggregation.

J.G. Brook et al., "Dietary Soya Lecithin Decreases Plasma Triglyceride Levels and Inhibits Collagen-and ADP-Induced Platelet Aggregation," *Biochem. Med. Metab. Biol.* 35, no. 1 (1986): 31–39.

A normal level of taurine increases resistance to platelet aggregation, and supplementation given to healthy subjects increases resistance 30–70 percent.

K. C. Hayes et al., "Taurine Modulates Platelet Aggregation in Cats and Humans," *American Journal of Clinical Nutrition* 49 (1989): 1211–16.

Flavonoids inhibit aggregation of blood platelets.

N. A. Nikolaev et al., [Therapeutic Efficacy of Laser and Electropuncture Reflexotherapy in Correcting the Initial Manifestations of Cerebral Circulatory Insufficiency], *Zh. Nevropatol. Psikhiatr.* 86, no. 1 (1986): 60–64.

A study of rats reveals that *eleutherococcus* activates the anticoagulating system and protects against thrombogeneration.

G. G. Bazaz'ian et al., [Effect of *Eleutherococcus* on the Functional Status of the Anticoagulation System in Older Animals], *Fiziol. Zh. SSSR* 73, no. 10 (October 1987): 1390-1395.

Ginkgo biloba was shown experimentally to have an anticlotting action.

R. H. Bourgain et al., "Thrombus Induction by Endogenic Paf-Acether and its Inhibition by *Ginkgo Biloba* Extracts in the Guinea Pig," *Prostaglandins* 32, no. 1 (July 1986): 142-144.

Ginkgolides can fully inhibit platelet aggregation.

P. Nguyen et al., "Mechanisms of the Platelet Aggregation Induced by Activated Neutrophils and Inhibitory Effect of Specific PAF Receptor Antagonists," *Thrombosis Research*, 78, no. 1 (1995): 33-42.

Olive oil inhibited platelet aggregation experimentally.

A. Petroni et al., "Inhibition of Platelet Aggregation and Eicosanoid Production by Phenolic Components of Olive Oil," *Thrombosis Research* 78, no. 2 (1988): 141–60.

Bromelain had an anticlotting effect on heart patients in two large-scale tests.

G. E. Felton, "Fibrinolytic and Antithrombotic Action of Bromelain May Eliminate Thrombosis in Heart Patients," *Medical Hypotheses* 6, no. 11 (1980): 1123–33.

Curcumin inhibits platelet aggregation.

R. Srivastava et al., "Effect of Curcumin on Platelet Aggregation and Vascular Prostacyclin Synthesis," *Arzneim. Forsch.* 36 (1986): 715–17.

Garlic normalizes plasma lipids and inhibits platelet aggregation, studies have shown.

E. Ernst, "Cardiovascular Effects of Garlic (*Allium sativum*): A Review," *Pharmatherapeutica* 5, no. 2 (1987): 83–89.

The best garlic product would be one that is rich in all garlic compounds, including the one responsible for its odor: allicin.

M. T. Murray, "Cardiovascular Effects of Commercial Garlic Preparations," *American Journal of Natural Medicine* 2, no. 5 (June 1995): 5–7.

A dried garlic preparation (containing 1.3 percent allicin) was given to 12 healthy volunteers at a level of 900 mg/day and was shown to have an anticlotting effect.

C. Legnani et al., "Effects of Dried Garlic Preparation on Fibrinolysis and Platelet Aggregation in Healthy Subjects," *Arzneim. Forsch.* 43, no. 1 (1993): 119–21.

Aqueous extracts of garlic produced dose-dependent inhibition of platelet aggregation.

K. C. Srivastava, "Aqueous Extracts of Onion, Garlic and Ginger Inhibit Platelet Aggregation and Alter Arachidonic Acid Metabolism," *Biomed. Biochem. Acta* 43, no. 8/9 (1984): S335–46.

Ajoene, a product derived from garlic, has an anticlotting effect.

K. C. Srivastava and O. D. Tyagi, "Effects of a Garlic-Derived Principle (Ajoene) on Aggregations and Arachidonic Acid Metabolism in Human Blood Platelets," *Prostaglandins, Leukotrienes and Essential Fatty Acids* 49 (1993): 587–95.

Ajoene inhibits fibrinogen binding.

R. Apitz-Castro et al., "Effect of Ajoene, the Major Antiplatelet Compound from Garlic, on Platelet Thrombus Formation," *Thrombosis Research* 68 (1992): 145–55.

Gingerol isolated from *Zingiber officinale* has been shown to inhibit clotting.

J. Tao and K. Y. Feng, "Experimental and Clinical Studies on Inhibitory Effect of *Ganoderma Lucidum* on Platelet Aggregation," *Journal Tongji Med. Univ.* 10, no. 4 (1990): 240–43.

Hsien-Ho-Tsao (HHT), a traditional Chinese medicine, has been proven effective for acute pulmonary thromboembolism due to its antiplatelet action.

M. F. Hsu et al., "Effect of Hsien-Ho-Tsao (*Agrimonia Pilosa*) on Experimental Thrombosis in Mice," *American Journal of Chinese Medicine* 15, no. 1–2 (1987): 43–51.

The traditional Chinese medicine xinmaining has been shown effective as an antithrombotic treatment.

P. Nguyen et al., "Mechanisms of the Platelet Aggregation Induced by Activated Neutrophils and Inhibitory Effect of Specific PAF Receptor Antagonists," *Thrombosis Research* 78, no. 1 (1995): 33–42.

Traditional Chinese medicine, in combination with Western medicine, was shown effective in preventing clotting.

X. Jin, [Formation of Extrinsic Blood Thrombosis in 102 Cases of Thromboangiitis Obliterans], *Chung Hsi I Chieh Ho Tsa Chih* 10, no. 3 (March 1990): 152–54, 32.

Ganoderma lucidum was proven effective in inhibiting platelet aggregation in a study of 15 healthy volunteers and 33 patients with therosclerotic diseases.

J. Tao and K.Y. Feng, "Experimental and Clinical Studies on Inhibitory Effect of *Ganoderma Lucidum* on Platelet Aggregation," *Journal Tongji Med. Univ.* 10, no. 4 (1990): 240–43.

Electrical and laser acupuncture was used in 100 patients to treat cerebral circulation insufficiency. Prolonged clotting time resulted.

N. A. Nikolaev et al., [Therapeutic Efficacy of Laser and Electropuncture Reflexotherapy in Correcting the Initial Manifestations of Cerebral Circulatory Insufficiency], *Zh. Nevropatol. Psikhiatr.* 86, no. 1 (1986): 60–64.

13. HERPES

In the 1970s herpes was a cause for widespread concern, but it took a back seat to AIDS in the 1980s. While not as deadly, herpes is more prevalent, causing pain to most of those afflicted. Over half the population get cold sores from time to time, the result of herpes simplex virus 1 (HSV1). Others become afflicted with shingles, a herpes zoster infection, years after they get chicken pox. Additionally, people get Epstein-Barr, the form of herpes that causes mononucleosis. Still others break out in genital herpes, an infection caused by herpes simplex virus 2 (HSV2). All in all, the number of men and women with herpes is greater than 80 percent.

Causes

Herpes is a contagious virus that lives at the base of the spine in the nerve cells. Periodic attacks occur whenever the immune system is below par. Any kind of emotional, mental, or physical stress can lower the body's defense system and create the perfect climate for an outbreak. Common physical stressors include illness, menstrual periods, vaginal yeast infections, too much sunlight or friction (which breaks down skin cells), allergies, and certain foods. Genital herpes can be sexually transmitted. Pregnant mothers can transmit the virus to their unborn children via blood or through direct contact with infected tissue during delivery. Prescription drugs that lower immunity can set off an attack: such medications include antibiotics, steroids, and antidepressants.

Symptoms

Genital herpes causes surface sores on the skin and lining of the genital area. In women, sores can appear on the cervix, vagina, or perineum, which may be accompanied by a discharge or vaginal blisters. There is often a burning sensation, especially at the onset of an outbreak. Other symptoms may include urinary problems, fever, and lymphatic swelling. Intercourse is painful and should be avoided during an outbreak to prevent sexual transmission. HSV2 occurs intermittently and usually lasts from five to seven days.

As the name implies, oral herpes tends to attack the skin and mucous membranes on the face, particularly around the mouth and nose. These cold sores tend to appear as pearl-like blisters. Although they are short-term, they can be irritating and painful. Herpes zoster, the result of the varicellazostervirus (VZV), causes agonizing blisters on one side of the body, usually the chest or abdomen. Pain is usually felt before effects are seen, the result of overly sensitive skin covering the affected nerve. Symptoms may last from a few days to several weeks.

Clinical Experience

There is no conventional medical cure for herpes, although drugs are commonly given to lessen symptoms. The most famous of these is acyclovir, also known as Zovirax, which supposedly reduces the rate of growth of the herpes virus. Herpes medications have many potential side effects, including dizziness, headaches, diarrhea, nausea, vomiting, general weakness, fatigue, ill health, sore throat, fever, insomnia, swelling, tenderness, and bleeding of the gums. In addition, acyclovir ointment can cause allergic skin reactions.

Herpes sufferers will be glad to learn that natural remedies are often highly effective in shortening the length of outbreaks and in diminishing their frequency. These are some of the important ones to know about:

NUTRITION AND LIFESTYLE
When herpes strikes, it s always a good idea to rest and eat lightly. Short fruit fasts, with plenty of pure water and cleansing herbal teas, can be very helpful. Good herbs to include are sage, rosemary, cayenne, echinacea, goldenseal, red clover, astragalus, and burdock root. Beneficial bacteria, such as those found in yogurt, or supplements of lactobacillus and acidophilus, support the digestive processes necessary for the maintenance of the immune system. Other nutrients that directly enhance the immune system include garlic, quercetin, zinc gluconate, buffered vitamin C, and beta carotene or vitamin A. In addition, 500 mg of the amino acid L-lysine, taken 2 to 4 times a day, can produce excellent results. Bee propolis is anti-inflammatory, while B vitamins combat stress. Also good are bee pollen, blue-green algae, and pycnogenol.

Nervous system stressors, such as caffeine, alcohol, and hard-to-digest foods like meat, should be avoided, especially at the onset of an attack. Foods high in the amino acid arginine, such as chocolate, peanut butter, nuts, and onions, are also associated with higher incidences of outbreaks.

Since stress promotes outbreaks, it is important to make time for activities that alleviate tension. Many possibilities include biofeedback, yoga, meditation, deep breathing, and exercise. Toothbrushes should be changed frequently, and completely dried before reuse to prevent reinfection. Soaking them in baking soda also fights germs.

HOMEOPATHY

According to Dr. Erika Price, classical homeopathy is the most effective form of treatment for people with the herpes virus: "The properly chosen remedy will motivate and empower the individual's own defense systems to fight back against anything harmful to it," she claims. Unlike orthodox medicine, homeopathy does not suppress ailments. This is very important because when you suppress a disease, it doesn't go away but goes somewhere else deeper inside of you. Deeper means it goes to a more important organ than the skin. Homeopathy has no adverse effects and can only be of benefit. When the patient's physical, mental, and spiritual nature are taken into account, a cure can be found. The following remedies may prove extremely helpful:

FOR COLD SORES

Natrum muriaticum. When sores are on the lips, especially in the middle of the lips, the 30c potency should be taken twice a day.

Phosphorus. Cold sores that manifest above the lips, accompanied by itching, cutting, and sharp pain, need the 30c potency twice a day.

Petroleum. For cold sores that erupt in patches and become crusty and loose around the lips and mouth, petroleum is indicated. A 9c potency is needed 3 times a day.

Apis. Apis helps cold sores around the mouth and lips that are accompanied by stinging, and painful blisters that itch and burn. A 6c potency is needed 3 to 4 times daily.

FOR FEMALE GENITAL HERPES

Natrum muriaticum is indicated when the herpetic lesions are pearl-like blisters and the genital area feels puffy, hot, and very dry. A 6c potency may be beneficial when taken 4 times a day.

Dulcamara. Women who tend to get a herpes outbreak in clusters on the vulva or on the hair follicles around the labia and vulva every time they catch a cold or get their period probably need dulcamara in a 12c potency 2 to 3 times a day.

Petroleum. This may help if herpes eruptions form in patches and the sores become deep red and feel tender and moist. Outbreaks usually occur during menstrual periods, and most often affect the perineum, anus, labia, or vulva. A 9c potency should be taken 3 times a day.

FOR SHINGLES

Arsenicum album benefits most cases of shingles, especially when the individual feels worse in the cold, worse after midnight, and better with warmth. If taken at the onset of an attack, it is best taken in a 30c potency twice a day for 2 to 3 days. After the first three days, arsenicum album is indicated if there is a burning sensation in the areas that were affected by the zoster eruptions (typically the chest and abdomen). At this point 12c, taken 2 to 3 times a day, is best. This remedy is excellent for the getting rid of the burning sensation that is often present.

Hypericum perforatum is a wonderful remedy for any kind of nerve pain. It is indicated whenever there is intense neuritis and neuralgia, with burning, tingling and numbness along the course of the affected nerves. Hypericum perforatum should be taken in a 30c potency, 2 to 3 times a day, as needed.

When taking homeopathic remedies, Dr. Price reminds patients to not touch them directly, as that may disturb the vibration of the medicine. Rather, they should be placed under the tongue until dissolved. Coffee, mint, camphor, and chamomile must be avoided, as they work against the remedies. It is also important to note symptoms; as they change, so must the remedy.

AROMATHERAPY

The use of essential oils has recently gained popularity in the United States, where it is used widely in skin and body care products. But its medicinal value has long been accepted in other countries, particularly France, where, in many instances, its antimicrobial properties make it an acceptable replacement for drug therapy. Aromatherapist Valerie Cooksley, author of *Aromatherapy: A Lifetime Guide to Healing with Essential Oils*, says that pure essential oils, properly used, can heal cold and canker sores. One mouthwash she recommends combines 5 drops each of peppermint, bergamot, or tea tree oil to raw honey, which is used as a carrier. This is important, as oils do not mix with water alone. The mixture is then added to a strong sage or rosemary tea. Rinsing with the formula several times a day balances the pH of the mouth and helps to heal infections. Using this daily may even prevent outbreaks.

Additional spot treatments alleviate pain and restore health. One that Cooksley recommends involves dabbing a cotton swab with myrrh oil and applying directly onto cold and canker sores. Another aromatherapist, Sharon Olson, dabs a cotton swab with diluted tea tree oil and places that on the cold sore to kill the virus. She follows this up later with lavender, which soothes the sore and stimulates the growth of new skin. The addition of fresh aloe vera gel further promotes healing. A side benefit of the therapy is its ability to lift the spirits. "When I get a cold sore, I get depressed," reveals Olson, "so I usually inhale some rosemary or basil to lift my spirits and clear my mind."

Herbal Pharmacy

Plants containing phytochemicals with antiherpes properties, in order of potency:

Myrciaria dubia (camu-camu)
Glycyrrhiza glabra (licorice), plant
Viola tricolor hortensis (pansy)
Sophora japonica (Japanese pagoda tree), bud
Oenothera biennis (evening primose)
Malpighia glabra (acerola)
Glycyrrhiza glabra (licorice), root
Sophora japonica (Japanese pagoda tree), flower
Coffea arabica (coffee)
Aesculus hippocastanum (horse chestnut)
Rhizophora mangle (red mangrove)
Citrus limon (lemon)
Camellia sinensis (tea)
Abrus precatorius (crab's eyes)
Podophyllum hexandrum (Himalayan mayapple)
Mangifera indica (mango)
Origanum vulgare (wild oregano)
Phyllanthus emblica (emblic)
Allium cepa (onion)

Hot News

Many studies have proven the effectiveness of zinc in combating herpes; one of these concludes that, specifically, zinc monoglycerate is the best zinc treatment. Other nutritional supplements found useful for herpes treatment are vitamin C, adenosine, L-lysine, and retinoic acid, a form of vitamin A found in breast milk. Herbal extracts that have lessened or eliminated herpes symptoms include glycyrrhizic acid, a component of licorice root; pine cone extracts; tannins; poplar bud extract; lemon balm cream; an infusion from flowers of *Sambucus nigra*, aerial parts of *Hypericum performatum*, and roots of *Saponaria officinalis;* peppermint; and extracts of *Cordia salicifolia, Geum japonicum, Rhus javanica, Syzgium aromaticum,* and *Terminal chebula.* Lithium, when used to treat psychiatric illnes, has also proven to reduce herpes infections, indicating that lithium ointment could be an effective treatment. And herpes outbreaks on the lips may be avoided by the use of sunscreen, one study concludes, since ultraviolet B light is a recognized stimulator of the herpes simplex virus. *(See below.)*

FROM THE MEDICAL LITERATURE ON HERPES

NUTRITION

Studies have shown the antiviral effects of zinc ions with respect to herpes, as well as the efficacy of topical zinc treatments and zinc salts on genital infections.

G. A. Eby and W. W. Halcomb, "Use of Topical Zinc to Prevent Recurrent Herpes Simplex Infection: A Review of Literature and Suggested Protocols," *Medical Hypotheses* 17, no. 2 (June 1985): 157–65.

A placebo-controlled study of patients suffering from cold sores found that after 13 days of treatment, 70 percent of the lesions in those treated with zinc monoglycerate had healed, compared to 9 percent of the lesions in those treated with zinc oxide. Aside from intravenous administration, the authors argue, zinc monoglycerate is the best means of zinc treatment.

A. Apisariyakulm et al., "Zinc Monoglycerolate is Effective Against Oral Herpetic Sores," *Medical Journal of Australia* 152 (January 1, 1990): 54.

Zinc sulfate inhibits herpes replication.

Y. J. Gordon et al., "Irreversible Inhibition of Herpes Simplex Virus Replication in BSC-1 Cells by Zinc Ions," *Antimicrobial Agents Chemother.* 8, no. 3 (1975): 377–80.

Herpes simplex I patients with recurrent eruptions were treated with 250 mg of vitamin C and 100 mg of zinc twice daily over a 6-week period. Results: Patients experienced either complete suppression of the viral eruptions, local tingling with or without limited eruption or local swelling and limited vesiculation lasting for less than one day, or one bout of serious eruption that was not repeated as long as the treatment was continued.

J. Fitzherbert, "Genital Herpes and Zinc," *Medical Journal Aust.* 1 (1979): 399.

A 0.25 percent zinc sulfate in saturated camphor water solution was administered to both Type I and Type II herpes patients beginning within one day of lesion appearance. When the solution was administered 8–10 times a day, the lesions generally receded within 3-6 days. When the solution was administered every 30–60 minutes, symptoms such as itching, burning, stinging, and pain generally receded within 2–3 hours. Administration of the solution as a douche also proved effective in cases of vaginal herpes.

E. F. Finnerty, "Topical Zinc in the Treatment of Herpes Simplex," *Cutis* 37, no. 2 (1986): 130–31.

A study found vitamin C to be an effective treatment for recurrent cold sores. When the vitamin was taken in doses of 1–2 g daily, 30 of 38 patients remained free of such sores for four years following the start of supplementation. The remaining 8 patients found it possible to suppress the herpes virus by ingesting vitamin C when symptoms started to appear.

S. Lewin, *Vitamin C: Its Molecular Biology and Medical Potential* (New York: Van Nostrand Reinhold, 1973).

In a placebo-controlled study, patients suffering from herpes labialis were treated with 200 mg of vitamin C and 200 mg of bioflavonoids 3–5 times a day beginning within two days of the appearance of symptoms. Results: Blisters appeared in only 14 out of the 38 patients receiving treatment, and only 20 of the 38 showed disruption of the vesicular membrane, compared to all 10 of the patients receiving a placebo in each case. Beginning treatment within 12 hours of initial symptoms proved to be even more effective. All differences between treatment and control groups were statistically significant.

G. T. Terezhalmy et al., "The Use of Water-Soluble Bioflavonoid-Ascorbic Acid Complex in the Treatment of Recurrent Herpes Labialis," *Oral Surg.* 45 (1978): 56–62.

Herpes labialis patients treated with 9–12 doses of adenosine on alternate days experienced the drying up of lesions in 24 to 36 hours and the disappearance of pain within 48. Of the 36 patients treated, 23 suffered from no recurrences for over 2 years, with the rest experiencing only one bout of recurrence.

S. H. Scklar and E. Buimovici-Klein,"Adenosine in the Treatment of Recurrent Herpes Labialis," *Oral Surgery* 48, no. 5 (1979): 416–17.

In a placebo-controlled study, herpes simplex patients suffering from either oral or genital recurrent infections (or both) were treated with 1 g three times daily of L-lysine and told to avoid certain foods, such as nuts, gelatin, and chocolate. Of those receiving treatment, 74 percent rated it as either effective or very effective after 6 months, compared to 28 percent of the controls. Treatment patients had an average number of outbreaks of 3.1, compared to 4.2 for controls over the same time period.

R. S. Griffith et al., "Success of L-lysine Therapy in Frequently Recurrent Herpes Simplex Infection," *Dermatologica* 175 (1987): 183–90.

Herpes patients treated with 1248 mg daily of L-lysine monohydrochloride were found to experience a decrease in the recurrence rate and a reduction of symptoms. Cutting the dose in half did not produce the same results.

M. A. McCune et al., "Treatment of Recurrent Herpes Simplex Infections with L-lysine Monohydrochloride," *Cutis* 34, no. 4 (1984): 366–73.

A controlled experiment gave genital herpes patients lithium ointment 4 times a day for one week, beginning within 2 days of the appearance of lesions. The treated patients experienced significant reductions in pain and quicker healing times than controls did. By the fourth or fifth day of treatment, only 14 percent of the treatment group was excreting virus, compared to 55 percent of controls. Further, those in the control group who were still excreting virus at this point showed a mean excretion rate 30 times greater than those excreting virus in the treatment group.

G. R. Skinner, "Lithium Ointment for Genital Herpes," *Lancet* 2 (1983): 288.

Patients receiving lithium for psychiatric illness experienced a significantly lower rate of recurrent labial herpes infections compared to pretreatment, while rates for those taking other antidepressants were not affected.

J. D. Amsterdam et al., "A Possible Antiviral Action of Lithium Carbonate in Herpes Simplex Virus Infections," *Biological Psychiatry* 27, no. 4 (1990): 447–53.

Researchers have discovered that retinoic acid, a form of vitamin A found in breast milk, slows the growth of the herpes simplex virus I after 48 hours.

J. Kahn, "Vitamin A May Help Suppress Herpes Outbreaks," *Medical Tribune* (May 18, 1995): 10.

HERBS/PLANT EXTRACTS

An extract of *Cordia salicifolia*, COL 1-6, was found to inhibit herpes simplex virus type 1.

K. Hayashi et al., "Antiviral Activity of an Extract of *Cordia Salicifolia* on Herpes Simplex Virus Type 1," *Planta. Med.* 56, no. 5 (October 1990): 439–43.

A review article examined the antiviral effect of 472 traditional medicinal herbs on herpes simplex type 1. The ten most effective herbs against the virus are *Aristolochia debilis, Artemisia anomala, Lindera strychnifolia, Patrinia villosa, Pinus massoniana, Prunella vulgaris, Pyrrosia lingua, Rhus chinensis, Sargussum fusiforme,* and *Taraxacum mongolicum.*

M. Zheng et al., [Experimental Study of 472 Herbs with Antiviral Action Against the Herpes Simplex Virus], *Chung Hsi I Chieh Ho Tsa Chih* 10, no. 1 (January 1990): 39–41.

Researchers showed that, at high concentration in vitro, glycyrrhizic acid, a component of licorice root, inhibits the growth and effects of the herpes simplex virus.

R. Pompeii et al., "Antiviral Activity of Glycyrrhizic Acid," *Experientia* 36 (1980): 304.

Glycyrrhizin, in experiments on mice, aided immune-system resistance to herpes simplex type 1.

T. Utsunomiya et al., "Glycyrrhizin Improves the Resistance of Thermally Injured Mice to Opportunistic Infection of Herpes Simplex Virus Type 1," *Immunology Letters* 44 (1995): 59–66.

A double-blind, placebo-controlled study found that 75 percent of those taking 4 g of *Eleutherococcus senticosus* extract for 6 months experienced significant improvements in the duration, frequency, and severity of herpes simplex type II attacks, compared to only 34 percent of controls.

M. Williams, "Immuno-Protection Against Herpes Simplex Type II Infection by Eleutherococcus Root Extract," *International Journal of Alternative and Complementary Medicine* 13, no. 7 (July 1995): 9–12.

A study demonstrated the ability of pine cone extracts to inhibit plaque formation of herpes simplex virus types I and II strains in human adenocarcinoma cells.

K. Fukuchi et al., "Inhibition of Herpes Simplex Virus Infection by Pine Cone Antitumor Substances," *Anticancer Research* 9, no. 2 (March–April 1989): 313–17.

Several chemically defined plant extracts were investigated for their anti–herpes simplex virus activity on both infected human adenocarcinoma cells and infected kidney cells from the African green monkey. Extracts with the greatest such activity included monomeric hydrolyzable tannins, oligomeric ellagitannins, and condensed tannins.

K. Fukuchi et al., "Inhibition of Herpes Simplex Virus Infection by Tannins and Related Compounds," *Antiviral Research* 11, no. 5–6 (June–July 1989): 285–97.

Combining acyclovir with historically used herbal medicines resulted in strong therapeutic anti-HSV-1 activity in mice, especially reduction of virus yield in the brain. The herbs demonstrating the most effectiveness were *Geum japonicum, Rhus javanica, Syzgium aromaticum,* and *Terminal chebula.*

M. Kurokawa et al., "Efficacy of Traditional Herbal Medicines in Combination with Acyclovir Against Herpes Simplex Virus Type 1 Infection in Vitro and in Vivo," *Antiviral Research* 27 (1995): 19–37.

Genistein inhibits the replication of herpes simplex virus type I.

Y. Yura et al., "Inhibition of Herpes Simplex Virus Replication by Genistein, an Inhibitor of Protein-Tyrosine Kinase," *Archives of Virology* 132 (1993): 451–61.

A poplar bud extract was found to inhibit herpes simplex virus type I in vitro.

M. Amoros et al., "Comparison of the Anti-Herpes Simplex Virus Activities of Propolis and 3-Methyl-but-2-Enyl Caffeate," *Journal of Natural Products* 57, no. 5 (May 1994): 644–47.

A placebo-controlled study demonstrated that lemon balm cream significantly reduces herpes labialis lesion size and symptoms such as skin redness and swelling.

H. J. Vogt et al., "Melissa Extract for Herpes Simplex," *Verlag Kirchheim* 13, no. 11 (1991).

A dried extract taken from lemon balm leaves, when administered via a topical cream, has antiherpes effects. Results of a double-blind, placebo-controlled study showed that treatment was most effective when initiated at the early stages of infection.

R. H. Wolbing and K. Leonhardt, "Local Therapy of Herpes Simplex with Dried Extract from *Melissa Officinalis*," *Phytomedicine* 1 (1994): 25–31.

Peppermint has been shown to inhibit and kill the herpes simplex virus, among many other microorganisms.

D. B. Mowrey, *The Scientific Validation of Herbal Medicine* (New Canaan, Conn.: Keats Publishing, 1986): 73.

In a study, an infusion from flowers of *Sambucus nigra*, aerial parts of *Hypericum performatum*, and roots of *Saponaria officinalis* exhibited an anti–herpes simplex virus type I effect in vitro. The preparation contains flavonoids, triterpene saponins, phenolic acids, tannins, and polysaccharides, which could be responsible for its antiviral properties.

J. Serkedjieva et al., "Antiviral Activity of the Infusion (SHS-174) from Flowers of *Sambucus Nigra L.*, Aerial Parts of *Hypericum Perforatum L.*, and Roots of *Saponaria Officinalis L.* Against Influenza and Herpes Simplex Viruses," *Phytotherapy Research* 4, no. 3 (1990): 97–100.

The Chinese herbal medicine kanzo-bushi-to was shown, in mice, to help the immune system fight herpes.

R. Matsuo et al., "Effects of a Traditional Chinese Herbal Medicine, Kanzo-Bushi-to, on the Resistance of Thermally Injured Mice Infected with Herpes Simplex Virus Type 1," *International Journal of Immunopharmacology* 16, no. 10 (1994): 855–63.

ENZYME THERAPY

A study found that herpes zoster patients suffering from skin lesions who were adminstered enzyme combination preparations fared just as well as those administered acyclovir after a 14-day period.

P. Billigmann, [Enzyme Therapy–An Alternative in Treatment of Herpes Zoster: A Controlled Study of 192 Patients], *Fortschr Med.* 113, no. 4 (February 10, 1995): 43–48.

ACUPUNCTURE

Electro-acupuncture was shown effective in treating herpes zoster patients, with minimal side effects.

C. J. Coghlan, "Herpes Zoster Treated by Acupuncture," *Central African Journal of Medicine* 38, no. 12 (December 1992): 466–67.

RELAXATION

In a study, 10 sessions of applied relaxation treatment were proven to be an effective means of herpes simplex virus reduction in four subjects diagnosed with frequent recurrences.

K. A. Koehn et al., "Applied Relaxation Training in the Treatment of Genital Herpes," *Journal of Behavior Therapy & Experimental Psychiatry* 24, no. 4 (1993): 331–41.

ULTRAVIOLET LIGHT PROTECTION

Ultraviolet B light is a recognized stimulator of the herpes simplex virus. In a double-blind, placebo-controlled study, a solution containing sunscreen was placed on the lips of patients suffering from labial herpes and was found to prevent the recurrence of virus in all but one of 35 patients who received the treatment following ultraviolet exposure. In comparison, 71 percent of the 38 controls experienced recurrence (with a mean recurrence time of 2.9 days).

J. F. Rooney et al., "Prevention of Ultraviolet-Light-Induced Herpes Labialis by Sunscreen," *Lancet* 338 (December 7, 1991): 1419–22.

14. INFERTILITY

Approximately two-and-a-half million American couples are unable to conceive. The question of what can and should be done to conquer infertility is not only a complex medical issue but, with the advent of more and more advanced techniques for getting around nature's roadblocks to conception, at times a thorny ethical dilemma as well, with high emotional stakes.

Causes

Reasons for infertility include endometriosis *(see chapter 9, Endometriosis)*; poor diet; deficiencies in folic acid, vitamin B6, vitamin B12, and iron; heavy metal toxicity; obesity; immature sex organs; abnormalities of the reproductive system; hormonal imbalances; and genetic damage from electromagnetic radiation. In men, saunas and excessive vigorous exercise can diminish sperm production.

It may be surprising to learn that the birth control pill, and other sources of estrogen, can add to the problem. Barbara Seaman, an advocate for women's health issues and author of *The Doctors' Case Against the Pill*, the publication of which led to detailed product warnings being included in birth control pill prescriptions, concludes that the chemicals in the pill may increase infertility in three ways: by suppressing the natural productions of hormones; increasing the risk of STDs, especially chlamydia; and upsetting the assimilation of nutrients.

LOSS OF CYCLES. "Fertility experts confirm that many women who have been on the pill for a long time have problems reestablishing their monthly cycles. In Switzerland, Fabio Bertarelli, the billionaire owner of the largest company to manufacture fertility drugs, publicly states that he owes his fortune to the birth control pill. In 1993, Bertarelli told the *Wall Street Journal* that his typical customer is a women over thirty, who has been taking birth control pills since she was a teenager or in her early twenties. When she got off the pill, her normal cycles did not come back."

Seaman adds: "Fact is, there are a lot of nutritional issues involved. If a woman has been on the pill for a long time, she may be very low in folic acid; vitamins B1, B2, B6, B12, C, and E; and trace minerals zinc and magnesium, all essential to normal fertility. Sometimes just getting on a really good diet with really good supplements can get her back into a fertile cycle without needing heavy-duty drugs. It should be noted, however, that any dietary supplements used should be low in vitamin A, niacin, copper, and iron, the levels of which tend to be elevated in pill users."

CHLAMYDIA. "Another reason the pill is bad for female infertility is that it promotes the growth of chlamydia. This condition has reached epidemic proportions in the United States, with over half a million new cases yearly. Chlamydia causes pelvic inflammatory disease, which can then cause sterility. Usually, the first time it strikes, chlamydia does not render a woman sterile. Woman who get the condition once should give up the pill at once."

Symptoms

After ten years of fertility tests and treatments, Carla Harkness, frustrated by the lack of consumer-oriented literature on the subject, consulted over a hundred medical specialists and put together *The Fertility Book*. Carla sees infertility as an emotional life crisis that is largely unacknowledged by society: "Reactions include grief and mourning, loss of self-esteem, and impaired self-image. Couples often have difficulties communicating with one another. Their sexual relationship is tested and damaged. All in all, it is a traumatic experience."

She adds that an early end to pregnancy, due to miscarriage, produces the same frustrations: "The failure of a fertilized egg to implant is amazingly common. Often up to 50 percent of fertilized eggs do not make it past the initial two-week period to implantation. Up to 20 percent of confirmed pregnancies are miscarried in the first trimester in women under thirty-five years old. As a woman approaches forty, that number can exceed 25 percent, and by the age of forty-five, the miscarriage rate is almost 50 percent. The emotional impact of miscarriage is similar to infertility. There is often grief and mourning that are not accepted as genuine mourning in our society. Couples often hear things like, 'I guess it was meant to be,' 'Something was wrong,' or 'You'll have another.' That is often of little solace to someone feeling this kind of loss."

Clinical Experience

ASSISTED REPRODUCTIVE TECHNOLOGY

"The laboratory options have just exploded in the past decade for infertile couples," Carla reports. "In 1978, the first 'test-tube' baby was born in England through a process called in vitro fertilization. Since then, the process has been instituted worldwide. There are now over 260 clinics practicing some form of that kind of laboratory fertilization, which is now called Assisted Reproductive Technology or ART.

"Now the boundaries have even exceeded menopause. Before you had the practice of donor sperm for artificial insemination. Now there is the ability to fertilize donor eggs from younger women with the husband's sperm, and to implant those eggs in an infertile woman who is over forty-five or fifty. She is able to carry a child to term that is not genetically related to her. These kinds of options have all become available, and they offer a great deal of hope to many couples."

ETHICAL ISSUES. While modern advances in fertility treatments offer a wealth of new possibilities, the other side of the coin is that they raise ethical concerns. "A number of religious groups have raised questions about the intervention of technology in the natural process of reproduction," Harkness explains. "There is also a theme of pronatalism at any cost here, emphasizing that to be complete as couples or as women, people absolutely must birth a biological child. Another big issue revolves around extending maternal age past nature's deadline of menopause. Before, women in their mid-forties probably weren't able to get pregnant because their bodies would stop that function. Now, it is possible for women in their fifties and sixties to become pregnant. This raises such questions as, Is that putting too much demand on their bodies? What about the age difference between them and their children? What about obligations to aging parents while having little ones in your midlife? Additionally, there is a legal and moral question revolving around the status of unused, frozen embryos in the event of death and divorce.

"There are further questions surrounding the availability of this expensive technology to those without the means or the medical insurance. Unfortunately, these treatments are quite expensive. From the moment you walk into a specialist's office asking for an evaluation, you start incurring costs in the hundreds of dollars for examinations and tests, all the way to thousands of dollars for the in vitro techniques. It's about $10,000 per cycle for a straight in vitro lab procedure, all the way up to $15,000 if egg donor in vitro fertilization is utilized."

Many women generally distrust scientific intervention. Problems with IUDs have caused pelvic inflammatory disease resulting in infertility. DES (diethystilbestrol, an estrogen replacement often used as a "morning-after" pill in the United States, even after it was linked to cancer and anomalies of the vagina and cervix) has been another big problem, as has thalidomide. Now there is a concern about using female hormones to stimulate ovulation. With most infertility treatments, whether the problem is due to the man or woman, it is mainly the women who undergo the drug treatments, the surgeries, and so forth. What are the long-term effects of exposing women to these drugs?

AN ALTERNATIVE APPROACH

Dr. Marjorie Ordene, a gynecologist from Brooklyn, New York, believes that while there is a place for technology in fertility, women are too quick to seek out these methods, and suggests trying these natural options first:

LEARNING TO RECOGNIZE OVULATION. Women should learn to recognize their time of ovulation by taking their temperature first thing in the morning, before getting out of bed: "Usually, temperature rises in the second half of the cycle, two weeks before menstruation. The mucus that is produced around the time of ovulation has a clear and slippery quality. This is the kind of mucus that is needed for the sperm to penetrate the cervix." *(See chapter 3, Birth Control.)*

HEALTHY LIFESTYLE. Women should follow a healthy diet and a basic exercise program.

EMOTIONAL AND SPIRITUAL WORK. Often, a woman has apprehensions about becoming pregnant that need to be addressed. It may be reassuring to talk to the inner child and let her know that even though there will be another child, the little girl in her will still get the attention she needs. This kind of spiritual work is often important in achieving pregnancy.

ORIENTAL NATUROPATHIC APPROACH

The traditional Eastern approach to fertility depends less on modern technology, and more on time-tested knowledge. Dr. Roger Hirsch, a naturopathic physician from Santa Monica, California, explains Chinese philosophy and infertility treatments based on this point of view: "We look at making the abdomen happy. This is an aphorism for correcting the digestion, menstruation, and hormones, so that women can conceive. Of course, raising the man's sperm count and sperm motility is important as well, because it is not just the woman who is infertile in an infertility situation. A key to this is the way the blood flows in the pelvic cavity."

INCREASING PELVIC BLOOD FLOW. A study of endometriosis-induced infertility was performed in China and published in the *Shanghai Journal of Traditional Chinese Medicine and Medicinals* in 1994. Forty patients were treated with neon laser acupuncture, retention enemas, and injection into the endometrial nodes with common sage root, which is a blood-vitalizing or blood-moving herb. In the forty patients treated, the size of lumps diminished and symptoms disappeared in seventeen. Thirteen women conceived. Among these, six had suffered from fallopian tube blockage and seven from ovulatory dysfunction. There was a total amelioration rate of 97.5 percent.

SEXUAL HYGIENE. Another important consideration in reversing endometriosis and infertility is good sexual hygiene. There was a study done with Israeli women several years ago that showed them to have a low percentage of endometriosis as a cultural group. This was related to sexual hygienic laws in the orthodox Jewish religion which says that you can't be with a man during menstruation. Chinese medicine says the same thing. Having intercourse during menstruation causes an imbalance of energy and results in the migration of endometrial tissue into the pelvic cavity.

HERBS. "In Chinese medicine, herbs are used to tone renal/adrenal function because reproductive function is related to the kidney and its related complex. The actual viability of the eggs for a woman over forty is related to kidney yang function.

One of the herbs very good for kidney yang is called *herba epimeti*, which translates in English to "horny goat weed." This is an aphrodisiac that the Chinese discovered by watching goats become sexually active after eating this particular plant. They put the plant into the herbal formula for women who are kidney yang deficient, and they noted that it increased sexual desire.

Deer antler is a renewable resource from the deer, which grows every year. *Lutaigou* is the gelatin that comes from boiling the deer antler. This is wonderful for helping women over forty who are trying to extend their egg-producing years. It helps slow down the biological clock.

In the European system, we have wormwood, which creates more circulation in the pelvic cavity. The Chinese use this along with daughter seed and fructose litchi, a little red berry.

A lot of people know about *dong quai*. This helps the circulation in the pelvic cavity. Also used is *cortex cinnamomi*, which is not the cinnamon you put in your mulled cider, but a thick bark cinnamon.

ACUPUNCTURE. In China, acupuncture has been used in the treatment of infertility for centuries. The first published account of this is seen in medical literature dating back to 11 A.D. The Chinese look at five principal organs—the liver, spleen, heart, lung, and kidney—and use acupuncture to release blockages from these systems so that energy or *chi* can move freely. This helps the body return to good health. Promoting fertility is one benefit that can be obtained.

Acupuncture to kidney points releases psychological blocks that interfere with reproduction. Dr. Hirsch uses the treatment to help patients overcome deep-rooted fears connected to sexual abuse: "If there has been early abuse, rape, or incest, there sometimes is a problem with hormone maturation. In other words, fear causes the hormones to become dormant. This is related to the kidney, as this organ controls reproductive function, endocrine function, and hormonal function. I needle points along the kidney meridian to help establish a connection between the heart and the uterus. I also use the Bach flower remedies walnut and crab apple. Walnut breaks links, and crab apple cleanses."

Dr. Hirsch connects another psychological issue—low self-esteem—to endometriosis and infertility: "In treating self-esteem issues, I work on the heart and kidney points. The acupuncture points that seem extremely valuable for this are pericardium 5 and 6. If a practitioner is having a problem with understanding whether or not a psychological issue is involved in the infertility, and the patient does not know what the issue is, pericardium 5 can be needled. If something is holding the person back, that will bring an event or dream to memory, and the patient will understand why she is stuck. In treating self-esteem issues, we may also release stress by needling the heart 7 point, heart 9, and sometimes heart 7 to heart 5.

"We also address conception vessel 17, which is between the breasts. This is a very important place for women because it opens their energy. It also helps relieve liver *chi* congestion or stuckness. Remember, the liver and the liver hormones, both in Chinese and Western medicine, govern the flow of blood in the pelvic cavity."

WESTERN NATUROPATHIC APPROACH

Dr. Joseph Pizzorno says that as a naturopath and midwife he saw numerous infertile couples and discovered two causes of the condition that were not generally recognized by the orthodox medical profession: "The first was pituitary insufficiency. The pituitary gland was not secreting enough of the hormones needed to stimulate the ovaries to mature, ripen and produce a viable ovum. Most of these women had been on birth control pills for long periods of time. Even though they had been off it for several years, their pituitary never functioned fully again.

"With these women I did two things. I gave them a herbal concoction using herbs that are commonly used for women's health problems, which are supposed to stimulate proper pituitary functioning. I also gave them raw pituitary gland from an animal. There were surprisingly good results with this treatment. A urine test beforehand measured the level of hormones from the pituitary. If a patient had low hormone levels, I would then use this protocol with them. A surprising number became pregnant once their urinary hormone levels returned to normal.

"The second major cause was pelvic inflammatory disease, where there were infections in the fallopian tubes, the little tubes that go from the uterus to the ovaries. Infections leave scars. Then the ovum cannot penetrate the tube and get into the uterus for fertilization.

"An age-old hydrotherapy procedure, called sitz bath, helps end this problem. A woman gets two big pots of water. (We use washtubs that are about three feet in diameter.) One tub gets filled with hot water (as hot as she can stand it). When a woman sits in it with her arms and legs out of the tub, the water level reaches her umbilicus. The other tub gets filled with ice cold water. That tub is filled to the point just below the umbilicus. In other words, there is more hot water than cold water. The woman sits in the hot water for five minutes, and then in the cold water for one minute. She alternates back and forth three times.

"The first time a woman does this, she will find it startling. But after a while she will actually start to like it. She does this every day. After a few treatments, she starts getting a discharge. As near as we can make out, this discharge is the body throwing off scar tissue and toxic material in the ovaries. This is a particularly dangerous time for a woman to have intercourse. The ovaries are starting to open up, and there is a high probability of an ectopic pregnancy. The egg will only be able to go partway down the tube since the tube is not yet open enough for it to get all the way into the uterus. We therefore tell women no unprotected intercourse for at least three months while doing these treatments every day. Again, a surprising number of them become pregnant."

RESTORING THYROID BALANCE. Even as far back as the 1930s, alleviating low thyroid conditions was found effective against infertility. Dr. Ray Peat says, "Over the last fifteen years, I have worked with quite a few women, some who have tried for as long as ten years to get pregnant. Several had spent as much as $100,000 on other treatments. Consistently, within a few weeks of correcting their thyroid, they get pregnant."

To keep thyroid levels up, women should snack frequently and eliminate unsaturated fats. Although touted as beneficial, recent studies show them to inhibit thyroid secretion. More high-quality protein may be needed, especially by women following a weight loss program or vegetarian diet. A daily minimum of 40 grams is recommended. Taking a thyroid supplement for a short period of time can greatly help. "People whose thyroid function is suppressed can benefit from a week or two of thyroid supplementation," Dr. Peat advises. "They don't need to take this indefinitely."

NATURAL HYGIENE. Anthony John Penepent, M.D. practices natural hygiene which he has known about his whole life. In fact, he says that it made his own birth possible: "Members of my family were natural hygienists before I was born. Back in the forties, my mother fasted for thirty days at Dr. Christopher John Cursio's hospital in Rochester, New York, the Castle of Health, so that she could conceive and retain pregnancy."

Today, Dr. Penepent follows the principles of natural hygiene when treating any medical condition: "Over the years, I have seen many wonderful things happen with natural hygiene which would not have been possible with allopathic medicine." Explaining infertility, Dr. Penepent says there are many causes, but that all of them can be treated similarly: "There are many mechanisms that can come into play. You can have basic amenorrhea or failure to ovulate. You can have any variety of hormonal imbalances, or fallopian tube obstruction. In 40 percent of the cases it is not the woman's fault, although she may take the blame to save her husband's ego. The man may have a low sperm count, depressed sperm motility, or abnormal sperm morphology. These are all possibilities. Then again, conception may occur but the egg or ovum may not have sufficient nutrients for the embryo to develop. What happens then is you have unrecognized spontaneous abortions that make it appear as if the woman is infertile, when in actuality she just has a nutritional deficiency.

"In many cases, an infertile woman can conceive and go on to have a successful pregnancy with a minor amount of dietary change. In the case of the fallopian tube obstruction, it may be necessary for her to fast for several days. I remember one patient, a rabbi's wife, who was childless. Because of their religious beliefs, it was absolutely essential for her to bear children. In her particular case, I put her on a fast for several days and followed that up with a nutritional regimen. She was able to conceive within six months."

SUPPLEMENTS. The right nutrients can make a difference in whether or not pregnancy is possible:

Colloidal silver. When chlamydia is causing infertility, colloidal silver helps to clean up the system.

Vitamin E. High doses of vitamin E balance hormone production. Under the guidance of a health care professional, an individual should start slowly and gradually increase dosage.

Zinc is particularly important for helping men to fertilize and mobilize sperm. Generally 50 mg are needed daily.

CONSUMER ADVOCACY GROUPS

Carla Harkness recommends becoming a part of a consumer advocacy group that can provide individuals and couples with support and information. One group, called Resolve, has its national office in Somerville, Massachusetts, and a string of chapters across the country: "Resolve is a great ally that provides literature, referrals, and legal advocacy to the infertile. Chances are, wherever you live, there's a chapter by you."

Herbal Pharmacy

Plants containing fertility-promoting phytochemicals, in order of potency:

> *Myrciaria dubia* (camu-camu)
> *Malpighia glabra* (acerola)
> *Cucurbita foetidissima* (buffalo gourd)
> *Rehmannia glutinosa* (Chinese foxglove)
> *Aloe vera* (bitter aloes)
> *Helianthus annuus* (sunflower)

Pinus pinea (Italian stone pine)
Ceratonia siliqua (carob)
Nigella sativa (black cumin)
Juglans cinerea (butternut)
Cnidoscolus chayamansa (chaya)
Citrullus vulgaris (watermelon)
Lupinus albus (white lupine)
Nasturtium officinale (berro)
Cucurbita pepo (pumpkin)
Cinamomum cassia (cassia)
Arachis hypogaea (peanut)
Momordica charantia (bitter melon)
Allium schoenoprasum (chives)
Sesamum indicum (sesame)

Hot News

Promising substances for the treatment of fertility are sarsaparilla root; kelp, which is used for this purpose in Asia; 6-methoxybenzoxazolinone (6-MBOA), a non-estrogenic component of young rapidly growing plants. Chinese drugs in combination with clomiphene citrate and progesterone have proved more effective than treatment with either Chinese or Western drugs alone, and a Chinese technique combining moxibustion and acupuncture has had some success in treating infertility. Factors shown to contribute to difficulty conceiving are smoking, even moderately; exposure to nitrous oxide; and environmental hazards like pesticides, methyl mercury, and lead in tap water. *(See below.)*

FROM THE MEDICAL LITERATURE ON INFERTILITY

NUTRITION

Vitamin C stimulates progesterone and oxytocin secretion, enhances the ovulation-inducing effects of clomiphene, and may reduce the frequency of birth defects.

M. R. Luck et al., "Ascorbic Acid and Fertility," *Biology of Reproduction* 52 (1995): 262–66.

Zinc is required in humans for ovulation and fertilization. Deficiencies of zinc during pregnancy can lead to growth retardation, toxemia, spontaneous abortions, prematurity, malformation, and complications during delivery. Studies have shown complications during pregnancy to be reduced by zinc supplementation.

A. Favier, "The Role of Zinc in Reproduction: Hormonal Mechanisms," *Biological Trace Element Research* 32 (1992): 363–82.

A study found that 48 infertile women had significantly lower copper concentrations than did controls. The authors suggest that low plasma copper concentrations can influence normal fertility in females.

M. H. Soltan and D. M. Jenkins, "Plasma Copper and Zinc Concentrations and Infertility," *British Journal of Obstet. Gynaecol.* 90, no. 5 (May 1983): 457–59.

Those countries with the greatest per capita milk consumption tend to show higher declines in female fertility with aging compared to countries consuming less milk.

D. W. Cramer et al., "Adult Hypoclasia, Milk Consumption, and Age-Specific Fertility," *American Journal of Epidemiology* 139, no. 3 (1994): 282–89.

Vitamin B12 therapy may help normalize reproductive function.

J. S. Sanfillippo and Y. K. Liu, "Vitamin B12 Deficiency and Infertility: Report of a Case," *International Journal of Fertility* 36, no. 1 (1991): 36–38.

A study documents the cases of three women suffering from infertility for years, two of whom were gluten-intolerant. All three became pregnant within 3 to 15 months following supplementation with 5 mg of folic acid 3 times a day, which normalized their blood chemistry.

D. W. Dawson and A. H. Sawers, "Infertility and Folate Deficiency: Case Reports," *British Journal of Obstet. Gynaecol.* 89 (1982): 678–80.

Supplementation with 100–800 mg of pyridoxine daily for 6 months, as treatment for PMS, resulted in the pregnancies of 12 out of 14 women who had been infertile for anywhere between 18 months to 7 years. B6 supplementation significantly increased progesterone levels in 5 of 7 women studied.

G. E. Abraham and J. T. Hargrove, *Medical World News* (March 19, 1979).

Iron and vitamin C play a role in fertility. Seven women who were part of a study of 113 women between the ages of 18 and 54 on hair loss became pregnant within 28 weeks after being treated with 35 mg of iron and 200 mg of vitamin C. Of these 7, 3 had suffered from infertility for 5 to 9 years, and none of the other 4 had become pregnant during the prior 30 months despite their efforts to do so and despite absence of menstrual problems.

D. H. Rushton et al., "Ferritin and Fertility," *Lancet* 337 (1991): 1554.

Fo-ti has been found to enhance fertility, according to the American Herbal Pharmacology Delegation.

Report of the American Herbal Pharmacology Delegation, National Academy of Sciences, 1975.

Steroid saponins and genins of sarsaparilla are similar to and are used in steroid sex hormone synthesis, which explains sarsaparilla root's use in treating infertility and venereal disease in many parts of the world. Another plant used to treat infertility is kelp, which is used for this purpose in Japan, China, and Malaysia.

D. B. Mowrey, *The Scientific Validation of Herbal Medicine* (New Canaan, Conn.: Keats Publishing, 1986): 153.

A study examined the effect of 6-methoxybenzoxazolinone (6-MBOA), a nonestrogenic component of young rapidly growing plants, on the reproductive responses of prepubertal and mature female rats, and found that it had a stimulatory effect in both.

G. M. Butterstein et al., "A Naturally Occurring Plant Compound, 6-Methoxybenzoxazolinone, Stimulates Reproductive Responses in Rats," *Biology of Reproduction* 32 (1985): 1018–23.

Fennel and anise are plants that have been used as estrogenic agents for millennia. They have been reputed to increase milk secretion, promote menstruation, facilitate birth, and increase libido. Research suggests the pharmacologically active agents of fennel and anise are polymers of anethole, such as dianethole and photoanethole.

M. Albert-Puleo, "Fennel and Anise as Estrogenic Agents," *Journal of Ethnopharmacology* 2 (1980): 337–44.

BODY WEIGHT

A study demonstrated that a 0.1-unit increase in waist-hip ratio in women seeking artificial insemination for the first time resulted in a 30 percent reduction in the likelihood of conception per cycle. Based on these results, the authors conclude that body fat distribution in reproductive-aged women is a more important factor in fertility than age or obesity.

B. M. Zaadstra et al., "Fat and Female Fecundity: Prospective Study of Effect of Body Fat Distribution on Conception Rates," *British Medical Journal* 306 (February 20, 1993): 484–87.

In a study involving 276 infertile women with evidence of ovulatory dysfunction, results showed that approximately 6 percent of primary infertility with the presence of ovulatory dysfunction is caused by being excessively underweight, and another 6 percent stems from being excessively overweight.

B. B. Green et al., "Risk of Ovulatory Infertility in Relation to Body Weight," *Fertility and Sterility* 50, no. 9 (1988): 621–26.

RELAXATION

In a study, 34 percent of infertile women completing a relaxation-response-based behavioral treatment program became pregnant within six months. Statistically significant improvements were also reported with respect to decreases in anxiety, depression, and fatigue, as well as to increased vigor.

A. D. Domar et al., "The Mind-Body Program for Infertility; A New Behavioral Approach for Women with Infertility," *Fertility and Sterility* 53, no. 2 (February 1990): 246-49.

TRADITIONAL CHINESE MEDICINE

When the herbal medicine Hachimijiogan was given orally to two hyperprolactinemic infertile women, a reduction in serum prolactin level was seen in both, and both became pregnant following a normalization of ovulatory cycle.

S. Usuki et al., "Treatment with Hachimijiogan, a Non-ergot Chinese Herbal Medicine, in Two Hyperprolactinemic Infertile Women," *Acta Obstet. Gynecol. Scand.* 68, no. 5 (1989): 475–78.

Zhibai dihuang pills were successfully used to treat 8 immunologically infertile couples with antisperm and/or anitzona pellucida antibodies in their blood serum. Study results: Over 80 percent of the couples achieved successful pregnancies within 9 months.

D. J. Li et al., [Treatment of Immunological Infertility with Chinese Medicinal Herbs of Ziyin Jianghuo], *Chung Kuo Chung Hsi I Chieh Ho Tsa Chih* 15, no. 1 (January 1995): 3–5.

Traditional Chinese herbs were used to treat infertility by regulating the menstrual cycle and tonifying the kidney. Basal body temperature was significantly increased by treatment, there was improvement in the hyperthermal phase 7–8 days following ovulation, and a 56 percent pregnancy rate was achieved in uncomplicated cases of luteal-phase defect.

F. Lian, "TCM Treatment of Luteal Phase Defect–An Analysis of 60 Cases," *Journal of Traditional Chinese Medicine* 11, no. 2 (June 1991): 115–20.

Treatment of sterility with Chinese drugs in combination with clomiphene citrate and progesterone proved to be significantly more effective than treatment with either Chinese or Western drugs alone. The combination resulted in a 57 percent pregnancy rate.

Z. Wang, "Clinical Observation on the Effects of Combined Traditional Chinese and Western Medicine Therapy for Excessive Suppressive Syndrome," *Journal of Traditional Chinese Medicine* 14, no. 4 (December 1994): 247–53.

ACUPUNCTURE

A study found that auricular acupuncture was capable of producing results comparable to those of drug therapy in the treatment of infertility.

I. Gerhard and F. Postneek, [Possibilities of Therapy by Ear Acupuncture in Female Sterility], *Geburtshilfe Frauenheilke* 48, no. 3 (March 1988): 165–71.

A study examined the effects of moxibustion and acupuncture on 30 cases of infertility in women ranging from 24 to 37 years of age. Results showed that after just one course of treatment 9 women conceived, with another 8 conceiving after 2 courses of treatment.

Shi Zhen-dong and Shi Ya-ping, [The Acupuncture and Moxibustion Treatment of 30 Cases of Female Infertility,] *Shang Haie Zhen Jiu Za Zhi* 1 (1994): 17–18.

RISK FACTORS

A study of 45 infertile women with a mean age of 31 and a mean infertility duration of 4 years found that smoking was associated with a two-thirds reduction in the normal rate of egg fertilization.

S. K. Rosevear et al., "Smoking and Decreased Fertilization Rates in Vitro," *Lancet* 340 (November 14, 1992): 1195–96.

A study showed there to be a 31 percent difference in fertility rates between nonsmoking couples and couples in which both the man and the woman smoke.

D. J. Rowlands et al., "Smoking and Decreased Fertilization Rates in Vitro," *Lancet* 340 (December 5, 1992): 1409–10.

Smoking reduced the fertility of women who drank a minimum of 8 cups of coffee or tea per day, whereas no such effects of caffeine were found in nonsmokers, a study found.

Jorn Olsen, "Cigarette Smoking, Tea and Coffee Drinking, and Subfecundity," *American Journal of Epidemiology* 133, no. 7 (1991): 734–39.

Smokers—regardless of coffee consumption—had only half the fertility of women who neither smoked nor drank coffee, a study revealed. Such effects were seen in women smoking as few as 1 to 9 cigarettes daily.

Ethel Alderete et al., "Effect of Cigarette Smoking and Coffee Drinking on Time to Conception," *Epidemiology* 6 (1995): 403–8.

Cigarette smoking can lead to diminished ovarian reserve.

F. I. Sharara et al., "Cigarette Smoking Accelerates the Development of Diminished Ovarian Reserve by the Clomiphene Citrate Challenge Test," *Fertility and Sterility* 62, no. 5 (August 1994): 257–62.

A study on the relationship between caffeine and fertility found that tea consumption had minimal effects compared to soft drinks, which showed a major relationship to decreases in fertility. Controlling for other factors, just one caffeinated soft drink per day was associated with a reduced monthly chance of conception of 50 percent.

A. J. Wilcox and C. R. Weinberg, "Tea and Fertility," *Lancet* 337 (May 11, 1991): 1159–60.

Noting the fact that 15 percent of all couples are infertile and more than 50 percent of conceptions result in spontaneous abortions, a study examined the relationship between infertility and stress. Women from a university medical school fertility and endocrinology center were evaluated relative to controls, with results suggesting that psychosocial stress is a significant factor in some types of infertility.

S. K. Wasser et al., "Psychosocial Stress as the Cause of Infertility," *Fertility and Sterility* 59, no. 3 (March 1993): 685–89.

Moderate alcohol consumption can increase the likelihood of certain kinds of infertility, and any alcohol greatly increases the risk of endometriosis, a controlled study indicated.

Francine Grostein et al., "Infertility in Women and Moderate Alcohol Use," *American Journal of Public Health* 84, no. 9 (September 1994): 1429–32.

Numerous environmental and endocrine factors influence reproduction. Examples include stress, smoking, drug addiction, obesity, nutrition, alcohol, pharmaceutical agents, pesticides, and industrial toxins.

Alex Vermeulen, "Environment, Human Reproduction, Menopause and Andropause," *Environmental Health Prospectives Supplements* 101, suppl. 2 (1993): 91–100.

There are numerous environmental hazards that women planning to conceive should be aware of, such as pesticides, methyl mercury, and lead in tap water. The following telephone hot lines can be called for more information: the National Pesticides Telecommunications Network, at 800-858-7378; the U.S. Environmental Protection Agency Safe Drinking Water hot line, at 800-426-4791; and the National Institutes for Occupational Safety and Health hot line, at 800-356-4674.

"Environmental Hazards May Endanger Conception," *Medical Tribune* (June 2, 1994): 12.

A study documents the association between nitrous oxide exposure and fertility difficulties. Results from questionnaires mailed to 7,000 dental assistants in California showed that high-level exposure to nitrous oxide was significantly related to problems with fertility.

A. S. Roland et al., "Reduced Fertility Among Women Employed as Dental Assistants Exposed to High Levels of Nitrous Oxide," *New England Journal of Medicine* 327, no. 14 (October 1, 1992): 993–97.

Smoking marijuana results in an increase in fertility risk, especially among women using the drug within a year of trying to conceive. Cocaine significantly increases the odds of tubal abnormality as a cause of infertility.

B. A. Mueller et al., "Recreational Drug Use and the Risk of Primary Infertility," *Epidemiology* 1, no. 3 (May 1990): 195–200.

DES (DIETHYLSTILBESTROL)

Five to 10 million U.S. women received DES during pregnancy or were exposed to it in utero. Many of the mothers were unaware of their exposure. There is an increased risk of clear-cell cervicovaginal cancer (ccc) in DES daughters.

R. M. Giusti, "Diethylstilbestrol Revisited: A Review of the Long-Term Health Effects," *Annals of Internal Medicine* 15, no. 122 (1995): 778–88.

A study of the records of 186 women with vaginal cancer, compared to the records of 1,772 women without cancer, showed that vaginal bleeding during pregnancy reduced the effect of DES and decreased the risk of vaginal tumors.

G. B. Sharp and P. Cole, "Vaginal Bleeding and Diethylstilbestrol Exposure During Pregnancy: Relationship to Genital Tract Clear Cell Adenocarcinoma and Vaginal Adenosis in Daughters," *American Journal of Obstetrics and Gynecology* 162 (April 1990): 994–1001.

It is possible that the cancer-causing effect of DES could be inherited from generation to generation. A study on mice showed that the cancer-causing effects of DES resulted in increased cancer levels in the third generation. The DES could affect the animals' germ cells—the cells with reproductive function.

"Does the Legacy of DES Continue?" *Cancer Biotechnology Weekly* (July 10, 1995): 6–7.

A study of 2,500 exposed and 2,500 unexposed females over 20 years showed that the relative risk of breast cancer from DES was approximately 1.35 (a modest but statistically signficant increased risk).

Theodore Colton et al., "Breast Cancer in Mothers Prescribed Diethylstilbestrol in Pregnancy: Further Follow-up," *JAMA* 269, no. 16 (April 28, 1993): 2096–2100.

Vitamin C reduced tumors from estradiol or DES by 50 percent in hamsters. This vitamin prevents tumors that would otherwise have been induced by estrogen.

J. G. Liehr, "Vitamin C Reduces the Incidences and Severity of Renal Tumors Induced by Estradiol and Diethylstilbestrol," *American Journal of Clinical Nutrition* 54 (1991): 1256–60S.

The National Institutes of Health recommendations for DES mothers are as follows: monthly breast self-exam, annual breast exam, follow established recommendations for mammography. Their recommendations for DES daughters: careful inspection of cervix and vagina using half-strength aqueous Lugol and palpation of entire vaginal wall, annual Pap smear, vaginal cytologic tests and colposopy if results warrant it, biopsy as indicated, and treat as high-risk obstetric patients because of increased risk of spontaneous abortions, ectopic pregnancy, early cervical effacement, and premature labor.

R. M. Giusti, "Diethylstilbestrol Revisited: A Review of the Long-Term Health Effects," *Annals of Internal Medicine* 15, no. 122 (1995): 778–88.

15. LUPUS

Lupus, an autoimmune disorder affecting four times more women than men, can be mild or life-threatening; it affects 1 out of 130 women between the ages of 20 and 40. Females of African, Native American, and Asian descent develop the condition more frequently than those of European ancestry.

Causes

Although the exact cause of this swelling disease is unknown, hormones are believed to aggravate it, particularly estrogen, which is why so many women are affected. Symptoms may be exacerbated by infections, extreme stress, antibiotics, and certain other drugs.

Symptoms

Initial signs include arthritis, a red skin rash across the bridge of the nose and on the cheeks, weakness, prolonged and extreme fatigue, and weight loss. There may also be fever over 100 degrees, light sensitivity, skin sores on the neck, hair loss, chest pain, Raynaud's disease (a constriction of circulation in the extremities that causes fingers to turn white or blue in the cold), anger, depression, anemia, and seizures if the central nervous system is involved. Additional symptoms include mouth or nose ulcers, and a nail fungus, which is an outgrowth of *Candida albicans*. Often lupus sufferers have headaches. If skin sores spread to other tissues in the body, tissue wasting may occur.

Clinical Experience

TRADITIONAL WESTERN TREATMENT
Steroid drugs are usually prescribed for internal and external use. Long-term use of these medications can damage the liver and weaken the bones.

NATUROPATHIC TREATMENT

HERBS AND SUPPLEMENTS. To lessen inflammation: pycnogenol, cat's claw, black walnut, omega-3 fatty acids, and flaxseed oil. Pau d'arco and aloe vera juice act as blood cleansers. A good nervous system tonic is gota kola. Colloidal silver is antibacterial, antifungal, and antiarthritic.

ACUPUNCTURE. Acupuncturist and massage therapist Gina Michaels, of New York City, explains that she attunes her acupuncture treatments to the patient's unique profile: "The Chinese recognize that there are different kinds of arthritis. One type is from heat and wind, another from cold and damp. Western pharmacopeia treat them all the same, but we make a differentiation according to the symptoms that the client is displaying. Then a strategy is formed.

"Each decision an acupuncturist makes looks at the large picture. For example, if the person has a headache, along which meridian is that headache located? Is it the gallbladder channel? The stomach channel? Are they having other symptoms, such as fever or sweat? Is the central nervous system affected? All of this is very, very important in deciding what treatment protocol to choose.

"There are eight meridians formed during conception that go to a very deep constitutional level. Treating these is very useful for illnesses that are systemic or of a much deeper nature."

DIET. The diet should be high in vegetables and low in grains. Wheat grass is excellent for reducing inflammation. Foods detrimental to healing include alfalfa sprouts, which can produce inflammation, as well as peanuts, bread, corn, soybeans, and other foods that can produce fungi and molds. In addition, alcohol, spinach, and carrots may aggravate the condition. Acid-producing foods, such as orange juice, meat, and dairy, can also be harmful.

EXERCISE. Regular exercise is important, because it helps to keep the joints moving.

STRESS MANAGEMENT. Lupus can flare up during times of dire stress. Working at a job one dislikes can be a contributing factor, for example. It is important for people to examine their lives and to create circumstances that promote health and happiness.

AROMATHERAPY. Essential oils can help calm the emotions and eliminate flare-ups. Rubbing tree oils, such as pine and cedar, directly onto the joints can diminish swelling. A drop of chamomile, lavender, lilac, or neroli can be placed on the palms and breathed in for relaxation. When there is chest congestion, eucalyptus is excellent for clearing the nasal passages and lungs.

Herbal Pharmacy

Plants containing phytochemicals with antilupus properties, in order of potency:

>*Portulaca oleracea* (purslane)
>*Triticum aestivum* (wheat)

Ipomoea aquatica (swamp cabbage)
Morinda citrifolia (Indian mulberry)
Chrysanthemum coronarium (garland chrysanthemum)
Rumex acetosa (garden sorrel)
Luffa aegyptiaca (luffa)
Mimosa pudica (sensitive plant)
Peperomia pereskiifola (perejil)
Hibiscus rosa-sinensis (Chinese hibiscus)
Zizyphus jujuba (black date)
Basella alba (vinespinach)
Daucas carota (carrot)
Tropaeolum majus (nasturtium)
Hordeum vulgare (barley)
Symphytum offinale (comfrey)
Cinnamomum cassia (cassia)
Centella asiatica (gota kola)

Hot News

Lupus has responded well to dietary supplementation, especially of fatty acids; also fish oil, MaxEPA (eicosapentaenoic acid), selenium, flaxseed oil, alpha-linolenic acid, and large doses of vitamins A and E. Skin lesions of discoid lupus patients have responded to IV injections of nicotinamide and to beta carotene supplementation. *(See below.)*

FROM THE MEDICAL LITERATURE ON LUPUS

NUTRITION/DIET

Mice with lupus were helped to live longer by being fed diets supplemented with flaxseed and rich in alpha-linolenic acid and plant lignans.

A. V. Hall et al., "Abrogation of MRL/lpr Lupus Nephritis by Dietary Flaxseed," *American Journal of Kidney Diseases* 22, no. 2 (August 1993): 326–32.

In a double-blind, placebo-controlled crossover study, lupus erythematosus patients received 20g per day of MaxEPA (eicosapentaenoic acid) as part of a low-fat isoenergetic diet. Results showed that after 34 weeks, 14 of the 17 patients receiving the MaxEPA benefited significantly from the treatment, as opposed to the 13 patients who received the placebo.

A. J. Walton et al., "Dietary Fish Oil and the Severity of Symptoms in Patients with Systemic Lupus Erythematosus," *Annals of Rheumatism Disease* 50, no. 7 (July 1991): 463–66.

A study found that autoimmune lupus is suppressed in mice by fish oil supplementation as the exclusive source of lipid.

V. E. Kelley et al., "A Fish Oil Diet Rich in Eicosapentaenoic Acid Reduces Cyclooxygenase Metabolites, and Suppresses Lupus in MRL-lpr Mice," *Journal of Immunology* 134, no. 3 (March 1985): 1914–19.

A study looked at the effect of dietary fatty acids on systemic lupus erythematosus in mice following the onset of disease. Results showed that dietary restriction improved survival and that mice receiving a fish oil diet benefited significantly.

J. Watson et al., "The Therapeutic Effects of Dietary Fatty Acid Supplementation in the Autoimmune Disease of the MRL-mp-lpr/lpr Mouse," *International Journal of Immunopharmacology* 10, no. 4 (1988): 467–71.

Selenium, administered in doses of 4 parts per million in drinking water, improved the survival time for autoimmune mice with lupuslike disease, relative to controls. Selenium increased the natural killer cell activity in the treated mice.

J. R. O'Dell et al., "Improved Survival in Murine Lupus as the Result of Selenium Supplementation," *Clinical Exp. Immunology* 73, no. 2 (August 1988): 322–27.

Studies of diet in mice models of systemic lupus erythematosus have established the beneficial effects of a low-calorie, low-fat diet, as well as the importance of the specific sources of dietary fat.

L. C. Corman, "The Role of Diet in Animal Models of Systemic Lupus Erythematosus: Possible Implications for Human Lupus," *Seminars in Arthritis and Rheumatism* 15, no. 1 (August 1985): 61–69.

A study found that doses of 100,000 IU daily of vitamin A, taken for 2 weeks, enhanced the immune systems of lupus patients.

C. V. Vien et al., "Effect of Vitamin A Treatment on the Immune Reactivity of Patients with Systemic Lupus Erythematosus," *Journal of Clinical Laboratory Immunology* 26, no. 1 (May 1988): 33–35.

Lupus erythematosus patients given daily IV injections of nicotinamide were shown to experience improvement in skin lesions as soon as one day following the first injection. Lesions continued to improve over time with the treatment, but never disappeared entirely.

I. Dainow, "Recherches Clinques Sur Certaines Proprietes Anti-Allergiques de la Nicotinamide," *Z Vitaminforsch* 15 (1944): 245–50.

Three SLE patients who had previously not benefited from oral and intramuscular vitamin E experienced a total disappearance of lesions following 6 weeks of intramuscular B12 supplementation.

M. T. Block, "Vitamin E in the Treatment of Diseases of the Skin," Clinical Medicine, January 1953, pp. 31–34.

Lupus erythematosus patients given 10–15 g daily of pantothenic acid and 1,000–2,000 mg daily of vitamin E experienced major benefits from the treatment, with discoid lupus patients demonstrating improvement after 4–6 months, disseminated discoid lupus patients in 2 months, and subacute disseminated patients in 1 month.

A. L. Welsh, "Lupus Erythematosus: Treatment by Combined Use of Massive Amounts of Pantothenic Acid and Vitamin E," *Arch. Dermatol. Syphilol.* 70 (1954): 181–98.

Fifty milligrams of beta carotene administered daily was shown to effectively clear all lesions within a week in three patients with treatment-resistant chronic discoid lupus bothered by sun exposure.

P. C. H. Newbold, "Beta Carotene in the Treatment of Discoid Lupus Erythematosus," *British Journal of Dermatology* 95 (1976): 100–101.

A study showed the efficacy of nutritional supplementation and food eliminations in bringing on remissions in patients with systemic lupus erythematosus and in those suffering from lupus-like symptoms.

H. M. Cooke and C. M. Reading, "Dietary Intervention in Systemic Lupus Erythematosus: 4 Cases of Clinical Remission and Reversal of Abnormal Pathology," *Int. Clin. Nutr. Rev.* 5, no. 4 (1985): 166–76.

Results of a placebo-controlled study showed that women suffering from mild to moderate lupus who were administered 200 mg/day of DHEA for 3 months experienced fewer flare-ups and showed more overall improvement than did controls.

"DHEA May Be Effective in Systemic Lupus Erythematosus," *American Family Physician* 49, no. 1 (1994): 197.

Ten women with systemic lupus erythematosus took 200 mg of DHEA for 3 months. Improvements were seen in the SLE Disease Activity Scores, and general assessments from physicians were improved as well, in all cases. Cortiscosteroid dosages decreased also.

R. F. Vollenhoven et al., "An Open Study of Dehydroepiandrosterone in Systemic Lupus Erythematosus," *Arthr. Rheum.* 37 (1994): 1305–10.

TRADITIONAL CHINESE MEDICINE

Preliminary studies have produced evidence supporting the use of the following herbs in the treatment of systemic lupus erythematosus: *Atractylodes ovata, Angelic sinensis, Cordyceps sinensis, Ligustrum lucidum, Codonopsia pilosula.*

J. R. Chen et al., "The Effects of Chinese Herbs on Improving Survival and Inhibiting Anti-ds DNA Antibody Production in Lupus Mice," *American Journal of Chinese Medicine* 21, no. 3–4 (1993): 257–62.

A study examined the efficacy of combining Western medicine and traditional Chinese medicine in treating lupus nephritis. Results: Treatment with the combined approach was superior to that with just Western medicine alone.

R. G. Ye et al., [Therapy of Integrated Traditional Chinese Medicine and Western Medicine on 74 Lupus Nephritis Patients], *Chung Kuo Chung Hsi I Chieh Ho Tsa Chih* 14, no. 6 (June 1994): 343–45, 324.

Lupus nephritis patients received cyclophosphamide (CTX) and traditional Chinese medicine (TCM) in a study in which controls received only the CTX. After six months, the CTX and TCM group experienced significantly more therapeutic benefits than did the controls.

J. Ruan and R. G. Ye, [Lupus Nephritis Treated with Impact Therapy of Cyclophosphamide and Traditional Chinese Medicine], *Chung Kuo Chung Hsi I Chieh Ho Tsa Chih* 14, no. 5 (May 1994): 276–78, 260.

A study showed that preincubation of peripheral blood mononuclear cells with *Astragalus membranaceus* and *Tripterygium hypoglaucum*, or a combination of the two, stimulated natural killer cell cytotoxicity in both healthy volunteers and systemic lupus erythematosus patients.

X. Z. Zhao, [Effects of Astragalus Membranaceus and Tripterygium Hypoglaucum on Natural Killer Cell Activity of Peripheral Blood Mononuclear in Systemic Lupus Erythematosus], *Chung Kuo Chung Hsi I Chieh Ho Tsa Chih* 12, no. 11 (November 1992): 669–71, 645.

Findings of researchers working with autoimmune-prone mice support traditional Chinese herbal medicines, specifically sairei-to, as a promising systemic lupus erythematosus treatment.

H. Kanauchi et al., "Evaluation of the Japanese-Chinese Herbal Medicine, Kampo, for the Treatment of Lupus Dermatoses in Autoimmune Prone MRL/Mp-lpr/lpr Mice," *Journal of Dermatology* 21, no. 12 (December 1994): 935–39.

In a study, 24 of 27 discoid lupus patients who received 30–60 g in divided doses of *Tripterygium wilfordi* roots and stems over a 14-day period experienced improvement, the majority within 2–4 weeks of treatment.

Q. Wanzhang et al., "Clinical Observations on *Tripterygium Wilfordi* in Treatment of 26 Cases of Discoid Erythematosus," *Journal of Traditional Chinese Medicine* 3, no. 2 (1983): 131–32.

In a study, 103 patients with systemic lupus erythematosus were successfully treated with daily doses of 20–45 g of the Chinese herb *Triptergyium ilfordii* over one month. Over 90 percent showed improvements of symptoms, laboratory findings, and immunologic changes.

Q. Wanzhang et al., "*Tripterygium Wilfordii* Hook F in Systemic Lupus Erythematosus: Report of 103 Cases," *Chinese Medical Journal* 94 (1981): 827–34.

16. MENOPAUSE

Menopause marks the end of the female reproductive cycle, which typically occurs between the ages of forty-five and fifty but can happen anywhere from forty to sixty, or earlier as a result of surgery or illness. Perimenopause, the beginning stage, normally occurs over a period of years, and may take as long as a decade. Many women harbor misconceptions about the nature and effects of menopause; in cultures where menopause is less feared, symptoms are virtually nonexistent, and in fact menopause is anticipated as a rite of passage into a stronger, wiser time of life.

Causes

During menopause, the ovaries shut down, and estrogen, a hormone produced by the ovaries, diminishes and eventually stops. The symptoms of menopause are the result of the body's readjustment to the absence of estrogen.

Symptoms

One of the first symptoms perimenopausal women experience is a change in the frequency of their menstrual cycle. The time between cycles may increase or decrease, or it may skip a month. Usually blood flow is reduced, but, occasionally, women experience heavy, irregular bleeding. Another common symptom is hot flashes. Additionally, women may experience dry skin, mood swings, depression, irritability, vaginal dryness, night sweats, bladder infection, fatigue, and sleep disturbances.

Before menopause, estrogen is produced by the ovaries; afterward the adrenal glands take over. Women with healthy adrenal glands at menopause therefore experience less traumatic changes.

Clinical Experience

MISCONCEPTIONS ABOUT MENOPAUSE

MENOPAUSE CAUSES A LOSS OF SEX DRIVE. According to clinical psychologist Dr. Janice Stefanacci, society expects menopausal women to lose their sex drive, but this does not have to be the case. "Many women fear that they are going to lose their passion and sexuality. Really, only a small portion of women who go through menopause have their sex drive adversely affected. For these women who lose their sexual desire or have difficulty becoming and staying aroused, help is available. But most women do not experience sexual arousal problems, and many report feeling more sexual because the risk of pregnancy is gone."

MENOPAUSE CREATES PSYCHOLOGICAL PROBLEMS. Dr. Linda Ojeda, author of *Menopause Without Medicine*, says many women see menopause as the beginning of the end. "They believe that life is going to be downhill from this point on. They no longer think of themselves as youthful, as able to contribute to society. They fear that their behavior will become erratic, hysterical, and out of control. This is not true. When we reach fifty, we do not turn into these raging maniacs, and we are not more susceptible to clinical depression. In some women, however, lowered levels of estrogen, endorphins, and serotonin, the hormones that affect mood, can create mood swings. Levels can be raised naturally in these women.

"We know that beliefs and attitudes affect the transition," she continues. "In Asian countries, symptoms are virtually nonexistent. In these countries, menopause is looked at as an important event in a woman's life. She now has more prestige and is viewed as a wise, older woman. Women anticipate this time of life with relish. If you are approaching menopause with fear and trepidation, you need to examine your attitude."

MENOPAUSE IS A DISEASE. The medical community has created this belief by stressing the need for hormone replacement therapy. In reality, menopause is not a disease but a natural transition that should be dealt with naturally. Dr. Ojeda wants women to know that there is a science behind safe, effective, holistic methods for helping women through this transition period easily.

DANGERS OF HORMONE REPLACEMENT THERAPY

Dr. Bruce Hedendal of Boca Raton, Florida, expresses concern regarding hormone replacement therapy as it is practiced in this country today. "The powers that be would like us to believe that they are using hormones. They are if your own body is making them, or if they are from plant estrogen sources, like soy products and yams. But Premarin, the most commonly given synthetic, is actually from pregnant mares' urine. Ten million women take Premarin in pill or patch form.

"Most people are told that estrogen prevents osteoporosis. This is true to some degree. Around menopause, the benefits of synthetic estrogen replacement therapy is effective for five to seven years only. It slows down the bone loss, but it does not reverse it in any way, shape, or form. The studies have shown that eight to ten years after menopause is finished, there are no benefits to estrogen replacement therapy on bone loss.

"The average woman would be surprised to learn that synthetic estrogen has some very serious side effects. I've talked with a lot of holistic doctors. Their opinion is that synthetic estrogen has definitely been shown to increase the risk of cancer of the breast. They have been toying with this concept for years. Of course, the makers of Premarin and other synthetics say no, but the research now confirms this as true. A recent study published in the *New England Journal of Medicine* proves an increased risk of breast cancer, almost 33 percent, in post-menopausal women using hormone replacement therapy."

Dr. Robert Atkins, director of the Atkins Centers for Complementary Medicine, adds that estrogen therapy has one side effect that people don't talk about: insulin resistance. "This syndrome is characterized by low blood sugar, high blood pressure, or high insulin levels. But the most frightening one of all to most women has to do with upper body obesity." The good news is that natural therapies often make the need for synthetic estrogens unnecessary.

NATURAL THERAPIES THAT WORK

DIET. Jane Guiltinan, a naturopathic physician from Seattle, Washington, says, "A lot of women don't know that there may be alternatives to estrogen replacement therapy. There are some very good plant sources of estrogens in some of our foods. In fact, you can get significant amounts of plant estrogens. They have been shown in several research studies to improve menopausal symptoms.

"The food that has the highest content of estrogen is soy. Soybeans, tofu, tempeh—anything made with soy—will contain plant estrogens. Oats, cashews, almonds, alfalfa, apples, and flax seeds contain smaller amounts of estrogen. A woman emphasizing those foods in the diet can experience significant decreases in her hot flashes."

Studies suggest that too little magnesium in the diet causes hot flashes. Magnesium can be found in whole grains and beans and soy products.

Sugar, which can cause hot flashes and other menopausal symptoms, should be avoided. Sugar, coffee, and alcohol adversely affect the blood sugar and can disturb the emotions.

VITAMINS AND MINERALS. The following nutrients provide an additional boost to good health in the menopausal years:

Multivitamins. Women need a natural multivitamin/mineral supplement containing higher amounts of magnesium than calcium, and high amounts of B and C vitamins. A good multiple vitamin helps build the adrenal glands, which lessens emotional symptoms.

Vitamin E. This vitamin is known for its ability to rejuvenate the reproductive system and alleviate hot flashes. Low amounts of FSH and LH are related to hot flashes, and Vitamin E helps to increase levels of these brain hormones. It also helps lessen vaginal thinning and dryness. Mixed (beta, delta, and gamma) tocopherols are best as they are found together in nature. D-alpha tocopherol is also preferred over synthetic vitamin E. Generally, 400 IU per day should be taken in the beginning. The dosage can be gradually increased to 600 IU, although some women may need up to 800 IU.

Zinc. This mineral supports ovarian function. A good source is zinc picolinate. It can also be taken as an amino acid chelate or as zinc methionine. Twenty-five to 30 mg per day is generally needed.

B complex. B-complex vitamins are important throughout life, but there is an extra need for these during menopause. They can be obtained from whole grains, and green vegetables. B5 and B6 are especially helpful during menopause (300–400 mg B5, 150 mg B6 per day). Folic acid, in prescription doses, is a valuable replacement for female hormones, according to Dr. Carlton Fredericks.

Essential fatty acids. EFAs, which are precursors to the natural hormones in the body, are very important for both men and women. People on low-fat diets should pay special attention to this. A diet too low in fats can lead to an increased risk of cancer and aging. Omega-6 fatty acids can be found in flaxseed, sesame, pumpkin, and safflower oils. Omega-3 fatty acids are found in fish oil capsules or fish. Both are needed. EFAs help prevent or treat vaginal dryness.

Vitamin D. The best source of vitamin D is sunlight. It can also be taken in supplementation (400–600 IU per day), although caution should be taken not to get too much of this vitamin. Another source of vitamin D is salmon oil. People living in polluted environments need more vitamin D.

Calcium. Calcium is essential for the prevention of osteoporosis; supplementation should begin before the onset of menopause. There are many forms to choose from. Dairy is a poor source because many people have an intolerance to it. Calcium citrate is easy to digest, as it is already in an acidic medium. Calcium carbonates are alkaline and therefore more difficult to digest. Amino acid chelate is an excellent source of calcium. Calcium lactate is another good source. Calcium gluconate can be made into a powder and mixed into drinks; 1300 mg per day, from food and supplemental sources, is the recommended dosage. If it is not being absorbed well, more may be required. Each person should be analyzed to see the amount needed.

Gammalinolenic acid (GLA). This is available as evening primrose oil, borage oil, or blackcurrant-seed oil; 200 mg per day is recommended.

Boron. Research shows boron to be a precursor of both female and male hormones.

OTHER SUPPLEMENTS. Additional products that help create hormones:

Pregnelalone. Taking 25–30 mg a day serves helps the body create female hormones.

DHEA. Natural DHEA, found in wild yam extract preparations, rejuvenates the body.

Progesterone cream or serum. Progesterone is a woman's rejuvenating hormone, which protects against cancer and fibrocystic cysts and increases the beneficial effects of thyroid hormone. In addition, it guards against osteoporosis by putting calcium back in the bones. After menopause, progesterone can be taken three or four weeks out of the month. Wild yam cream contains progesterone, and can be purchased over the counter. Oral natural progesterone can also be taken.

Estriol. This is a natural, friendly estrogen that has been shown to inhibit breast tumors in animals. Some gynecologists are beginning to recommend Estriol for menopausal women, as being safer and more effective than synthetics.

Triple Estrogen. This formula is 80 percent estriol. The remaining 20 percent is made from estrone and estradiol. Estriol provides protection from breast tumors. Together, estrone and estradiol help protect against osteoporosis and cardiovascular problems. There are no negative side effects.

HERBS.

Chaste berry. Sold under the trade name, Vitex, chaste berry is commonly referred to as the menopausal herb because it alleviates many symptoms, including hot flashes, vaginal dryness, and mood swings. It works by raising the progesterone level.

Ginkgo biloba. Studies demonstrate ginkgo's effectiveness in leveling mood swings.

Ginseng normalizes brain hormones. It balances body temperature and is effective in preventing hot flashes.

Wild yam contains beneficial progesterone, the precursor of estrogen. This gives a woman the building blocks needed to create more hormones.

The following herbs may also prove beneficial: licorice root, black cohosh, *dong quai*, alfalfa, red clover, sarsaparilla, and blessed thistle.

HOMEOPATHY

The homeopathic remedy chosen should correspond to the symptoms described. According to Ken Korins, a classically trained homeopathic physician in New York City, only one should be used for best results. Sometimes it's a matter of trial and error; if one does not work, another can be tried. These are some of the remedies Dr. Korins recommends for menopause:

REMEDIES FOR HOT FLASHES:

Lachasis. Heat is felt all day long, while cold flashes may be experienced at night. Once the flow begins, all the symptoms disappear. Symptoms are worse with pressure and heat, and better with the onset of discharges or flows. Increased sexual desire is also associated with a need for lachasis.

Belladonna. There are many hot flashes. The face looks red and feels hot, and there is hot perspiration coming from the face and a pounding, throbbing, congested feeling in the head. Often there is dryness. Condition improves with resting quietly in the dark. Symptoms worsen with light, cold air, and sudden jolts. Emotionally, the state can border on hysteria with rages.

Glonine. Hot flashes are focused, with pressure in the head and feelings of congestion. There may be an associated rise in blood pressure at the time of the flashes. Symptoms are worse with heat and better with cold air. Emotionally, there is a fear of death and mental agitation.

Amyl nitrate. Flashes of heat are accompanied by headaches. Often they are associated with anxiety and heart palpitations.

Manganum. Hot flashes are associated with nervous system depression. The body does not want to move. Symptoms improve when patient is lying down. Emotional state is peevish and fretful. There is a loss of pleasure in joyful music, but a profound reaction to sad music.

REMEDIES FOR FLOODING (irregular periods which stop for awhile and return very heavy); these remedies may also help younger women with extremely heavy periods:

China. There is heavy bleeding, with dark, clotted blood. This leads to debilitating fatigue. Symptoms get worse with drafts and light pressure, but better with strong pressure and heat. Emotional symptoms are apathy with a strong disposition toward hurting other people's feelings (not the normal state).

Sabina. Characterized by heavy, bright red, clotted blood. Expelling the clots is painful, and radiates from the sacrum to the pubis. Emotional symptoms are irritability and a dislike for music.

Secale. Periods are profuse and prolonged. Blood is almost black. Symptoms worsen with heat and improve with cold.

Phosphorus. There is easy, frequent bleeding of bright red blood, often with no clots. The emotional state is low-spirited, with multiple fears. Also, memory may decrease. Another symptom is constant chilliness.

REMEDIES FOR VAGINAL DRYNESS AND THINNING:

Sepia. The vaginal area is itchy and dry. There is a sense that the uterus is falling out of the vagina. There is also a loss of libido. Symptoms tend to be worse with standing, cold and rest, anything that causes venous congestion. Symptoms are improved with anything that increases venous flow, such as motion. Emotionally, there is an indifference to loved ones, sadness, and a tendency to weep easily.

Natmur. Vaginal dryness makes sexual intercourse very painful. Discharges tend to be acrid and burning. There is often a loss of pubic hair. Emotional state is one of depression and irritability, which is worse with consolation. Symptoms also tend to worsen around ten o'clock in the morning.

Bryonia. Vaginal dryness is accompanied by severe headaches. Any motion is painful and distressful. Condition gets better with rest.

Nitric acid. Vaginal dryness reaches the point where the mucosa fissures, causing splinterlike sensations in the vaginal area.

EXERCISE

Regular exercise can reduce the frequency and severity of hot flashes. This is because follicle stimulating hormones decrease. For best results, it is a good idea to begin exercising before menopause begins. Otherwise, it may trigger hot flashes. Exercise also alleviates mood swings and depression by naturally raising serotonin and endorphin levels in the brain. The best exercises to engage in are dancing, brisk walking, running, swimming, biking, and tai chi. Additional benefit is derived from cross-training, doing different exercises on different days. The advantage is that it prevents any one part of the body from becoming overdeveloped.

AROMATHERAPY

"Aromatherapy is truly holistic because it is a mind and body treatment," states Ann Berwick, author of *Holistic Aromatherapy and Women's Health.* "I think this is part of the secret of its power." Berwick uses essential oils to help alleviate a number of conditions, including hormonal imbalance in women going through menopause. "Cyprus, fennel, and clary sage are believed to have estrogen-like effects. For overall balancing, I recommend to my clients that they use these oils in a lotion or body oil, and apply to their body two or three times a day. When women are experiencing hot flashes, I also suggest that they breathe in peppermint or basil on a Kleenex throughout the day. I find that a great help for most of my clients."

AYURVEDIC MEDICINE

Ayurveda means "the science of life." It is a system of medicine widely used in India for the past 4,000 years. Menopausal women report relief and rejuvenation from Ayurvedic formulas using herbal phytoestrogens and phytoprogesterones. Ayurveda believes that balance is the key to perfect health. It basically determines which body/mind type a person is and, based on that system, helps people choose the type of foods they should eat and the type of exercise best for them. For more information, read *Perfect Health* and *Ageless Body, Timeless Mind* by Deepak Chopra.

REFLEXOLOGY

In the chapter 22, on pre-menstrual syndrome, Laura Norman outlines reproductive system reflex points. Here she gives additional information on specific ways to relieve menopausal symptoms: "For menopause, in addition to working the reproductive organs, I also would encourage you to work your thyroid gland, as this will help take over when the ovaries stop producing estrogen. This is how to find this point: the base of the toes reflects the neck area where the thyroid is located. At the base of your toes, press your thumbs and thumb-walk across that ridge, particularly in the base of the big toe.

"Another area to massage is the adrenal gland reflex point. You are on the big toe side of the foot. Go about a third of the way down your foot. You are under the ball of the foot, in line with the big toe. If you press your thumb into that area, it will provide energy when you feel fatigued.

"Also, the pituitary gland, which helps all the other glands to work, is located in the center of the big toe. Pressure applied there helps stimulate that area. Both feet should be massaged equally."

Hormonal Imbalance

The disturbance of a woman's unique hormonal cycle can play a major role in the development of various medical conditions. Women are affected both by their monthly hormonal cycle and by the hormonal phases associated with the life cycle of adolescence, maturity, pregnancy and childbirth, and menopause, so an understanding of these natural cycles is invaluable in understanding and treating a multitude of symptoms.

Causes

Dolores Perri, a nutritionist from New York City, lists several diet and lifestyle factors that can interfere with normal hormonal production and balance:

ALCOHOL blocks the body's gammalinolenic acid (GLA) production, thus preventing the manufacture of natural hormones. This quickens the aging process. Alcohol creates deficiencies in B vitamins, magnesium, and calcium, which upsets hormone imbalance. Further, alcohol damages the liver, which then interferes with hormone metabolism.

ANIMAL PROTEINS are loaded with hormones and synthetic antibiotics that throw our own hormone levels out of balance.

BIRTH CONTROL PILLS deplete the body's B vitamins, which are needed for natural hormone production. The pill increases the tendency toward allergies and liver problems, which can affect hormonal balance.

CAFFEINE is found in coffee, tea, chocolate, soft drinks, and certain medications. Like alcohol, it blocks GLA production. In addition, chocolate inhibits the liver's breakdown of hormones, and tea interferes with the absorption of iron and zinc, particularly if drunk with meals. Caffeine also raises adrenaline levels and increases stress.

EXERCISE. Athletes and those training vigorously have a tendency to upset their hormonal balance and upset their periods. The physical demands of training may use up so many vitamins and minerals that the body has insufficient means to maintain hormonal production.

PHOSPHATES AND POLYPHOSPHATES—found in many food products, such as soft drinks, processed meats, and cheese—can interfere with the absorption of nutrients.

CIGARETTES contribute to hormonal problems by increasing the need for vitamins and minerals to detoxify the poisons in tobacco smoke. This reduces the amount of nutrients available for hormone production.

STRESS is a major contributor to hormonal imbalance. This includes any type of stimuli that requires the body to change and adapt, such as day-to-day hassles, psychological trauma, financial problems, and environmental pollution. Stress can cause hormones to decline, which creates an internal stress, and further diminishes hormonal production. This can interfere with immune function and result in allergies or autoimmune illnesses, such as thyroiditis or lupus. Conversely, stress can create problems by causing the body to secrete too many hormones.

SUGAR interferes with the absorption of nutrients, particularly B vitamins. It also reduces hormone transport around the body.

EXCESS WEIGHT adversely affects hormonal balance. The ratio of fat to lean body mass is critical in the initiation and continuation of the ovarian cycle. Being too thin is equally undesirable. If you fall below a certain weight, the pituitary hormone stops sending the message to the ovaries, and ovulation and menstruation stop.

OTHER FACTORS that contribute to hormonal imbalance include food sensitivity, allergy, chronic illness, candida, menstrual and gynecological problems, drugs taken over long periods of time, and low levels of thyroid hormone.

Symptoms

Dr. Elizabeth Vleit, founder and medical director of the Women's Center for Health Enhancement and Renewal at All Saint's Hospital in Fort Worth, Texas, and author of *Screaming to Be Heard: Hormonal Connections Women Suspect and Doctors Ignore*, describes some of the conditions that hormonal imbalance can trigger and tells when they are likely to occur: "Women's body's are cyclic in their response to hormones. They have a monthly rhythm of hormonal changes from puberty to menopause, which have a critical bearing on many dimensions of health. Men's bodies, on the other hand, have a tonic pattern of secretion, which means that the same amount of key hormones are produced every day. They vary within 24 hours in terms of their hormone production. But basically each day is similar to the day before and the day after.

"For women, the first half of the menstrual cycle is dominated by a rise in ovarian estradiol. This is the primary estrogen that is active at receptor sites through all the cells in the brain and body, from puberty to menopause. This rise in estrogen allows the ovary to prepare the follicle that will become the egg released at ovulation.

"At ovulation, when the egg is released, the estradiol level drops briefly. The egg then takes over and produces progesterone for the second half of the cycle. Progesterone levels rise, and estrogen levels rise again, though not as high as in the first half of the menstrual cycle. Progesterone and estrogen drop prior to bleeding, when the egg is not fertilized. The body sheds the lining of the uterus and starts over.

"When hormones fall, right before bleeding, that triggers a drop in certain critical brain neurotransmitters, such as serotonin and endorphins. This is associated with mood changes women describe—feelings of irritability, insomnia, depression or anxiety. This may be a time in the cycle when women get migraines. The drop in estrogen that triggers changes in serotonin, norepinephrine, and endorphins sets off a cascade of blood vessel spasms that are involved in migraine headaches. That also affects chemical messengers involved in regulating the immune system, the gastrointestinal tract, the heart, heart rate, blood vessels, and as many as four hundred other functions.

"We also see hormonal connections in women who have the diffuse muscle aches of fibromyalgia. These women often develop aches and pains and tender points after some type of hormonal change, such as postpartum or post tubal ligation, or following a hysterectomy, even if the ovaries are left in place. We see this in menopause too. If we look at the patterns of this type of pain in women, we see that 80 percent of fibromyalgia patients are female, and that the average age of fibromyalgia development is about 44 or 45 years."

Clinical Experience

TESTS

Dr. Vleit says women need to be aware of the relationship between hormonal cycles and medical conditions: "One of the ways to do that is to track patterns relative to cycles, and to test the blood for various hormones that women's bodies produce. I've developed an approach to doing that by measuring the hormonal levels at the right time of the menstrual cycle. This helps women know what is happening to their hormone levels at the time that they are having symptoms. I become frustrated when doctors tell me that we don't need to measure the female hormones because they vary. I say in response, That's the whole point. They do vary, and how they vary, relative to women experiencing problems, is what we must find out in order to offer them the most constructive options.'"

It is also important to check thyroid function. Thyroid hormone controls progesterone, cholesterol, and the ovaries. It acts as a cascading system. When not functioning properly, other hormones get out of balance.

NUTRITION

The typical American diet is high in fat, protein, caffeine, simple sugars, and salt, ingredients that interfere with optimal hormonal balance. These foods create a vicious cycle. They fuel pre-menstrual cravings for sweets and chocolate, and giving in to them worsens cravings.

Perri says not to reach for a prescription drug for hormonal problems. It is better to eat high-quality organic foods and avoid foods that throw the system off balance. Beans and legumes are better sources of protein than meats, which are loaded with hormones. In addition, Perri advises cold-processed oils, nuts, seeds, fatty fish, and beans. "These foods are all very high in GLAs," she advises. "The GLAs help us to make natural estrogen in our own bodies."

SUPPLEMENTS. Wild yam and DHEA promote the production of natural estrogens in the body, if it is needed by the body. If it is not needed, it is eliminated by the body, making it totally safe to use. Magnesium and calcium may also be beneficial, as most women do not get enough of these nutrients.

HERBS. Blue cohosh, black cohosh, yarrow, and chaste tree help to balance hormone production. Other herbs for balance include raspberry leaf, *dong quai*, wild yam, and passion flower.

Herbal Pharmacy

Plants that are helpful during menopause, in order of potency:

Oenothera biennis (evening primrose)
Helianthus annuus (sunflower)
Psophorcarpus tetragonolobus (asparagus pea)
Lablab purureus (bonavist bean)
Moringa oleifera (ben nut)
Nasturtium officinale (berro)
Sinapis alba (white mustard seed)
Cucurbita foetidissima (buffalo gourd)
Cicer arietinum (chickpea)
Sesamum indicum (sesame)
Phaseolus vulgaris (black bean)
Spinacia oleracea (spinach)
Cucurbita pepo (pumpkin)
Trigonella foenum-graecum (fenugreek)
Basella alba (vinespinach)
Corchorus olitorius (Jew's mallow)
Brassica nigra (black mustard)
Vigna radiata (green gram)

Hot News

Much of the recent research into causes and symptoms of menopause has focused on the value of a vegetarian diet, specifically one that provides phytoestrogens (natural plant estrogens) and that is rich in soy products. The plant estrogens found in legumes, such as peas and beans, provide the same benefit as estrogen replacement therapy without its cancer risks; boron also seems to mimic the results of estrogen replacement. Smoking, meat consumption, and alcohol consumption can bring about early menopause. Hesperidin, gamma-oryzanol, and vitamin C are effective in treating many menopausal symptoms. Plant extracts that have proven valuable are remifemin, an extract of *Cimicifuga racemosa;* ginseng; and wild yam and *dong quai,* especially for women just entering menopause. Other therapies of value include acupuncture, exercise, and relaxation techniques. *(See below.)*

According to Dr. Vicki Hufnagel, the use of NCHT (Natural Cyclic Hormone Therapy, an alternative to traditonal hormones using natural hormones in physiological doses) delays onset and reverses many of the symptoms of menopause, while also reducing the incidence of long term complications such as heart disease and osteoporosis.

FROM THE MEDICAL LITERATURE ON MENOPAUSE

NUTRITION/DIET

The Japanese diet incorporates high amounts of soybean products, which may explain why Japanese women tend to suffer less from hot flashes and menopausal symptoms in general than do women in other countries.

H. Adlercreutz and E. Hamalainen, "Dietary Phyto-Estrogens and the Menopause in Japan," *Lancet* 329 (May 16, 1992): 1233.

A study found that postmenopausal vegetarian women have lower urinary levels of estriol and total estrogens, lower plasma prolactin levels, and higher sex-hormone-binding globulin levels than do postmenopausal women who are not vegetarian. These findings could be a factor in why vegetarian women have lower rates of breast and endometrial cancers than do nonvegetarian women.

B. K. Armstrong et al., "Diet and Reproductive Hormones: A Study of Vegetarian and Nonvegetarian Postmenopausal Women," *Journal of the National Cancer Institute* 67, no. 4 (October 1981): 761–67.

In a placebo-controlled study, alphatocopherol (vitamin E) was shown to help women with vasomotor symptoms. Symptoms returned when treatment stopped.

R. S. Finkler, "The Effect of Vitamin E in the Menopause," *Journal of Clinical Endoctrinol. Metab.* 9 (1949): 89–94.

Hesperidin and vitamin C are useful in treating vasomotor symptoms, a study showed.

A. Horoschak, "Nocturnal Leg Cramps, Easy Bruisability and Epistaxi in Menopausal Patients Treated with Hesperidin and Ascorbic Acid," *Del. State Med. Journal* (January 1959): 19–22.

In a clinical trial, 100 mg of gamma-oryzanol were given 3 times a day to 40 women with vasomotor problems, insomnia, headaches, muscle or joint pain, and nervousness or depression. Results showed that after 4–8 weeks of treatment, 40 percent experienced excellent results, 35 percent had good results, 15 percent described the treatment as effective, and 10 percent received no benefit.

M. Ishihara, "Effect of Gamma-Oryzanol on Serum Lipid Peroxide Level and Climacteric Disturbances," *Asia Oceania Journal Obstet. Gynaecol.* 10, no. 3 (1984): 317.

Gamma-oryzanol was given daily to 8 menopausal women and 13 women who had had their ovaries removed. Sixty-seven percent of all patients and 75 percent of the menopausal patients experienced a 50 percent or greater reduction in their menopausal symptoms.

Y. Murase et al., "Clinically Cured Cases Per OS Gamma Oryzanol of Menopausal Disturbances or Menopausal-Like Disturbances," *Sanfujinka no Jissai* 12, no. 2 (1963): 147.

Thirty milligrams daily of gamma-oryzanol was shown to alleviate menopause-related symptoms after 2 weeks of administration.

N. Okuda et al., "Mechanism of Action of Gamma Oryzanol and Clinical Experience," *Sanka to Fujinka* 29 (1962): 1488.

In a study, three different supplements (45 g/day of soya, 10 g/day of clover sprout seeds, and 25 g/day of linseed) were each given to 25 postmenopausal women. Vagina cells sensitive to circulating estrogen levels were monitored, with changes being recorded after 6 weeks of supplementation. The results lead the authors to argue that heavy consumption of foods containing plant estrogens can reduce the severity of menopausal symptoms.

G. Wilcox et al., "Oestrogenic Effects of Plant Foods in Postmenopausal Women," *British Medical Journal* 301 (October 20, 1990): 905.

Consumption of high levels of phytoestrogens can result in significant estrogenic effects and is believed to be an important reason why women in cultures with predominantly plant-based diets rarely suffer from menopausal symptoms.

R. S. Kaldas and C. L. Hughes, "Reproductive and General Metabolic Effects of Phytoestrogens in Mammals," *Reprod. Toxicol.* 3 (1989): 81–89.

Animal studies lead researchers to conclude that phytoestrogens may be signficantly more effective in treating menopausal symptoms than estrogen, since the former have not been linked to estrogen's side effects.

D. P. Rose, "Dietary Fiber, Phytoestrogens, and Breast Cancer," *Nutrition* 8 (1992): 47–51.

HERBS/PLANT EXTRACTS

A study looked at the effects of remifemin, an extract of *Cimicifuga racemosa*, on the LH and FSH secretion of menopausal women. Levels of LH, but not FSH, were found to be reduced significantly in patients who received the extract. Subsequent animal experiments within the same study supported these results.

E. M. Duker et al., "Effects of Extracts from *Cimicifuga Racemosa* on Gonadotropin Release in Menopausal Women and Ovariectomized Rats," *Planta. Med.*, 57, no. 5 (October 1991): 420-424.

A case study showed that ingestion of Rumanian ginseng can have a strong estrogenic effect.

R. Punnonen and A. Lukola, "Oestrogen-Like Effect of Ginseng," *British Medical Journal* 281 (1980): 1110.

An article makes the following recommendations for treating the emotional and physical symptoms of menopause: Panax or American ginseng for hot flashes, especially in women who are nervous and high-strung or have reproductive problems; wild yam and dong quai for women just entering menopause and particularly for those with problems of the reproductive system; vitex for dry skin, dry vagina, or chapped lips; aloe vera gel and slippery elm powder for mucous membrane irritations in the vagina; and cleavers, chickweed, dandelion leaves, and nettles for water retention, and to restore potassium and cleanse the kidneys.

R. Gladstar, "Herbs for Menopause," *East West Natural Health* 22, no. 5 (September–October 1992): 46.

EXERCISE

An Australian study found that exercise had a beneficial effect on the emotional and physical symptoms of menopausal women, regardless of whether or not they were taking hormone therapy.

L. Carroll, "Exercise Helped Quell Symptoms of Menopause," *Medical Tribune* (April 20, 1995): 20.

Sweating and hot flashes were reported to be only half as common among menopausal women participating in organized physical exercise as among controls.

M. Hammar et al., "Does Physical Exercise Influence the Frequency of Postmenopausal Hot Flashes?" *Acta Obstet. Gynecol. Scand.* 69, no. 5 (1990): 409-412.

RELAXATION

Results of a study showed that paced respiration significantly reduced the frequency of hot flashes.

R.R. Freedman and S. Woodward, "Behavioral Treatment of Menopausal Hot Flashes: Evaluation by Ambulatory Monitoring," *American Journal of Obstet. Gynecol.* 167, no. 2 (August 1992): 436–39.

ACUPUNCTURE

Eight weeks of either electrostimulated acupuncture or superficial needle position acupuncture led to a significant decrease in hot flashes for more than 50 percent of a group of healthy women with natural menopause. Women receiving the electrostimulated acupuncture experienced benefits for up to 3 months after treatment was stopped.

Y. Wyon et al., "Akupunktur Mot Klimakteriebesvar? Farre Vegetativa Symptom After Menopaus" [Acupuncture Against Climacteric Disorders? Lower Number of Symptoms After Menopause], *Lakartidningen* 91, no. 23 (June 8, 1994): 2318–22.

EARLY ONSET

Among the factors found to be independently associated with early natural menopause are smoking, age of maternal menopause, meat consumption, and consumption of alcohol.

D. J. Torgerson et al., "Factors Associated with Onset of Menopause in Women Aged 45-49," *Maturitas* 19, no. 2 (August 1994): 83–92.

HOMEOPATHY

In a study of women with menopausal symptoms, half were treated with a hormone substitution and the other half received a complex homeopathic remedy. Results showed no differences between the two approaches in FSH levels, E2 levels, cytologic effects, or endometrium thickness. However, the women receiving homeopathic treatment reported significantly fewer subjective complaints. The authors suggest such findings support the use of homeopathic remedies in women objecting to hormone therapy.

A. M. Beer et al., "Der Einsats Eines Homoopathischen Syndrom im Vergleich zur Hormonsubstitution," *Erfahrungsheilkunde* 44, no. 5 (May 1995): 336–40.

ESTROGEN REPLACEMENT THERAPY (ERT)

Sixteen different studies show that after 15 years of ERT, there is a 30 percent increase in the risk of breast cancer. The risk does not begin to appear until after 5 years of the therapy.

K. K. Steinberg et al., "A Meta-Analysis of the Effect of Estrogen Replacement Therapy on the Risk of Breast Cancer," *JAMA* 265, no. 15 (April 17, 1991): 1985–90.

A study of over 1300 women showed 50 percent more breast cancer after 5 or more years of taking hormones.

"Progestin Added to Estrogen Replacement Therapy Doesn't Eliminate Increased Risk of Breast Cancer," *Network News* 20, no. 5 (September–October 1995): 3.

Soybean supplements can replace ERT, providing beneficial effects on lipids and lowering bone metabolism rates.

C. Bullock, "Soybeans: An Estrogen Replacement Alternative?" *Family Practice News* (April 6, 1995): 11.

The plant estrogens found in legumes, such as peas and beans, provide the same benefit as ERT without ERT's cancer risk. In fact, there are 60 studies showing that plant estrogens are as effective as ERT, or even more so. These plant-derived compounds increase blood levels of HDL (good cholesterol), lower LDL (bad cholesterol), and favorably affect vasomotor response, permitting arteries to constrict and dilate as they should.

"Data on Estrogens in Soybeans May Make ERT More Acceptable," *Cancer Biotechnology Weekly* (October 23, 1995): 10-11.

Boron, given in a dosage of 3 mg/day for 49 days, was shown to mimic the effect of estrogen.

F. H. Nielsen et al., "Boron Enhances and Mimics Some Effects of Estrogen Therapy in Postmenopausal Women," *Journal of Trace Elements in Experimental Medicine* 5 (1992): 237–46.

17. MENSTRUAL CRAMPS (Dysmenorrhea) and IRREGULAR MENSTRUATION

Painful and difficult periods are so commonplace in our society that some women have come to think of them as normal, but they are not normal at all. Many experts feel that the symptoms of dysmenorrhea are related to our dietary practices, as well as to unresolved emotional difficulties.

Causes

"What causes menstrual cramps?" asks Dr. Pat Gorman. "In addition to toxins found in foods with preservatives, additives, and caffeine, they are due to putrid proteins found in dairy and red meat. These foods contain a lot of hormones that upset the system. In addition, foods fried in heavy oils cause problems and should be cut out immediately by any woman interested in getting rid of dysmenorrhea."

Dr. Gorman adds that the Chinese attribute this condition in part to pent-up anger and frustration. "If you are not happy with your life, if you are angry with people, you must work this out. The liver, which stores blood and prepares it for the period, is also responsible for anger. That's not a Western concept, but with my patients I find that working out anger helps the liver to relax. As a result, there is far less of a problem with dysmenorrhea."

Dr. Marjorie Ordene, a gynecologist in Brooklyn, New York, agrees that hormonal and psychological factors cause painful periods and explains the underlying factors: "What causes dysmenorrhea is exagerrated uterine contractions. These contractions are mediated by receptors in the uterine lining that are stimulated by hormonal and psychological factors. Hormonal factors that stimulate the uterine receptors have actually been isolated. They are chemical messengers called prostaglandins. Two things are clear. People with menstrual cramps have an excess of prostaglandins, and there is an imbalance in the type of prostaglandin they produce."

She adds that eating foods we are allergic to can increase prostaglandin production: "For example, many women are sensitive to yeast, and eating baked foods, breads, pastries, and processed fruit juices, can cause an increase in prostaglandin production."

Symptoms

There are different types of menstrual pain. Usually it is experienced as a spasmodic cramp, but there can also be an achiness, a feeling of heaviness in the lower abdomen, or discomfort in the lower back or thighs. Other symptoms may include nausea, vomiting, loss of appetite, diarrhea, headache, dizziness, tiredness, anxiety, and depression.

Dysmenorrhea usually begins at the onset of menstruation, lasting a few hours, but it can begin premenstrually and remain several days. According to traditional Asian medicine, if the tongue has a thick white coating, the problem is the result of too many of the wrong type of proteins, while a thick yellow covering signals toxicity from protein.

Clinical Experience

CONVENTIONAL TREATMENT

Medical doctors often prescribe medications, such as ibuprofen, to inhibit prostaglandins. While these work to relieve menstrual cramps and accompanying symptoms, problems occur when drugs are taken month after month. Side effects can include gastrointestinal bleeding, decreased blood flow to the kidneys, and leaky gut syndrome, a condition that allows undigested food particles to enter the blood.

NATUROPATHIC TREATMENT

DIET. Changes in diet can decrease overproduction of prostaglandins and restore normal balance. Cool, green foods help reduce hot stabbing pains and inflammation. It is good to eat foods such as organic grains, legumes, oatmeal, and steamed green vegetables. Deep sea fish such as salmon, tuna, or mackerel can be included, as well as flaxseed oil. Hot spices should be avoided, as well as fried, greasy foods, sugar, salt, alcohol, and stimulating foods such as garlic and onions. Foods that produce allergies should be eliminated as well.

Women who have nerve-related menstrual pain can benefit from tofu, but should stay away from too many cold raw salads, hot spicy foods, and even white potatoes. Herbalist Letha Hadady suggests this soothing recipe: warm tofu cooked with sweet spices, like pumpkin pie spices or nutmeg. This quiets the nerves and helps a woman feel nurtured and relaxed.

FASTING. Dr. Anthony Penepent, a physician who practices natural hygiene, helps patients with painful menses by placing them on a strict hygienic regimen. "I put them on a fast one day before the onset of their period. In serious conditions, I might have them fast one day and then prescribe juices or juice blended with salad and fruit for the following days until they complete their menses." *(For a description of a typical hygienic regimen, see "Patient Stories" in chapter 9, Endometriosis.)*

SUPPLEMENTS.

Evening primrose oil. Taken throughout the month as a daily supplement, this prevents headaches and blemishes that occur just before the period.

Magnesium citrate. Magnesium deficiencies are common and result in the release of prostaglandins that cause spasm and pain. Magnesium is antispasmodic and helps relieve the problem. Take 300–500 mg daily and work up to bowel tolerance.

HERBS.

The following herbs help to alleviate menstrual problems:

Gardenia and philodendron are popular in Chinese medicine, and can be obtained by prescription from an herbalist.

Corn silk tea helps to get rid of the bloating that comes from too many hormones stored in the blood. Women's Rhythm also eliminates bloating. This Ted Kapchuk formula can be found in certain health food stores or ordered from Kahn Herbs.

Xiao Yao Wan. This wonderful remedy, which can be purchased at pharmacies in Chinatowns in major cities, such as Pearl River Pharmacy in New York City, helps digestive processes. Not only does this formula relieve painful periods, it also alleviates anger.

Green tea is cooling and satisfying, with very little caffeine. A pinch of tea can be added to a pot of boiled water, steeped for five minutes, and sipped throughout the day. People experience an energy pickup from digestion being activated, not from nerves being stimulated. Helps soothe sharp, stabbing pains.

Aloe vera juice or gel can eliminate headache, irritability, fever, stabbing pain, blemishes, and bad breath associated with menstrual cramps. Aloe also reduces acid from the stomach and liver, and is slightly laxative. Just add to juice, tea, or water.

Dandelion helps to break apart impurities in the system. Can be bought as capsules or tea.

Sarsaparilla helps hot, stabbing pains brought on by inflammation. Sarsaparilla is anti-inflammatory, antiseptic, diuretic, and soothing.

Valerian is a sedative herb that makes a woman feel quieter, more relaxed and grounded. It is especially good for nervous women who experience insomnia, anxiety, crying jags and emotional upsets, and other nervous problems. Valerian quiets the nerves that go to the uterus.

Yunnan Pai Yao. This combination of herbs helps reduce heavy bleeding and stabbing pain. By increasing the circulation, internal bleeding is healed, and swelling and pain are reduced.

HOMEOPATHIC REMEDIES. Homeopathy was developed in Germany over 200 years ago by Dr. Samuel Hahnemann, and means "like cures like." The same substances that cause a disease in a healthy individual can heal an ailment in a sick person, when diluted and given in minute proportions.

Homeopathic physician Ken Korins, M.D., explains that the dilution process is what makes homeopathic remedies so safe: "Homeopathy is a vibrational medicine. We are dealing with very subtle energies. Substances are given in extremely small dilutions that cannot possibly have any toxic effects. In fact, if you were to analyze these substances, you would not find a trace of the original material in the final dilution."

The correct homeopathic remedy is the one that most closely matches the symptoms that manifest themselves. Dr. Korins recommends that dysmenorrhea sufferers choose among the following:

Colocynthis. This frequently indicated remedy is useful when you have a severe onset of sudden cramps, particularly on the first day of menstruation. Emotionally, there is an intense irritability and anger associated with the menstrual cramps. A key indication is that you feel better when your knees are pulled up toward the stomach, and held with firm pressure.

Magnesia phosphorica. This helps spasmodic cramps with bloating. The key indication for this remedy is that you feel better from warmth. Magnesia phosphorica and colocynthis will help alleviate the symptoms in 85 percent of the cases.

Pulsatilla. A key indication for pulsatilla is variation; the cramps and the flow of bleeding are changeable. The pains themselves are typically cutting and tearing, and may be felt in the lower back or kidney region. Generally, you feel worse in warm stuffy rooms and better in the open fresh air. Emotionally, you tend to be mild, gentle, and weepy when entering the menstrual state and prefer the company of other people to being alone.

Viburnum. This is indicated when the menses are very scant and often late. In fact, they may only last a few hours. When you get cramps, the flow of the blood stops. Cramps tend to radiate to the sacrum and the thighs. You may feel faint or like passing out.

Cimicifuga. This is indicated for spasmodic, cramping pains. The pains radiate across the pelvis from one thigh to the other. It is often associated with a pre-menstrual headache. Increased flow results in more pain. Emotionally, you may feel nervous to the point of being scattered, and often somewhat depressed.

Chamomilla. This is helpful if you are either hypersensitive and insensitive to any pain. Emotionally, you tend to be irritable and contrary. Someone brings you something that you ask for, then you don't want it. During intense periods, you may become dependent on coffee and other stimulants and sedatives. Another symptom is anger. When you become angry, your symptoms become worse.

AROMATHERAPY. Marjoram, clary sage, and lavender are wonderful analgesics. Eighteen to twenty drops of oil added to a lotion or oil and massaged into the abdomen and lower back helps to relieve menstrual pain. Breathing in the cooling fragrances of rose, lavender, or sandalwood can alleviate sharp, stabbing pain.

STRESS MANAGEMENT. Deep abdominal breathing, meditation, tai chi, and other mind/body disciplines eliminate frustrations and anger that bring on pain. Additionally, it is helpful to slow down the pace of life from the time of ovulation to the period.

Amenorrhea and Menorrhagia

Amenorrhea and menorrhagia are medical terms for abnormal blood flow. Amenorrhea refers to the cessation of bleeding, or very light and infrequent periods, most often caused by an abnormally functioning hypothalamus, pituitary gland, ovary, or uterus as a result of drugs or surgery that removes the ovaries or uterus. "Bulemics and anorexics also exhibit this pattern," notes Dr. Pat Gorman, an acupuncturist and educator from New York City. "Sometimes this is caused by excessive dieting and overexercise driven by self-hatred. Not accepting who she is, a woman thinks, 'I've got to make myself thin, beautiful, and perfect.' If this is going on at the end of the cycle, when toxins are being released into the system, the woman is aggravating her body to the point of saying, We're not going to give up this blood. We desperately need it. Forget ovulation, forget periods." *(See chapter 8, Eating Disorders, for more information.)*

With menorrhagia the opposite scenario occurs, and there is profuse bleeding. The condition can be debilitating, sometimes bad enough to warrant immediate attention at a hospital's emergency ward. "The Chinese say menorrhagia is caused by excess toxins and heat in the blood from foods containing preservatives, additives, and caffeine, especially coffee. It's like water in your car radiator becoming low," Dr. Gorman says. "The engine will overheat and explode. Alcohol adds more toxicity because it constantly removes water from the blood. As water diminishes, it heats up the blood. When the blood is what we call 'hot,' or fast-moving, it's very hard for the body to hold it in. It can't stop the bleeding."

The emotional profile of the menorrhagic individual is someone who sees herself as a victim. Dr. Gorman explains, "This person feels the need to serve everybody. She does not know how to set boundaries. Whatever anybody wants, they get. She keeps pouring out her energy and pouring out her blood."

Dr. Vicki Hufnagel, a gynecological surgeon and activist for women's health rights, adds that heavy bleeding is often a sign of an underlying problem in the female system, especially when it is accompanied by pain. The problem is frequently due to a hormonal imbalance. "Anything can throw off a cycle," says Dr. Hufnagel. "Emotional stress, insomnia, too much estrogen in the system, or too little light, as in the winter. Other physical problems that can cause menorrhagia are fibroids, polyps, and a malfunctioning thyroid gland."

Symptoms

Oriental medicine can diagnose amenorrhea and menorrhagia by examining the skin. Amenorrhea manifests as pale, sallow, slightly yellowish skin from a deep lack of blood and nutrients. Often this is accompanied by a great deal of emotional anxiety. With menorrhagia, the tongue has a red tip and tiny red dots. When the condition is long-term, a woman can become anemic.

Clinical Experience

Before you can restore the blood flow in patients with amenorrhea or menorrhagia, you must discover the reason for the problem. Once the cause is addressed, periods should return to normal.

HORMONAL BALANCING FOR MENORRHAGIA

Dr. Hufnagel says that hormonal dysfunctions in women with menorrhagia can be corrected with oral doses of natural progesterone. "Often, the creams women are using are not adequate because they don't cause a rise in the blood level. We often have to give what we call oral physiological levels of progesterone. I give women natural hormones, in a cyclic manner, the way her body should be getting them."

Hormone balancing is also accomplished through diet. Fatty diets cause higher levels of estrogen in the system, which, in turn, can cause menorrhagia. Lean diets, and exercising with weights, produce more testosterone, which, in turn, helps to balance hormones and put an end to menorrhagia.

NATURAL HYGIENE APPROACH TO AMENORRHEA

Anthony Penepent, M.D., a natural hygienist from New York, says amenorrhea is one of the easiest conditions to correct. Mostly it stems from undernourishment and can be corrected with a diet that includes two green salads daily, using romaine lettuce, fresh lemon juice, olive oil, and some brewer's yeast. You should also include two pieces of fresh fruit and two soft boiled eggs in the daily menu. Where amenorrhea is caused by a thyroid condition, a thyroid supplement is needed. Additionally, if stress is in the picture, the stressful situation must be remedied. For more serious cases, additional dietary intervention is necessary. Usually, small changes in diet are all that are needed. Dr. Penepent says, "Even if the woman doesn't follow a completely natural hygienic regimen and is not vegetarian, she still can get tremendous results simply by increasing the amount of green leafy vegetables in the diet and providing concentrated nutritional sources, such as eggs and unsalted raw milk cheese."

HERBS. The following Chinese herbs have specific effects on the blood and are needed at different times of the monthly cycle. Dr. Gorman recommends working with a health practitioner to create an individual protocol and to monitor progress, but offers these general guidelines:

At the beginning of the cycle:

Dong quai. High in vitamins A, E, and B12, this blood-builder can be taken most days of the month, up to the point of menstruation, or just before it begins if there are strong pre-menstrual symptoms. "You don't want to be build-ing blood if you are having trouble moving that blood," Dr. Gorman warns.

Women's Precious. This formula is a tremendous blood builder, taken after the period ends for about three weeks. Women's Rhythm is then used the following week.

At the end of the cycle:

Gardenia. This is taken when PMS symptoms arise. By moving blood that is stuck, gardenia helps to relieve that heavy, bloated feeling. *(See also chapter 22, Pre-Menstrual Syndrome.)*

Women's Rhythm helps release a woman's blood. This is usually taken a week before the period to help move toxins out of the organs. (Women's Precious and Women's Rhythm are Ted Kapchik formulas that can be found in some health food stores and ordered directly from Kahn Herbs.)

Can be taken every day:

Floradix with iron. This wonderful product is available in most health care stores. Liquid Floradix is superior over the dry form because it contains more live nutrients.

Toxic Shock Syndrome (TSS)

Toxic shock syndrome is a rare, but serious—and sometimes fatal—disease. The victims tend to be tampon users under the age of thirty—and especially those between fifteen and nineteen. This sudden and serious disease affects persons with severely compromised immune systems, who are poisoned by a strain of bacteria, called *Staphylococcus aureus*, phage group I. This type of staph produces a substance called enterotoxin F, which can overpower and destroy a weak body.

Toxic shock syndrome is linked to the introduction of tampons with four new ingredients, in the early 1980s. Before then, tampons were made primarily of cotton. In the 1980s, though, highly absorbent polyester cellulose, carboxymethyl cellulose, polyacrylate rayon, and viscose rayon came into use. Three of these new ingredients were soon taken off the market; today, only one of the new ingredients, viscose rayon, is in use. Today's tampons are either entirely viscose rayon or a blend of cotton and viscose rayon. In addition, the tampons on the market today may contain an assortment of chemicals, including pesticides used in growing cotton, chemicals used in the manufacture of viscose rayon (lye, sodium sulfate, and sodium hydroxide), and dyes (some of which have been considered carcinogenic since the 1950s).

One theory of the reason for TSS is that the vagina is normally an oxygen-free environment, which limits growth of dangerous bacteria. However, air is trapped between the fibers that make up tampons. When that air is inserted in the vagina along with the tampon, the possibility of toxin production increases. Even after the tampon is removed, some of its fibers may remain.

TSS was originally thought only to affect women who wore high-absorbency tampons. But now it is known to affect newborns, children, and men as well. Initial indications can include a high fever, headache, sore throat, diarrhea, nausea and red skin blotches. These signs can be followed by confusion, low blood pressure, acute kidney failure, abnormal liver function, and even death.

A severe case of TSS is a medical emergency that may necessitate hospitalization. However, there are many natural ways to support the system once a crisis is over for quick recovery and prevention of recurrence.

NATUROPATHY

Dr. Linda Rector-Page, author of *Healthy Healing: An Alternative Healing Reference*, developed a protocol for healing from TSS out of necessity: "I actually came close to death on an operating table from TSS. I had to bring my body back, and I did it herbally. It took a couple of years, and now I can speak from experience."

Dr. Rector-Page's personal ordeal gave her a great deal of confidence in the power of natural remedies. The following herbs helped her to overcome toxicity, restore immunity, and return to health:

Ginseng. Both Panax and American varieties are general tonics that balance and tone all body systems, as well as improve circulation. Ginseng should not be used when there is a high fever.

Cayenne and ginger. These nervous system stimulants can help the body recover from shock. They can either be taken internally or applied to the skin in compresses.

Hawthorn extract. Hawthorn speeds up and normalizes the circulation, and restores a sense of well-being.

In addition to herbs, Dr. Rector-Page ate supernutritious foods that could be easily digested and quickly utilized by her failing system. These foods included high-potency royal jelly, bee pollen, wheat germ, brewer's yeast, and unsulfured molasses. The addition of green drinks, including chlorella, barley grass, spirulina, and wheat grass, supplied her with high potencies of vital minerals. "All these go into the body very quickly and help it to recover, even from a death situation," explains Dr. Rector-Page. "By going on a program of concentrated nutrients, I was eventually able to create a state of health that was better than before."

PREVENTION

Alternatives to tampons have included sea sponges. However, sea sponges are no longer sold as menstrual products. A 1981 report alleged risks from embedded sand, chemical pollutants, bacteria, and fungi. No additional studies were done, but the FDA halted menstrual sponge sales. Another alternative is called the Keeper, a rubber cup that sits in the lower vagina. The Keeper may hold an ounce of menstrual blood, and should be emptied several times a day. This device does not promote the growth of bacteria in the vagina. However, the Keeper is not widely available. Tampons that are 100 percent cotton, and thus present less risk than modern superabsorbent tampons that may also contain added chemicals, are available in many health food and natural goods stores.

Patient Stories

CLAUDIA

There are two basic areas of concerns that I had. Number one, I had a very troublesome menstrual cycle. Number two, I have certain characteristics that place me at a slightly higher risk for breast cancer than other women. Because of these two factors, I wanted to go beyond the traditional Western medical approach. Certainly, I wanted to use what Western medicine had to offer, like getting regular examinations, but I also wanted to take an additional step. That's why I sought herbal remedies and holistic health care.

Back in November 1993, I went to a health care seminar given by Letha Hadady on breast health. I was very impressed by the information that was given. I made an appointment with Letha after that, and the remedies she gave me were very helpful.

Before I had the herbal remedies, my menstrual cycles were extremely heavy, I had mood swings, and I was very prone to exhaustion. I was extremely irregular. When I started taking the herbal remedies, the menstrual cycle became very regular again, approximately every thirty days. The flow was more regular, the cramping was easier to deal with. The mood swings disappeared, and I became balanced. My own body told me that this was certainly working for me. The herbs have made a fundamental difference in my life.

The Chinese herbs are different from American herbs because they are given in combination. They address a number of symptoms at one time, and they are also cost-effective, which I think is important for many people today.

This is something that a woman can choose to use in conjunction with regular health care approaches: self-exams, medical care, proper nutrition, and addressing emotional health.

SUSAN

I had a job I loved, but it was very stressful. I wound up with amenorrhea for a few weeks. Since I am not yet premenopausal or even perimenopausal, I was upset by that.

I heard of a product from a friend called Eternal, a herbal tincture that contains damiana leaf, saw palmetto, and a lot of other wonder substances that help with hormonal rejuvenation. My friend had been on Premarin for almost twenty years because of hot flashes after a hysterectomy, and found great relief from Eternal. I tried it, and to my relief, it counteracted the effect the stress was having, and brought my periods back. Everything is back to normal, and I no longer have a problem.

Hot News

Additional substances that have been shown in scientific studies to relieve menstrual cramps include vitamin E, magnesium, black haw bark, and palmetto berry. Acupuncture and high-frequency transcutaneous electrical nerve stimulation (TENS) also produced pain relief in studies.

Vitamin A deficiency, which impairs enzyme activity, may be an important cause of menorrhagia. Papaya leaf seems to reduce the severity of bleeding and hemorrhage, thus inhibiting menorrhagia; shepherd's purse is another promising treatment. Hyperthermia is a new treatment for menorrhagia, using a technique of heating the uterus cavity with a probe. *(See below.)*

NUTRITION

Injections of vitamin E relieve pain in dysmenorrhea within 10 to 15 minutes.

G. M. Kryzhanovskii et al., "A-Tocopherol-Induced Activation of the Endogenous Opioid System," *Bulletin of Experimental Biology and Medicine* 108, no. 11 (November 1989): 566–67.

A study of patients with primary dysmenorrhoea showed that treatment with magnesium was effective in reducing the symptoms of most of them. The magnesium has a muscle-relaxant and vasodilatory effect.

B. Seifert et al., [Magnesium—A New Therapeutic Alternative in Primary Dysmenorrhea], *Zentralbl. Gynakol.* 111, no. 11 (1989): 755–60.

HERBS/PLANT EXTRACTS

Black haw bark is effective for dysmenorrhea. Saw palmetto berry can also be effective.

D. B. Mowrey, *The Scientific Validation of Herbal Medicine* (New Canaan, Conn.: Keats Publishing, 1986): 111.

OSTEOPATHIC MANIPULATION

A study of 12 subjects with lower back pain from dysmenhorrhea shows that osteopathic manipulation on the lower back can provide immediate relief.

D. Boesler et al., "Efficacy of a High-Velocity Low-Amplitude Manipulative Technique in Subjects with Low-Back Pain during Menstrual Cramping," *Journal of the American Osteopathic Association* 93, no. 2 (February 1993): 203–214.

HIGH-FREQUENCY TRANSCUTANEOUS ELECTRICAL NERVE STIMULATION (TENS)

For 14 out of 21 patients, high-frequency TENS (100 Hz) produced a pain reduction level of over 50 percent.

T. Lundeberg et al., "Relief of Primary Dysmenorrhea by Transcutaneous Electrical Nerve Stimulation," *Acta. Obstet. Gynecol. Scand.* 64, no. 6 (1985): 491–97.

When 61 women with primary dysmenorrhea were treated with TENS for two menstrual cycles, 10 percent reported that TENS had no effect on the pain, 60 percent reported moderate pain relief, and 30 percent reported marked relief.

B. Kaplan et al., "Transcutaneous Electrical Nerve Stimulation (TENS) as a Relief for Dysmenorrhea," *Clin. Exp. Obstet. Gynecol.* 21, no. 2 (1994): 87–90.

FROM THE MEDICAL LITERATURE ON AMENORRHEA

Amenorrhea may be induced by exercise, and so modifying the exercise program may be helpful. Other lifestyle factors correlated with the incidence of secondary amenorrhea are being single, being underweight, having an intellectual occupation, experiencing stress, and using sedatives and hypnotics.

"Infertility Can Stem from Lifestyle Factors," *Medical Aspects of Human Sexuality* (March 1991): 19.

Thirty-four patients with ovulatory dysfunction were treated an average of 30 times with acupuncture. All showed improvement, and there was a marked effectiveness rate of 35 percent.

X. Mo et al., "Clinical Studies on the Mechanism for Acupuncture Stimulation of Ovulation," *J. Tradit. Chin. Med.* 13, no. 2 (June 1993): 115–19.

Combining Western and traditional Chinese medicine treatment for amenorrhea produced significantly better results than using Western treatment alone.

X. L. Ge, "Treatment of Secondary Amenorrhea and Oligohypomenorrhea with Combined Traditional Chinese and Western Medicine," *Chung Hsi I Chieh Ho Tsa Chih* 11, no.11 (November 1991): 661–663, 645.

Black haw bark is effective in treating amenorhhea, as well as dysmenorrhea and threatened abortion.

Mowrey, *The Scientific Validation of Herbal Medicine* (New Canaan, Conn.: Keats Publishing, 1986): 111.

FROM THE MEDICAL LITERATURE ON MENORRHAGIA

NUTRITION

Vitamin A supplementation alleviated menorrhagia in 92 percent of the patients in a study. Vitamin A deficiency seems to be an important cause of menorrhagia; deficiency impairs enzyme activity.

D. M. Lithgow and W. M. Politzer, "Vitamin A in the Treatment of Menorrhagia," *South African Medical Journal* 51, no. 7 (February 12, 1977): 191–93.

HERBS/PLANT EXTRACTS

Papaya leaf is known as a digestive aid, but recent research shows that it reduces the severity of bleeding and hemorrhage, thus inhibiting menorrhagia. Shepherd's purse is effective when menorrhagia is characterized by lengthy, frequent, almost colorless flow.

D. B. Mowrey, *The Scientific Validation of Herbal Medicine* (New Canaan, Conn.: Keats Publishing, 1986): 187.

TRADITIONAL CHINESE MEDICINE

Shen-qian gu-jing granules are reported to be highly effective in stemming excess menstrual flow. Of 72 cases treated in a study, the amount of menstrual blood loss was significantly decreased in over 87 percent of the cases, and the level of fibrin degradation products in menstrual fluid and peripheral blood was also reduced.

L. X. Cao et al., [Effect of Shen-Qian Gu-Jing Granule on Fibrin Degradation Products in Serum and Menstrual Fluid of Patients with Menorrhagia], *Chung Kuo Chung Hsi I Chieh Ho Tsa Chih* 11, no. 7 (July 1991): 409–10, 389.

The Chinese remedy called Triple Action Hemostatic Decoction was shown experimentally to be effective in treating menorrhagia.

J. Gao, "TCM Treatment of Adolescent Functional Uterine Hemorrhage—A Clinical Report of 105 Cases," *Journal of Traditional Chinese Medicine* 10, no. 2 (June 1990): 118–21.

HYPERTHERMIA

Hyperthermia is a relatively simple-to-perform new technique of heating the endometrial cavity of the uterus using a probe. In a study of 32 patients given a single 20-minute hyperthermia treatment, a success rate of 84 percent in treating menorrhagia was seen.

M. V. Prior, "Treatment of Menorrhagia by Radio Frequency Heating," *International Journal of Hyperthermia* 7, no. 2 (April–March 1991): 213–20.

18. MIGRAINES

Twenty-three million Americans suffer from migraines. One in five women are affected, as compared to only one in twenty men, making women four times more susceptible to this widespread health problem.

Causes

It is now believed that these headaches occur when sudden dilation of blood vessels create pressure on the brain. There are numerous triggers for migraines. Dr. Mary Olsen, a chiropractor from Huntington, New York, who specializes in craniosacral adjustments and applied kinesiology, gives the eight most common reasons for their occurrence:

ALLERGIC REACTIONS

"Allergies can be dietary or environmental. Dietary triggers can be to foods, food combinations, or additives in foods. Alcoholic beverages, particularly red wine and beer, are among the most common causes of migraines. Tyramine, a chemical found in cheese, smoked fish, yogurt, and yeast extracts, may be involved. MSG, which we find in Chinese cuisine and most processed foods, is often implicated, as is sodium nitrate, found in cold cuts and hot dogs. Aspartame, a commonly used artificial sweetener, may lower serotonin levels in the body. Some researchers believe that this contributes to severe headaches. Chocolate and other foods containing caffeine can also be dietary triggers. In addition, people can have allergies to such common foods as wheat, dairy, corn, and eggs. A person can have environmental allergies to toxic fumes emitted from modern products found in the home."

HORMONAL FLUCTUATIONS

"Women suffer from migraines to a much greater extent than do men. Of these women, approximately 60 percent correlate headaches to their menstrual cycle. The major contributing factor is the hormone estrogen. We know that women who take oral contraceptives are more susceptible to severe migraines, and that women experience less frequency and severity of headaches after menopause, when there is a sharp reduction of estrogen. Unfortunately, the widespread use of estrogen replacement therapy has resulted in many women having a return of these headaches. Although the exact relationship between migraines and estrogen is unknown at this time, we do know that estrogen affects the central nervous system, including the systems involving serotonin, which can be involved in the development of migraines."

CRANIAL FAULTS

"Malposition in cranial bones or cranial faults is another factor contributing to migraines. Trauma to the head, such as striking the head on a car door, or birth trauma, may be enough to lock a bone into a particular position. A whiplash injury may also result in cranial faults."

MERIDIAN IMBALANCE

"The applied kinesiologist or acupuncturist checks for a meridian imbalance. Meridians are twelve bilateral electromagnetic channels of energy in the body, identified within the Chinese science of acupuncture. Blocked energy or *chi* (or *qi*) within a meridian causes dysfunction, including migraine headaches."

UPPER CERVICAL SUBLUXATION

"Another common cause of migraine is the cervical subluxation in the upper part of the neck. This is especially prevalent among people who use the telephone as a regular part of their work. The tendency to hold the phone between the neck and the shoulder forces the vertebrae in the opposite direction. You also see this with people who tend to read in bed. Propping the head up in one direction causes the vertebrae to shift, which puts stress on the nerves and contributes to the migraine."

LOW MAGNESIUM LEVELS

"A number of studies have noted that many people suffering from migraines have low levels of magnesium in their blood. This is true too of people who suffer from fibromyalgia, a myofascial condition that can cause severe pain to the head, mimicking a migraine."

OVER-THE-COUNTER AND PRESCRIPTION MEDICATIONS

"If you use aspirin, acetaminophen, mixed analgesics, or other acute care medications to get rid of your headaches, you actually may be causing them. The use of these painkillers is the single most common reason for migraines. They are called rebound headaches, and this is why they occur. When you take a painkiller often, the body gets used to having a certain amount of that drug in the bloodstream. When the level falls below that threshold, the body begins to experience withdrawal symptoms. One of these symptoms is headaches. If this situation exists, any preventive treatment for migraine will be undermined."

STRESS

"Although stress is not a cause in itself, it can exacerbate the effects of the headache or cause an increase in frequency."

Symptoms

Migraines differ from regular headaches in that they usually occur on one side of the head. They can be accompanied by nausea, vomiting, sensitivity to light and sound, fatigue, weakness, irritability, and vision problems. An aura sometimes precedes a migraine. Usually, this is a visual phenomenon that may appear as a flash of light. However, other sensory systems can be disturbed, causing the aura to appear as numbness, tingling, odor hallucinations, language difficulties, confusion, or disorientation.

Clinical Experience

Although exact treatment depends on a patient's individual needs, Dr. Olsen suggests general guidelines for treating migraines brought on by different factors. Of course, combination approaches are often indicated as well.

MIGRAINES CAUSED BY FOOD ALLERGIES. "Since migraines don't necessarily follow immediately after ingesting a food, it may be difficult to make a connection between a particular food and the resultant headache. We often have patients keep a food diary to record what is eaten and physical reactions. That makes it easier to correlate foods with delayed reactions. If we suspect that a particular food is troublesome, the patient is asked to place a sample of that food under the tongue. If there is a sensitivity, a muscle that tested strong previously will weaken. Pulse is also evaluated for such changes as increases in intensity or frequency. Treatment can be as simple as removing the offending food from the diet."

MIGRAINES CAUSED BY ENVIRONMENTAL ALLERGIES. "If the migraines appear to be caused by environmental allergies, the British Migraine Association recommends keeping houseplants. Different plants have the ability to absorb different toxins. For example, spider plants absorb the formaldehyde released from particle board, plywood, synthetic carpeting and new upholstery, while chrysanthemums protects against the toxic effects of lacquers, varnishes and glues. If you don't feel like keeping a lot of chrysanthemums around the house, the same effect comes from drinking an herbal tea made with this flower."

MIGRAINES CAUSED BY HORMONAL IMBALANCE. "To keep hormones in balance, supplementing the diet with vitamin B6 and evening primrose oil around the time of the menstrual period may help restore hormonal balance enough to forestall migraine attacks."

MIGRAINES CAUSED BY CRANIAL FAULTS. "Since migraines involve the cranial nerves, patients suffering from migraines should always be examined for cranial faults. These faults are extremely difficult to evaluate, due to the subtle movement of bones, but correcting them can be key to healing.

"One of my patients only partially responded to treatment after we corrected other findings that contributed to her headaches. Although the frequency decreased, she still reported migraines. At first, she had a general examination for cranial faults with no positive findings. Finally, after examining every single sutral point (or area of articulation) along the frontal bone in the forehead, we found the problem and corrected it. Her headaches stopped. In this case, the patient had an internally rotated frontal bone. Applied kinesiologists find this to be the most common cause of migraines from a cranial fault. This is particularly true if the patient reports eye pain with the migraine.

"The correction for this is done in three steps. First, pressure is applied to the posterior aspect of the palate on the side of internal rotation. Then a light pressure is applied on the lateral pterygoid muscle, located behind the upper molar in the mouth. Next pressure is applied to the medial pterygoid on the opposite side. That completes the treatment."

MIGRAINES CAUSED BY MERIDIAN IMBALANCE. "The task of the practitioner is to balance the energy by stimulating the meridians. There are various ways of accomplishing this. Acupuncturists use needles, while applied kinesiologists prefer to stimulate the meridians with a finger.

"There are three acupressure or acupuncture points helpful in treating migraines. Lung 7 is located about two finger-widths from the crease in the wrist, on the thumb side of the anterior part of the arm. Bladder 67 is found at the nail point of the little toe, and gall bladder 20 is located between the mastoid and the occipital protuberance in the skull. These are stimulated in a circular or tapping motion until there is an effective change."

MIGRAINES CAUSED BY UPPER CERVICAL SUBLUXATION. "The chiropractor can remove the subluxation with an adjustment to the proper area."

MIGRAINES CAUSED BY LOW MAGNESIUM. "I have found a combination of magnesium and malic acid helpful. A health care practitioner should be consulted because the dosage varies with each patient."

MIGRAINES CAUSED BY MEDICATION. "These individuals must gradually wean themselves away from drugs, with the help of their doctor. When they are no longer dependent on these medications, treatment can begin."

MIGRAINES CAUSED BY STRESS. "Studies in England suggest that the herbal remedy feverfew can reduce the frequency of migraines. Feverfew has sedative qualities and can be taken as a tea. One cup per day is usually effective. In addition, relaxation techniques, such as meditation, progressive muscle relaxation, and yoga can help to reduce stress. Regular moderate exercise, such as swimming or walking, also lowers tension and creates a psychological sense of well-being."

Dr. Jennifer Brett, of Stratford, Connecticut, also comments on the benefits of feverfew: "An important study reported by the *British Medical Journal* back in 1983 found that one to two capsules of a freeze-dried extract of feverfew would prevent most migraines from occurring."

SUPPLEMENTS

In addition to feverfew, Dr. Brett makes the following recommendations: "When feverfew is taken with magnesium, in doses of 250 to 500 mg daily, and *Ginkgo biloba*, most people notice a significant reduction in the number of migraines, even to the point of disappearance. This includes people who suffered daily. Many people come to me who have had no success with more conventional treatments. After starting them on feverfew and magnesium, they get a significant reduction in the number of headaches and the severity of pain. Even when they have headaches, they tend to be less frequent and less painful. In my experience, this combination will work for more than 70 percent of migraine sufferers.

"Some people find that they need to add the nutrient niacin. Niacin causes flushing in many people, and it is exactly this flushing that stops the migraine headache. By taking the blood out of the head and into the skin in the form of a flush, the migraine can be aborted before it even starts."

REFLEXOLOGY

Applying pressure to the feet can alleviate migraines because specific reflex points correspond to the head area. Reflexologist Gerri Brill says the most benefit comes from a routine that encompasses all body systems. Here she gives a detailed description of her program:

CREATING A COMFORTABLE ENVIRONMENT. "I start off by getting you to feel relaxed. Sometimes I use a foot basin to soften and warm up the feet. Then I have you lie down on my massage table while I explain the anatomy of the foot and the idea that each part corresponds to an area of the body. The big toe relates to the head and the little toes relate to the head and sinus. Under the toes is a ridge that corresponds to the neck and shoulders. The chest/lung area corresponds to the ball of the foot. The narrow part is the waist area, and at the heel you have the small and large intestines, the sciatic nerves, and the lower back."

RELAXING BREATHING. "There is a special place on the foot that corresponds to the solar plexus. This is a little notch just below the ball of the foot. The solar plexus is the seat of the emotions. By placing my thumb in this little notch, as you inhale, and releasing as you exhale, I help you to let go of a lot of stuck feelings held inside. It helps promote relaxation and is good to do at the end of the session as well."

WRINGING THE FOOT. "As you lie down, I wring out your foot three times or so, as if I were wringing out a washcloth. That helps the foot relax."

LUNG PRESS. "This is where I press the fist of my right hand into your chest/lung reflex, while holding your foot with my left hand. This area is on the pad of your foot, directly beneath the ridge of the toes. As I press, I slowly bring the flat of my fist down to the heel. I repeat this action three times. It is another relaxation technique."

FOOT-AND-TOE BOOGIE. "Next I do what is called the foot boogie. That means rocking your foot back and forth to loosen it up. Then I do the same with your toes. I place my hands around each toe as I shake your toes back and forth. It sounds silly but it feels great."

ZONE WALKING. "Zone walking is performed with the outer aspect of the thumb. If you place your thumb on your lap, it is the area that rests on your lap. It's important to keep fingernails short so as not to dig into anyone. Using the outer aspect of my thumb, I start way down at the heel. I mentally divide the foot into five zones, with each zone leading to a different toe. Starting at the outside portion of the foot, the fleshier part, I bend the working thumb at a 45 degree angle, and apply pressure as I creep up the foot ever so slightly. Each move is no more than a sixteenth of an inch. There are a lot of nerve endings in the feet, and I want to hit all of them. Applying a steady pressure, I work my thumb upward, all the way to the tip of the toe. When I reach the top of the toes, I go back down to the heel again to repeat the process. These steps are repeated for all five zones. By covering the whole body in this way, I help to create an equilibrium."

SPINE REFLEX. "Now I am at the inside aspect of the foot. That's the spine reflex, and it is very important because the spine supports you and holds you erect. I start at the bottom by your heel with my thumb. Again, I work with the outside corner of my thumb held at a 45 degree angle, and walk up your spine. I go all the way up to the big toe. Then, I turn around and thumb-walk down, using little steps and steady pressure. I don't want to hurt you, but I do want to exert a good amount of pressure since this is pressure therapy."

SHOULDER AND NECK REFLEX. "Now I move to the ridge underneath the toes. This corresponds to the neck and shoulder line, and it is important for headache relief because when people have tension and headaches, their neck and shoulders are usually tense. Again, I use the thumb-walk. I start at the outside of the big toe and thumb-walk to the ridge. I bend the toes back slightly to get inside. This is repeated until I get to the little toe. Then I turn around and thumb-walk back."

HEAD AREA. "The big toe relates to the head, so of course I want to work this area. I place the fingers of my right hand over my left hand, and thumb-walk down the fleshy part of your big toe. I divide the big toe into five zones and work down each area using very, very tiny bites or steps. My aim is for twenty-five bites on that big toe. That covers the whole area. I do that five times. This is very important."

BRAIN REFLEX. "Rolling my index finger over the top of the big toe stimulates the brain and relieves aches caused by migraines. Often this area feels sensitive because of crystal deposits that accumulate. These deposits need to be broken up."

HEAD AND SINUSES. "After finishing the big toe, I move to your little toes. Again, using my thumb, I divide each toe into three zones and thumb-walk, using little bites. This is repeated three times on each toe. This is another place that I feel tiny grains of sand. Breaking these up is the main way to relieve migraines."

CLOSING THE SESSION. "Just to make the session complete, I go back to the top of the foot while supporting the heel with the fist. I finger-walk with the right hand between the little bones on the top of the feet. This area helps the lymphatics, chest, breast, and also part of the back. Massaging here helps you to achieve a state of balance. Then I work around the ankle areas. The ankles relate to the reproductive organs and alleviate headaches caused by PMS. That's just one foot. Now I wrap up the foot that was worked on and start over on the other side. Afterward, I massage both feet at the same time, which is very soothing. At this point, you know that the session is coming to an end. Once again, I massage your solar plexus area and have you take a deep breath. Finally, I do a nerve stroke to soothe the feet. This is where I ask you to imagine taking in peace and balance with each breath. This promotes a profound sense of relaxation. At this point your session is over, but you should rest a few moments instead of getting up quickly. Just relax and acknowledge how great you feel. Be sure to drink some water after your session to flush out the deposits."

Patient Story

DR. OLSEN ON ONE PATIENT'S TREATMENT:
A patient of mine complained of headaches once a month, two days prior to her period. They occurred on the left side of her head and were debilitating, resulting in extreme fatigue and irritability. During this time, she felt that she was of no use to herself or her family, and she would go into a depression.

We made several recommendations. The first was a regular program of exercise, which for her meant walking daily. Exercise helps raise the level of endorphins in the body. Endorphins are the body's natural pain reliever and tend to elevate mood.

Our diet recommendations included the restriction of salt, caffeine, alcohol, and sugar. We added 200 mg of magnesium glyconate and a gram of fish oils each day. Many patients respond well to this.

It is also important to allot extra sleep at this time, particularly for women who have hormonally related migraines.

Her treatment was completed with a balancing of the cranial bones, which allowed the pituitary, the master gland that influences the menstrual cycle, to function properly.

Herbal Pharmacy

Plants containing phytochemicals with antimigraine properties, in order of potency:

>*Myciaria dubia* (camu-camu)
>*Malpighia glabra* (acerola)
>*Momordica charantia* (bitter melon)
>*Portulaca oleracea* (purslane)
>*Phyllanthus emblica* (emblic)
>*Rosa canina* (rose)
>*Capsicum annuum* (bell pepper)
>*Capsicum frutescens* (cayenne)

Carya glabra (pignut hickory)
Nasturtium officinale (berro)
Spinacia oleracea (spinach)
Phaseolus vulgaris (black bean)
Carya ovata (shagbark hickory)
Oenothera biennis (evening primrose)
Helianthus annuus (sunflower)
Allium schoenoprasum (chives)
Chondrus crispus (Irish moss)
Basella alba (vinespinach)
Brassica chinensis (Chinese cabbage)

Hot News

A hot treatment—literally—for cluster headaches is capsaicin, the substance that makes chili peppers hot, which has shown great promise in trials. Other natural treatments that have been the focus of research include a combination of vitamin D and calcium; magnesium supplementation; riboflavin; pyridoxine, used to combat medication-induced migraines; lithium, which raises choline levels (low in cluster-headache sufferers); omega-3 fatty acids; and feverfew.

Research has borne out many patients' claims that red wine, coffee, cow's milk, and chocolate are indeed migraine triggers. The effectiveness of an elimination diet, commonly avoiding preserved foods, dairy foods, and citrus, among others, has been shown in several studies.

Biofeedback is another effective treatment for migraines, along with chiropractics, relaxation techniques, and exercise. Most startling in its simplicity is the use of an elastic band around the head to ease migraine symptoms, which showed remarkable effectiveness in one recent study. *(See below.)*

FROM THE MEDICAL LITERATURE ON MIGRAINES

NUTRITION/DIET

A case study reports on two postmenopausal women with severe migraines who were successfully treated with a combination of vitamin D and calcium.

S. Thys-Jacobs, "Alleviation of Migraines with Therapeutic Vitamin D and Calcium," *Headache* 34, no. 10 (November–December 1994): 590–92.

Low magnesium levels were statistically associated with migraines in a case-control study, prompting the author to argue that magnesium supplementation would probably be effective in a significant number of migraine sufferers.

B. Baker, "New Research Approach Helps Clarify Magnesium/Migraine Link," *Family Practice News* (April 14, 1993): 16.

Italian researchers found a link between migraines and low magnesium levels.

G. Virgilio et al., "Magnesium Content of Mononuclear Blood Cells in Migraine Patients," *Headache* 34, no. 3 (March 1994): 160–65.

Daily supplementation with 400 mg of riboflavin over three months resulted in an approximately 70 percent drop in the severity of headaches in migraine-prone individuals.

J. Schoenen et al., "High-Dose Riboflavin as a Prophylactic Treatment of Migraine: Results of an Open Pilot Study," *Cephalalgia* 14, no. 5 (October 1994): 328–29.

Clinicians found that pyridoxine is an effective agent for combating medication-induced migraines when combined with a gradual detoxification from the offending medications.

A. L. Bernstein, "Vitamin B6 in Clinical Neurology," *Annals of the New York Academy of Sciences* 585 (1990): 250–60.

A case-control study found that red-blood-cell choline concentrations were low in patients suffering from cluster headaches during and between cluster periods, and that choline levels increased by 78 times as a result of treatment with lithium.

J. de Bellerche et al., "Erythrocyte Choline Concentrations and Cluster Headache," *British Medical Journal* 288 (1984): 268–70.

Omega-3 fatty acids were given as daily supplements to 15 severe migraine patients after other medications had failed to relieve their symptoms. The result was significant reductions in the frequency and intensity of the headaches.

C. J. Glucek et al., "Amelioration of Severe Migraine with Omega-3 Fatty Acids: A Double-Blind, Placebo-Controlled Clinical Trial," *American Journal of Clinical Nutrition* 43 (1986): 710.

A placebo-controlled study found that 20 g of fish oil per day in two 6-week treatment periods significantly reduced headache intensity and frequency in 5 of 6 patients.

T. McCarren et al., "Amelioration of Severe Migraine by Fish Oil Omega-3 Fatty Acids," *American Journal of Clinical Nutrition* 41 (1985): 847a.

Experimenters found that 33 out of 45 subjects placed on a histamine-free diet who had a history of wine or food intolerance and chronic headaches showed marked improvement after 4 weeks. Eight experienced a complete remission. Foods avoided in the diet included alcohol, cheese, hard-cured sausages, fish, and pickled cabbage. Reintroduction of such foods into the diet produced the resumption of symptoms.

F. Wantke et al., "Histamine-Free Diet: Treatment of Choice for Histamine-Induced Food Intolerance and Supporting Treatment for Chronic Headaches," *Clinical and Experimental Allergy* 23 (1993): 982–85.

Red wine can cause migraines, an experiment proved. Migraine patients believing that red wine specifically—rather than alcohol in general—provoked their headaches were tested for the effects of red wine or a diluted vodka mix disguised to taste and look like red wine and controlled for equivalent alcohol content. Nine of 11 patients experienced migraines following the consumption of red wine, while none of the 8 vodka consumers experienced migraines.

T.J. Littlewood et al., "Red Wine as a Cause of Migraine," *Lancet* 1 (March 12, 1988): 558–59.

A study found that patients with a history of migraines caused by diet have lower platelet levels of phenolsulfotransferase P compared to healthy controls or those whose migraines were not the result of food. This may explain the migraine-inducing effects of red wine, since it has been shown to cause 100 percent inhibition of phenolsulfotransferase P.

J. Littlewood et al., "Platelet Phenolsulfotransferase Deficiency in Dietary Migraine," *Lancet* 1 (1982): 983-86.

Removal of cow's milk from the diet of 48 patients suffering from either migraine or nonseasonal asthma resulted in clinical alleviation in 22. Of the patients experiencing a benefit, all showed signs of lactase deficiency.

D. Ratner et al., "Milk Protein-Free Diet for Nonseasonal Asthma and Migraine in Lactase-Deficient Patients," *Israeli Journal of Medical Science* 19, no. 9 (September 1983): 806–9.

A study found a significant association between daily caffeine intake and the prevalence of headache.

M. J. Shirlow and C. D. Mather, "A Study of Caffeine Consumption and Symptoms: Indigestion, Palpitations, Tremor, Headache, and Insomnia," *International Journal of Epidemiology* 14, no. 2 (1985): 239–48.

About 500 patients with classical or common migraines were asked about what brought their symptoms on. Twenty-nine percent reported headaches could be precipitated by alcohol, 19 percent by chocolate, 18 percent by cheese, and 11 percent by citrus fruit, with a significant number of patients reporting sensitivities to each.

R. C. Peatfield et al., "The Prevalence of Diet-Induced Migraine," *Cephalalgia* 4, no. 3 (September 1984): 179–83.

A study put 4 classic and 3 common migraine patients on a carbohydrate-rich diet, low in protein-trypophan. Improvements were seen in 3 of the 4 patients with classic migraines but in none of those with common migraines. The authors suggest these findings could be the result of increased brain serotonin levels or a restricted consumption of migraine-inducing foods.

L. Hasselmark et al., "Effect of a Carbohydrate-Rich Diet, Low in Protein-Tryptophan, in Classic and Common Migraine," *Cephalalgia* 7, no. 2 (June 1987): 87–92.

A study showed that women with recurrent migraines, flushes, urticaria, and itching excoriation experienced a reduction in all symptoms when placed on a diet eliminating serotonin-rich foods and restricting foods with a high tryptophan-to-protein ratio.

G. Unge et al., "Effects of Dietary Protein-Tryptophan Restriction upon 5-HT Uptake by Platelets and Clinical Symptoms in Migraine-Like Headache," *Cephalalgia* 3, no. 4 (1983): 213–18.

Foods often associated with migraine attack include cow's milk, which in a study was recorded as a problem in 10 out of 17 patients; eggs, flour, and cabbage (in 5 patients), cottage and Swiss cheese, preservatives, and pork (in 4 patients), chocolate and colorants (3 patients), and beef, strawberries, lemons, and butter (3 patients). Elimination diets were shown to be effective in limiting migraine attacks.

D. Mylek, "Migrena Jako Jedenz Objawow Alergii Pokarmowej" [Migraine as one of the Symptoms of Food Allergy], *Pol.Tyg. Lek.* 47, no. 3–4 (January 20–27, 1992): 89–91.

Migraine patients were surveyed as to whether they suspected specific triggers of their attacks. Seventy-nine percent were able to identify precipitating factors to their migraines such as fatigue, hormones, stress, and missing meals. Common foods that caused problems included chocolate, cheese, and alcohol.

"Migraine and Food Allergy," *Occupational Safety and Health* 25, no. 2 (February 1995): 38.

Double-blind studies have shown that monosodium glutamate can cause migraines in some individuals. The problem is that it's hard to eliminate this additive from the diet, since MSG is used in so many foods. Examples of everyday foods that often contain MSG without necessarily saying so on their labels are salad dressings, sauces, soups, and many frozen and prepared foods.

"MSG in Foods," *Nutrition Research Newsletter* 10, no. 5 (May 1991): 52.

In a study, 5-hour 100 g glucose tolerance tests were performed on 74 migraine patients who believed their attacks were brought on by fasting in midmorning or midafternoon. Fifty-six of the patients had test results suggestive of reactive hypoglycemia, and 6 were diagnosed as diabetic. Dietary therapy resulted in a 75 percent or greater improvement in 63 percent of the patients, between 50 and 75 percent improvement in 40 percent, and improvement of 25 to 50 percent in 9 percent of the patients.

J. D. Dexter et al., "The Five-Hour Glucose Tolerance Test and Effect of Low Sucrose Diet in Migraine," *Headache* 18 (1978): 91–94.

Foods like chocolate, nuts, wheat germ, and shellfish may be migraine inducers because they contain large amounts of copper. Also, citrus fruits can be a problem because they increase intestinal absorption of copper. The flavor-enhancer MSG, which binds transport copper between blood and tissue, is another potential migraine-inducing agent. The copper-migraine link seems to stem from copper's role in the metabolism of vasoneuroactive amines.

D. P. Harrison, "Copper as a Factor in the Dietary Precipitation of Migraine," *Headache* 26, no. 5 (1986): 248–50.

Approximately 30 to 40 percent of patients suffering from migraines experience relief by eliminating specific foods from the diet.

L. E. Mansfield, "Food Allergy and Migraine: Whom to Evaluate and How to Treat," *Postgraduate Medicine* 83, no. 7 (1988): 46–55.

Elimination diets can provide relief for a significant number of migraine-sufferers.

L. E. Mansfield, "Food Allergy and Adult Migraine: Double-Blind and Mediator Confirmation of an Allergic Etiology," *Annals of Allergy* 55 (1985): 126.

In a study of 171 headache patients, 8.2 percent identified aspartame as a cause. Aspartame was reported as a cause three times more often by migraine patients than by those suffering from other kinds of headaches.

R. Lipton et al., "Aspartame as a Dietary Trigger of Headache," *Headache* 29 (1989): 90–92.

A placebo-controlled study revealed that aspartame ingestion is significantly associated with an increased frequency of migraines.

S. M. Koehler and A. Glaros, "The Effect of Aspartame on Migraine Headache," *Headache* 28, no. 1 (1988): 10–14.

HERBS/PLANT EXTRACTS

Italian researchers found that 11 of 16 cluster headache patients experienced a cessation of headaches after being treated with a squirt of a capsaicin solution in the nostril on the same side of the face as that with the headache. Two additional patients experienced a decrease in headaches of 50 percent.

J. Raloff, "Hot Prospects for Quelling Cluster Headaches," *Science News* (July 13, 1991): 20–21.

Patients with cluster headaches who received treatment with intranasal capsaicin experienced a significant decrease in headache severity relative to controls who had received placebos, a double-blind study showed.

D. R. Marks et al., "A Double-Blind Placebo-Controlled Trial of Intranasal Capsaicin for Cluster Headache," *Cephalalgia* 13, no. 2 (1993): 114–16.

A randomized, double-blind, placebo-controlled crossover study examined the effects of feverfew (*Tanacetum parthenium*) on migraine patients. Results showed that one capsule of dried feverfew leaves taken daily for 4 months resulted in a reduction in the mean number and severity of migraine attacks.

J. J. Murphy et al., "Randomised Double-Blind Placebo-Controlled Trial of Feverfew in Migraine Prevention," *Lancet* 2, no. 8604 (July 23, 1988): 189–92.

Results of a double-blind, placebo-controlled trial demonstrated that 17 migraine patients who ate fresh feverfew leaves daily prevented the worsening of attacks.

E. S. Johnson et al., "Efficacy of Feverfew as Prophylactic Treatment of Migraine," *British Medical Journal* 291, no. 6495 (August 31, 1985): 569–73.

Noting that most migraine drugs have side effects that limit their use, some researchers propose ginger as an alternative since it is known in Ayurvedic and Tibb systems of medicine to be helpful in treating neurological disorders.

T. Mustafa and K. C. Srivastava, "Ginger (*Zingiber officinale*) in Migraine Headache," *Journal of Ethnopharmacology* 29, no. 3 (July 1990): 267–73.

BIOFEEDBACK

A study demonstrated that migraine patients treated with biofeedback experienced decreases in pain, need for medication, and systolic and mean cerebral flood flow velocity relative to a control group that practiced self-relaxation.

A. McGrady et al., "Effect of Biofeedback-Assisted Relaxation on Migraine Headache and Changes in Cerebral Blood Flow Velocity in the Middle Cerebral Artery," *Headache* 34, no. 7 (July–August 1994): 424–28.

Clinicians examined the effects of the home practice of hand-warming biofeedback therapy on migraine in 17 female patients. Results: a significant decrease in headaches in women who participated in home practice versus those who received biofeedback without the home practice.

J. Gauthier et al., "The Role of Home Practice in the Thermal Biofeedback Treatment of Migraine Headache," *Journal of Consul. Clin. Psychol.* 62, no. 1 (February 1994): 180–84.

Biofeedback is equally effective in reducing menstrual and nonmenstrual migraine, doctors found.

J. G. Gauthier et al., "The Differential Effects of Biofeedback in the Treatment of Menstrual and Nonmenstrual Migraine," *Headache* 31, no. 2 (February 1991): 82–90.

RELAXATION

Significant relief from migraines was achieved following 8 sessions of relaxation training, a study showed.

J. J. Wisniewskie et al., "Relaxation Therapy and Compliance in the Treatment of Adolescent Headache," *Headache* 28, no. 9 (October 1988): 612–17.

CHIROPRACTIC

Spinal manipulative therapy proved to be an effective means of treating tension headaches in a clinical trial.

P. D. Boline et al., "Spinal Manipulation vs. Amitriptyline for the Treatment of Chronic Tension-Type Headaches: A Randomized Clinical Trial," *Journal of Manipulative Physiological Therapy* 18, no. 3 (March–April 1995): 148–54.

EXERCISE

Results of a study confirmed that patients suffering from classical migraines experienced a reduction in headaches following a 6-week cardiovascular exercise program.

D. M. Lockett and J. F. Campbell, "The Effects of Aerobic Exercise on Migraine," *Headache* 32, no. 1 (January 1992): 50–54.

TRADITIONAL CHINESE MEDICINE

Over 50 patients with migraines were treated with the traditional Chinese herbal medicine *Radix puerairae*, in tablet form. Results demonstrated an efficacy rate of 83 percent, and no side effects. Based on these and previous findings, the authors believe that *Radix puerairae* works on migraines because it can lead to increased cerebral blood flow and a decrease in cerebrovascular resistance.

G. Xiuxian and L. Xiuqin, "*Radix Puerariae* in Migraine," *Chinese Medical Journal* 92, no. 4 (1979): 260–62.

HOMEOPATHY

Homeopathy offers help with migraines, researchers showed. In a randomized, double-blind, placebo-controlled study, they gave 60 patients either belladonna, ignatia, lachasis, silicea, gelsemium, cyclamen, natrium muriaticum, or sulphur, based on individual circumstances. After 2 weeks there was a significant decrease in the frequency and length of migraine attacks.

B. Brigo and G. Serpelloni, "Homeopathic Treatment of Migraines: A Randomized Double-Blind Controlled Study of Sixty Cases (Homeopathic Remedy Versus Placebo)," *Berlin Journal of Res. Homoeopath.* 1, no. 2 (March 1991): 98–106.

An article comments on the progress of a group of 54 migraine patients treated by one practitioner who treated them with homeopathic remedies and diet and then followed up 18 months later. Results showed that of the 43 respondents, 35 reported improvement in symptoms within a week of the treatment, and that they continued to do well.

A. D. Fox, "An Assessment of Treatment of Migraine-Headache Syndrome in Patients Seen in Private Practice," *British Homeopathic Journal* 79, no. 4 (October 1990): 221–23.

19. OSTEOPOROSIS

Osteoporosis (the word means "porous bones") is a serious problem in which the skeletal system weakens and fractures easily. More females than males become afflicted, with postmenopausal women being at greatest risk. Osteoporosis is attributed to the gradual loss of calcium, a process which begins in a woman's mid-thirties at a rate of 1–2 percent a year, and which can increase during menopause to a rate of 4–5 percent a year.

Causes

According to Dr. Jane Guiltinan, the most likely candidates for osteoporosis share a number of characteristics:

Northern European ethnic origin
Small frame
Family history of osteoporosis
Diet high in meat, caffeine, sugar, refined carbohydrates, and phosphates (found in sodas and processed foods)
Cigarette smoking
Alcohol use
Sedentary lifestyle

It may surprise some people to learn that dairy foods, while rich sources of calcium, can also contribute to the condition of osteoporosis. Registered nurse and acupuncturist Abigail Rist-Podrecca notes, "When I was in China, we noticed that no dairy was used. We expected to see a high incidence of osteoporosis, rickets, and other bone problems. In fact, we saw the lowest incidence. In the West, dairy is used a lot and osteoporosis is rampant. Something is not quite right here." Two main factors responsible for the Chinese not getting osteoporosis, she learned, are diet, weight-bearing exercise, and acupuncture. (*See below.*)

Symptoms

Osteoporosis is accompanied by pain, especially lower back pain, frequent, spontaneous fractures due to decrease in bone mass, loss in height, and body deformity.

Clinical Experience

CONVENTIONAL APPROACH

Synthetic estrogen is the traditional drug of choice for postmenopausal osteoporosis prevention, but controversy surrounds its safety and effectiveness. *(See chapter 4, Breast Cancer).*

NATUROPATHIC APPROACH

RISK ASSESSMENT. The first step in osteoporosis prevention is noting whether or not you are at high risk for the condition, says Dr. Guiltinan. Obviously, certain risk factors cannot be changed, but many can be addressed, and will prevent the destructive effects of the disease.

DIET. A diet that is low in animal products and high in plant foods promotes bone growth and repair. Green leafy vegetables contain vitamin K, beta carotene, vitamin C, fiber, calcium, and magnesium, which enhance the bones. Other calcium-rich foods include broccoli, milk, nuts, and seeds. Sesame seeds have high calcium content. The Chinese, who as mentioned earlier have low rates of osteoporosis, use sesame often in their foods, and cook with sesame seed oil.

Foods to avoid include sugar, caffeine, carbonated sodas, and alcohol, as these contribute to bone loss. Too much protein from chicken, fish, eggs, and meat are also contraindicated. These are high in the amino acid methionine, which the body converts into homocysteine, a substance that causes both osteoporosis and atherosclerosis.

VITAMINS AND MINERALS. Women over 25 need adequate calcium, approximately 1,000 mg in supplement form, and an additional 500–1,000 mg from the diet. After 40, 1,500–2,000 mg is needed. Women on estrogen replacement therapy require between 1,200 and 1,500 mg.

In addition to calcium, the following nutrients are critical for keeping bones strong:

> Magnesium (500–600 mg in citrate form)
> Vitamin D (400 IU)
> Vitamin C (1,000 mg)
> Vitamin K (100 mcg)
> Beta carotene
> Selenium (75–150 mcg)
> Boron (3 mg)
> Manganese (5 mg)
> Strontium
> Folic acid (1 mg)

Silica

Copper

Zinc

A balanced vitamin/mineral supplement will provide most of these nutrients. It is best to take zinc separately, however; otherwise, it can have an adverse effect on vitamin and mineral absorption.

NATURAL HORMONES

NATURAL PROGESTERONE. Research indicates that natural progesterone from wild yams is safer and more effective than estrogen in that it builds strong bones and has no harmful side effects. Dr. Guiltinan notes that "Estrogen minimizes calcium loss from bones, but progesterone can actually put calcium back into bones." Natural progesterone can be taken in pill form. It also comes in a cream form. Half a teaspoon should be rubbed into the skin over soft tissue and the spine, twice a day, for two weeks out of every month.

DHEA. This precursor to estrogen and testosterone is important in the prevention of numerous chronic conditions associated with aging. As we get older, there is often a drop in DHEA. If blood levels are low, 5 mg a day can safely be taken as a supplement.

EXERCISE

Dr. Howard Robins, director of the Healing Center in New York City and coauthor of *Ultimate Training* and *How to Keep Your Feet & Legs Healthy for a Lifetime,* stresses the importance of weight-bearing aerobic and weight-lifting exercises for osteoporosis prevention.

AEROBICS. Aerobic exercises use major muscle groups in a rhythmic, continuous manner. Weight-bearing aerobic exercises such as brisk walking, jogging, stair climbing, and dancing produce mechanical stress on the skeletal system, which drives calcium into the long bones. Non-weight-bearing aerobic exercises such as biking, rowing, and swimming are not as helpful in osteoporosis prevention, but they do promote flexibility, which is useful for women prone to arthritis.

"Women as well as men need to perform aerobic exercises anywhere from three to five or six times a week," says Dr. Robins. "You need a day off every third or fourth day so that the body can heal and reenergize."

WEIGHT TRAINING. "Most women stay away from weight training because they are afraid of developing, huge muscles like Arnold Schwarzenegger," says Dr. Robins. "The good news is, that won't happen. No matter how hard you train, you will never get huge muscles as a woman unless you take steroids to alter your body's metabolism."

Not only is weight training safe, it is important for preventing osteoporosis. As muscles are pulled directly against the bone, with gravity working against it, calcium is driven back into the bones. It also stimulates the manufacture of new bone. This adds up to a decrease in the effects of osteoporosis by 50–80 percent. Women need to do weight training two to three times per week for fifteen to thirty minutes. All the different muscle groups should be worked on. Twenty-four hours should lapse between sessions to rest muscles. For best results, an exercise program should be started long before the onset of menopause.

WARM-UPS AND COOL-DOWNS. A complete routine is more than aerobic and weight training exercises only. It incorporates warm-ups at the beginning and cool-downs at the end of a routine. Warm-ups are not to be confused with stretches. Rather, they are gentle exercises that produce heat by getting blood to flow into the muscles. To warm up leg muscles, for example, one could lie down on one's back and move the legs like a bicycle, or walk gently in place. Moving the arms and joints gently in all their ranges of motion will warm up the upper body. Warming up the body helps prevent injuries.

After exercise, when the body is loosest, stretching is performed. Stretches are long, continuous pulls, not bounces. Bouncing only tightens the muscles and can lead to injury. Robins's book *Ultimate Training* describes a holistic workout in detail. Aromatherapist Ann Berwick adds that essential oils enhance a warm-up and cool-down routine. "Before exercise, use warming and stimulating oils, such as black pepper, rosemary, ginger, and sage. Additionally, eucalyptus helps to deepen breathing. After exercise, you can apply a blend of lemon, rosemary, and juniper. These help to carry away waste products and to ease any stiffness."

YOGA. Yoga prevents osteoporosis in four ways: it builds and fortifies bone mass; it keeps muscles strong and flexible; it improves posture; and it helps balance and coordination. Physical therapist and yoga teacher Bonnie Millen explains why this is important: "With yoga, the old adage 'Use it or lose it' applies. Building and maintaining bone mass is most important for preventing osteoporosis. Remember, bone is alive. Yoga is unique in that it incorporates weight bearing on the upper extremities. Fractures of the wrist, forearm, and upper arm are common in women because as they fall they tend to reach forward with outstretched arms. Yoga has postures that involve weight bearing on the arms.

"Also important is building and maintaining muscle strength and flexibility. Let's keep the muscles strong so that they can receive the stress before the fracture happens. Also if the body is strong and flexible, it can cushion falls when they occur.

"Good posture improves overall functioning and prevents osteoporetic fractures of the spine. I teach yoga to a lot of older women who tell me they are afraid of getting a dowager's hump. This is where the body slouches forward and there is a hump on the back. Just take a moment to get into that posture where your chest caves in and your shoulders slump forward, with your head looking down toward the floor. Try to raise one arm up as if you wanted to touch the ceiling, and see how high the arm comes up. Now let the arm down and come into a nice seated posture, as if someone were going to take your picture. Sitting very tall, raise your arm up and see how high it goes. You can see from that little exercise that the slouched posture really decreases your range of motion. That makes it difficult to function. This is why you want to keep a good posture.

"By placing great pressure on the spinal vertebrae, the dowager's hump often leads to compression fractures of the spinal column. This is very painful, as you can well imagine, and you do not have to do anything special for it to happen. Just going up and down stairs or taking a step can cause breakage.

"The fourth way yoga helps is by improving balance and coordination. When you are balanced and coordinated, there is less chance of your falling in the first place. You are quicker to respond. And that can help prevent fractures."

Millen points out that there are several styles of yoga but that all systems have foundation poses that address the above needs. Here she outlines a few basic postures:

Downward-Facing Dog. This posture strengthens bone mass in the wrists and arms. In this pose, you stand and bring your hands to the floor so that the space beneath you is triangular. One part of the triangle is from your hands to your hips, and the other part is from your hips to your heels. The space on the floor between your hands and your feet is the third part. As you hold the position, you will feel that you are bearing weight on your arms.

Warrior poses. These poses increase muscle strength and flexibility, as well as balance. Here you are standing with your legs three to four feet apart, depending on your height. With your legs apart, you work at the hip to turn one leg out to the side. The other leg is turned slightly inward. That really works the hip muscles, which is important in helping to prevent the all-too-common osteoporetic hip fracture. The arms are either held out to the side or up over the head, depending upon which warrior posture it is.

Cobra. This is a back-bending pose that helps posture and gives flexibility and strength to the paraspinals, the muscles of the back of the spine. To begin, lie face down on the floor. Using the back muscles, sequentially lift the head and chest away from the floor.

Simple stretch for chest muscles. This is another exercise for improving posture that is especially helpful for women who tend to slouch forward. Take a blanket and fold it to resemble a box of long-stemmed roses. Lie down on this bolster, making sure that your head and your entire spine are completely supported. Place your arms out to the side or up to form a V-shaped position with the palms facing up toward the ceiling. Just allow gravity to relax the shoulders down to the floor (Shoulders should not be on the blanket). Breathe deeply. That will expand the intercostals, the muscles between the ribs. This is important because the intercostals become constricted with slouching. That, in turn, decreases lung capacity and causes all the organs to become compressed. This is a wonderful pose where you don't have to actually do anything. You just allow gravity to work for you and your breath to move through you.

Millen says that the best time to begin yoga is before osteoporosis sets in: "The time to begin a yoga practice, or any exercise, is not when you've gotten to menopause, and all of a sudden you realize, 'Oh my gosh! I'm at risk for osteoporosis.' You need to build bone mass throughout your whole life so that you have bone stored up. It's like preparing for retirement. You build up bone mass through exercise, you eat right, you maintain a healthy lifestyle. Then, when you reach your menopausal years, you've got a good store of bone mass to help protect you."

ACUPUNCTURE

As mentioned earlier, in China, osteoporosis is the exception rather than the norm. When it does manifest, women are treated with acupuncture. Rist-Podrecca explains how this works: "The Chinese use an electrical stimulus along the spine. The electrical impulse actually helps the bone stem cells, which are the reproductive cells of the bone, to reproduce, thereby strengthening the bone mass. It was very exciting to see this because we have some Western studies proving that peripheral stimulation by electricity, especially in the long bones in the leg, help this process also." She adds that women low in calcium need to take this supplement so that the body has the raw materials for making bones denser. When weight-bearing exercises are added, the benefits are remarkable.

HOMEOPATHY

Homeopathy can be used as an adjunct to the nutritional and lifestyle factors discussed above. These are some remedies to consider:

Calcarea phosphoric. This may help where the bones are weak, soft, curved, and brittle. It can be given for a long period of time.

Corticoid. Homeopathic corticoid is for painful posttraumatic osteoporosis, especially when it affects the hip. Consider this remedy for an elderly person who has fractured her hip because of osteoporosis.

Parathyroid. For diffuse pain in the bones, especially the long bones. Walking is very painful. Often, there is pain in the ankles, hips, and knees.

Regarding potencies, homeopathic physician Dr. Ken Korins says, "For acute conditions, meaning they come on suddenly, and they are very intense, use a 200c potency. That is a very dilute potency, but energetically speaking, it is very powerful. For more chronic conditions, where you will be giving the remedy for a longer period of time, you might want to start with 12c or 30c. In general, the remedies should be taken as three to four pellets placed under the tongue. Take them on an empty stomach. Wait fifteen to twenty minutes before or after eating. Avoid coffee and aromatic substances, such as mints, perfumes, and camphors, which can interfere with their effectiveness. Also, it is a good idea not to touch remedies with your hands because any residues from perfumes or other substances can interfere with their energy properties."

Hot News

The risk of osteoporosis is increased by alcohol, caffeine in coffee (although tea contains caffeine, it also contains fluoride, a bone-strengthening compound), animal fat, and a diet high in animal protein. Studies show that animal-based protein, which increases the amount of acid in the body, causes the body to use calcium as a pH buffer; since plant protein does not have this effect, vegetarians have a much lower incidence of osteoporosis. Potassium bicarbonate can neutralize the calcium-leaching acidity of the normal American diet, another study shows. Boron also can help keep calcium in the bones; it is supplied in a diet rich in fruit and vegetables, but can also be supplemented. Other supplements of value include essential fatty acids, arginine, and tochu bark extract, which speeds intestinal calcium absorption.

A promising nondietary therapy for osteoporosis is the use of pulsed electromagnetic fields; and study after study bears witness to the paramount value of exercise in maintaining bone density. *(See below.)*

FROM THE MEDICAL LITERATURE ON OSTEOPOROSIS

NUTRITION/DIET

Alcohol consumption increases the risk of osteoporosis. A study of almost 85,000 women showed that those drinking 25 g of alcohol or more per day had a risk of hip fracture over twice that of nondrinkers.

M. Hernandez-Avila et al., "Caffeine, Moderate Alcohol Intake, and Risk of Fracures of the Hip and Forearm in Middle-Aged Women," *American Journal of Clinical Nutrition* 54 (1991): 157–63.

Caffeine intake has been associated with an increased risk of hip fractures. However, according to one source, while coffee may increase the risk of osteoporosis, tea is not a problem, since it contains fluoride, a bone-strengthening compound. Also, tea drinkers tend to consume less caffeine than coffee drinkers do.

"Coffee Increases Risk of Osteoporosis," *East West Natural Health* 22, no. 5 (September–October 1992): 16.

A study of over 3,000 people showed that those drinking more than 2 cups of coffee or the equivalent amount of caffeine in tea on a daily basis were 53 percent more likely to fracture their hips than were abstainers from caffeine.

D. Kiel et al., "Caffeine and the Risk of Hip Fracture: The Framingham Study," *American Journal of Epidemiology* 132 (1990): 675–84.

A high-protein animal-based diet may cause osteoporosis in spite of an "adequate" dietary intake of calcium. The problem is that animal-based protein increases the amount of acid in the body, while plant-based protein does not. In response to acid, bones release calcium as a buffer. Then, rather than reabsorbing the calcium, the body excretes it because animal protein also inhibits reabsorption by lowering parathyroid activity. That "adequate" calcium intake may result in a negative calcium balance if diet is high in animal protein was seen in a study of women aged 50–64 that showed a negative calcium balance in most of those on a high-protein diet. A vegan diet is seen as being best in terms of osteoporosis prevention.

R. Pickarski, "The Protein Issue and Vegetarianism," *Total Health* 12, no. 3 (June 1990): 25–28.

Studies of various ethnic groups show that the higher the average protein intake, the greater the prevalence of osteoporosis. Americans have a high incidence: 26 percent of women have vertebral crush by age 65. And those on even higher animal-protein diets, i.e., North American Eskimos, have a higher risk of osteoporosis. By the time an Eskimo woman is in her early forties, chances are her bone density will be 85 percent less than that of an age-matched U.S. woman. On the other hand, those groups that eat vegetarian or vegan diets tend to have a low risk of osteoporosis. Examples include Bantu women, who have one-tenth as many hip fractures as white women, and Seventh Day Adventists, who tend to be lacto-ovo-vegetarians.

T. R. Watkins et al., "Urinary Acid and Calcium Excretion: Effect of Soy Versus Meat in Human Diets," in C. Kies (ed.), *Nutritional Bioavailability of Calcium* (Washington, D.C.: American Chemistry Society, 1985): 73–87.

The difference in bone mineral mass between lacto-ovo-vegetarian women compared to omnivorous women accelerates with age. At each decade after 50, omnivorous women had more osteoporosis. Between 60 and 89, omnivorous women lost 35 percent of their bone mass, while the lacto-ovo-vegetarian women lost 18 percent.

I. V. Sanchez et al., "Bone Mineral Mass in Elderly Vegetarian Females," *American Journal of Roentgenol.* 131 (1978): 542.

A study of 18 postmenopausal women showed that potassium bicarbonate neutralized the excess of acid—which results in calcium loss—of a normal American diet.

A. Sebastian et al., "Improved Mineral Balance and Skeletal Metabolism in Postmenopausal Women Treated with Potassium Bicarbonate," *New England Journal of Medicine* 330, no. 25 (June 23, 1994): 1776–1782.

Excess salt should be avoided because salt impairs the body's ability to use vitamin D.

C. Y. K. Pak, "Calcium Metabolism," *Journal of the American College of Nutrition* 8 (1989): 46S–53S.

In a study of 26 postmenopausal women receiving hormone replacement therapy, those receiving dietary counseling plus a multivitamin/multimineral supplement showed an 11 percent increase in bone density after 6-12 months, while those who received the dietary counseling alone showed only a 0.7 percent increase.

G. E. Abraham, "The Importance of Magnesium in the Management of Postmenopausal Osteoporosis," *Journal of Nutritional Medicine* 2 (1991): 165–78

Phosphorous supplements were shown to produce increases in bone surface involved in resorption.

R. S. Goldsmith et al., "Effect of Phosphorous Supplementation on Serum Parathyroid Hormone and Bone Morphology in Osteoporosis," *Journal of Clinical Endocrinology Metabolism* 43 (1976): 523–32.

The amount of boron usually found in diets high in fruit and vegetables (or a supplement of 3 mg daily) reduces urinary and magnesium excretion and helps the body keep calcium in the bones.

F. H. Nielsen et al., "Effect of Dietary Boron on Mineral, Estrogen, and Testosterone Metabolism in Postmenopausal Women," *Fed. Am. Soc. Exp. Biol.* 1, no. 5 (1987): 394–97.

Vitamin K was shown to decrease urinary calcium levels, and to increase calcium-binding capacity.

M. H. J. Knapen et al., "The Effect of Vitamin K Supplementation on Circulating Osteocalcin (Bone Gla Protein) and Urinary Calcium Excretion," *Annals of Internal Medicine* 111 (1989): 1001–5.

A study of 40 osteoporotic patients monitored the effectiveness of treatment with essential fatty acids (evening primrose oil, fish oil, and a mixture of the two). The therapeutic effect was measured by monitoring biochemical markers of bone turnover. The results were that EFAs reduced urinary excretion of calcium and increased calcium deposit in bones. Although the effects demonstrated by the study were modest, such incremental effects over years or decades add up. Another consideration is that EFAs are safe for long-term use by the elderly.

D. H. Van Papendorp et al., "Biochemical Profile of Osteoporotic Patients on Essential Fatty Acid Supplementation," *Nutrition Research* 15, no. 3 (1995): 325–34.

Pernicious anemia increases the risk of osteoporosis, but treatment with B12 and cyclic etidronate can help normalize bone density.

M. E. Melton and M. L. Kochman, "Reversal of Severe Osteoporosis with Vitamin B12 and Etidronate Therapy in a Patient with Pernicious Anemia," *Metabolism* 43, no. 4 (April 1994): 468–69.

Arginine supplementation may increase bone formation.

J. J. Visser and K. Hoekman, "Arginine Supplementation in the Prevention and Treatment of Osteoporosis," *Medical Hypotheses* 43, no. 5 (November 1994): 339–42.

Factors relevant to prevention of osteoporosis include calcium status, vitamin D, fluoride, magnesium, and other trace elements, especially copper, manganese, and zinc. All of these trace elements are necessary for optimal bone development and density.

P. D. Saltman and L. G. Strause, "The Role of Trace Minerals in Osteoporosis," *Journal of the American College of Nutrition* 12, no. 4 (August 1993): 384–89.

EXERCISE

High-impact aerobic exercise improves spinal bone mineral density by 7 percent in postmenopausal women. Jumping in place improves bone mineral density in thigh bones.

E. J. Bassey et al. "Exercise in Primary Prevention of Osteoporosis in Women," *Annals of the Rheumatic Diseases* 54, no. 11 (November 1995): 861-63.

A regular exercise period can be valuable in preventing osteoporosis. Bone mineral density (BMD) values increased almost 5 percent with regular exercise, researchers found, while in a control group BMD values decreased by almost 3 percent.

G. Dilsen et al., "The Role of Physical Exercise in Prevention and Management of Osteoporosis," *Clinical Rheumatology* 8, suppl. 2 (June 1989): 70–75.

HERBS/PLANT EXTRACTS

Results of a controlled study on female rats indicated that tochu bark extract accelerates intestinal calcium absorption, improving muscle weight and bone density.

L. J. Kiu et al., "The Effect of Tochu Bark on Bone Metabolism in the Rat Model with Ovariectomized Osteoporosis," *Journal of Nutritional Sci. Vitaminol.* 40, no. 3 (June 1994): 261–73.

TRADITIONAL CHINESE MEDICINE

Chinese medicinal herbs were proven effective against osteoporosis, studies with women have shown.

Y. H. Huang and X. Q. Ye, [Bone Metabolism and Chinese Medicinal Treatment of Menopausal Osteoporosis], *Chung Kuo Chung Hsi I Chieh Ho Tsa Chih* 13, no. 9 (September 1993): 522–24, 515.

ELECTROMAGNETIC FIELDS

Animal studies show osteoporosis can be prevented and reversed with a treatment of pulsed electromagnetic fields.

C. T. Rubin et al., "Prevention of Osteoporosis by Pulsed Electromagnetic Fields," *Journal of Bone Joint Surgery*, 71, no. 3 (March 1989): 411-417.

Osteoporosis in rat tibia was reversed with a 60-Hz symmetrical sinewave signal at 10V peak-to-peak.

M. Li, [Electrical Stimulation in the Treatment of Osteoporosis in Sciatic Denervated Rat Tibia], *Chung Hua Wai Ko Tsa Chih* 30, no. 8 (August 1992): 458–60, 508.

Pulsed electromagnetic fields were shown effective in slowing bone loss in rats.

T.W. Bilotta et al., "Electromagnetic Fields in the Treatment of Postmenopausal Osteoporosis: An Experimental Study Conducted by Densitometric, Dry Ash Weight and Metabolic Analysis of Bone Tissue," *Chir. Organi. Mov.* 79, no. 3 (July–September 1994): 309–13.

SMOKING

The more cigarettes smoked, the more bone mass reduces. On the other hand, quitting smoking (even in later life) should help preserve bone density.

K. A. Hollenbach, "Cigarette Smoking and Bone Mineral Density in Older Men and Women," *American Journal of Public Health* 83, no. 9 (September 1993): 1265–71.

20. PARASITES

Women who are getting no relief from chronic fatigue, urinary tract infection, pelvic inflammatory disease, vaginitis, and candida treatments should consider the possibility of this pervasive but underdiagnosed condition as the root cause of their problem. "Underestimated statistics suggest that approximately seven million Americans are infected with disease-producing parasites," states complementary physician Dr. Pavel Yutsis of New York, "which live at the expense of their hosts, human beings, and cause injury."

Parasites are represented by two main groups, one being worms and the other protozoa. Worms that invade the system include pinworms, hookworms, ringworms, roundworms, and tapeworms. They live off undigested food on the intestinal walls, especially sugar and refined carbohydrates. But the majority of people are affected by protozoa. Dr. Yutsis says these single-celled organisms multiply in the host and can survive and thrive in the face of the host's sophisticated defense forces: "Why are protozoa so resistant? It is because they live inside the cells, which make them immunologically untouchable. Although immunity to protozoa exists, it is unstable, often getting fooled and missing the target. This is why attention to protozoa is so important."

Causes

The fact that so many of us carry around everything from pathogenic microscopic organisms to large tapeworms may seem surprising in light of the fact that most Americans are generally attentive to sanitation. The prevalence of the condition is due to many factors, including eating in restaurants, where food handlers do not always wash their hands, drinking unfiltered water, traveling abroad, and sometimes sexual intercourse.

Dr. Yutsis says that to determine whether a patient might be a candidate for parasite treatment, a doctor should begin by asking the following questions. Yes responses build a case for the condition:

Do you or your sexual partners travel frequently?

Do you drink untested water?

Do you frequently eat out?

Do you like to eat raw fruits and raw vegetables?

Do you like undercooked meat or fish?

Do you work in a hospital, day care center, sanitation department, or garden?

Antibiotics and other immunosuppressive medications can also contribute to the problem: "These drugs derange the intestinal ecosystem, thereby creating an excellent breeding ground for both intestinal protozoa and *Candida albicans*," says Dr. Yutsis. "Here we come to a very interesting conclusion. If *Candida albicans* resists treatment, look for parasites."

Also important to consider is the state of the host. Complementary physician Dr. Robert Sorge believes that parasites cannot thrive in a healthy human: "A person who is nutritionally sound, with good bowel activity, cannot have parasites. Parasites, to a naturopathic doctor, are an indication of faulty lifestyle, poor elimination, and poor nutrition, especially the use of junk foods." He adds that parasite conditions have increased in recent years with the influx of imported foods and the increase in popularity of ethnic foods such as sushi.

Symptoms

Parasites produce a wide range of chronic, subclinical symptoms that create greater susceptibility to disease when left untreated. They affect intestinal, psychological and general systems:

INTESTINAL SYMPTOMS. These include flatulence, belching, abdominal bloating, abdominal pain, cramps, foul smelling stool, diarrhea, constipation, heartburn, anal itching, nausea, vomiting, and bloody or mucusy stools.

PSYCHOLOGICAL SYMPTOMS. Mental and emotional symptoms can include moderate to severe depression, nightmares, mood swings, irritability, spaciness, and hyperactivity.

GENERAL SYMPTOMS. Parasites may drain energy, causing intense fatigue. Patients with chronic fatigue syndrome should look into the issues of parasites. In women, cervicitis, vaginitis, pelvic inflammatory disease, and decreased libido may be present. Other general symptoms include rashes, hives, arthritis, allergy, Crohn's disease, colitis, food allergy, headaches, skin rashes and itching, anemia, insomnia, loss of appetite, weight loss, night sweats, and fever.

Dr. Marjorie Ordene, a complementary physician from Brooklyn, New York, tells why parasites can cause such diverse symptoms: "They interfere with the vital processes of the host by the various things that they produce. For example, they can produce enzymes that erode the intestinal wall. This can cause what we call a leaky gut, in which toxins can go across the barrier of the intestinal tract and cause symptoms in all parts of the body. Parasites can also confuse the immune system and trigger the body to react to its own tissues and destroy them, causing autoimmune disease, such as rheumatoid arthritis."

Clinical Experience

TESTING

Routine stool analysis tests are unreliable as they yield an unacceptably high false negative response for all parasites, according to Dr. Yutsis. "This is because parasites that adhere to the mucosal surface of the intestines and cannot be picked up by the fecal stream." Tests that biopsy part of the intestines also produce false negative results in many cases when the wrong part of the intestines are biopsied.

Dr. Yutsis adds that, fortunately, a highly accurate measure is available: "A test developed by Dr. Herman Bueno is the rectal swab technique. The recent development of fluorescent stains for numerous protozoan parasites has significantly enhanced and improved the sensitivity and specificity of the rectal swabs."

HERBS

Herbal treatments are more successful as long-term solutions than are commonly used drugs such as Flagyl and others. This is because long-term treatment is needed, and drugs can only be used safely for short periods of time: "Most textbooks convey the misinformation that protozoal infections can be successfully treated in five to fourteen days," says Dr. Yutsis. "Using repeated rectal swabs, we have never found conventional short-course therapies to produce cures in more than half of the cases. Successful therapy of chronic protozoal infection requires weeks or months of treatment. For this reason we prefer to use herbal preparations. It has been established that herbal treatments, especially with artemisia and citrus seed extract, are very effective. There are a lot of herbal combinations, some developed by leading protozotologists Dr. Buena and Dr. Parish, which have excellent results."

The following herbs should be considered in parasite-prevention or treatment programs:

Garlic. Garlic has the ability to kill most types of parasites, as well as fungi, microbacteria, and viruses. Eat raw garlic daily, or buy an odorless supplement in the health food store. Garlic can also be given intravenously by a health practitioner or added to colonics.

Goldenseal. Goldenseal has powerful antiparasitic action and has been proven effective against giardia. Research shows that berberine, one of goldenseal's active ingredients, increases macrophages that target this amoeba. Unlike garlic, goldenseal should not be taken for more than a month at a time.

Black walnut tincture. Excellent for expelling parasites throughout the body. Add a few drops to a glass of pure water, and drink first thing in the morning and at the end of the day.

Citrus seed extract. A small amount taken in water helps to prevent and remove
parasites.

Also consider Oriental herbs, which can be obtained in most Chinatowns:

Baibu. This Chinese herb helps get rid of pinworms. It is put on a piece of cloth
containing alcohol, and worn at night.

Ku shen. When used as a tea, cleanses lower intestinal and urogenital area.

Lei wan. A very strong Chinese herb for treatment of any parasitic infection.

La jiao (red pepper) and wu may eradicate tapeworms from the intestines.

DIET AND SUPPLEMENTS

Helpful foods for eliminating parasites include raw pumpkin seeds and lots of
raw garlic, onions, and horseradish. Avoid coffee, sugar, alcohol, milk and dairy,
which weaken the system, making the internal environment more conducive to
parasites. Even healthy foods such as fruit, honey, and tofu should be temporarily
cut out until the situation is brought under control.

The supplements B12, calcium, magnesium, and capsicum support the system while fighting off the problem.

ADJUNCTIVE THERAPIES

Colon therapy keeps the bowels clean and creates an unwelcome environment
for parasites. It is especially good for rebuilding a digestive system that has been
maligned by parasites. One colonic weekly is helpful during a parasite elimination program.

Other enhancements to treatment include ozone therapy, hydrogen peroxide
therapy, and the use of acidophilus, tea tree oil, probiotic homeopathic 59, and
colloidal silver.

PREVENTION

Dr. Sorge says preventive education is key to keeping parasites out of the body,
and teaches the following:

Avoid certain foods. Do not eat crustaceans, which include shrimp, lobster, and
crabs. Stay away from pork and pork products, as well as sushi and raw beef.

Take precautions when handling raw meat. Any time you handle raw meat before
cooking, millions of parasites are brought onto your hands. Separate your meat
cutting board from your vegetable board.

Reconsider eating out. Food establishments are not always as sanitary as your
home. Be especially wary of salads and other raw foods, which may be prepared by people who do not wash their hands after leaving the bathroom and
preparing your food.

Wash utensils carefully. Use food-grade hydrogen peroxide. Wash fruits and vegetables. Soak fruits and vegetables in food-grade hydrogen peroxide. Merely wiping fruits and vegetables does nothing to get rid of parasites.

Avoid tap water. This is a major source of parasites, despite the addition of fluoride and chloride.

Take precautions with your pets. Never sleep with pets and be sure to deworm them on a regular basis. Do not allow pets to lick your face or eat off your plate. Avoid walking barefoot around animals.

Wash hands every single time that you go to the toilet.

Keep bowel function optimal. When the normal eliminative channels are backed up, putrefaction occurs, creating a climate conducive to parasite growth.

Patient Story

LYNN

In 1990 I learned that I had parasites. I went to traditional doctors for treatments and received Flagyl, a drug commonly used for parasites, which can cause liver damage. I stayed on the treatment for two years, but was bedridden with chronic fatigue.

Then I found the Healing Center, where I was told I could get vitamin drips to help get over my chronic fatigue. This worked very well. During one of my treatment sessions, I met another patient who recommended Dr. Richard Bloom, a chiropractor who practices kinesiology. I was told he could rid people of parasites, Lyme disease, and candida within a few visits. After two visits, I felt better. After five, I tested negative for parasites. They haven't returned and I feel great. Dr. Bloom used several herbs, including black walnut tincture; all in all, the herbs only cost seven dollars.

21. PREGNANCY

A woman undergoes numerous internal changes during each stage of pregnancy. These physiological changes are described by nurse practitioner and massage therapist Susan Lacina:

FIRST TRIMESTER. "The fetus grows rapidly, and the mother's body changes to support this swift development. Hormonal balance changes. Human chorionic gonadotropin hormone (HCG) is needed for development. As it is released, it causes many discomforts, such as breast tenderness, digestive problems, nausea, and vomiting. Progesterone levels increase and may cause mild hyperventilation, heartburn, indigestion, and constipation. Increased blood flow and its change in composition contribute to fatigue, overheating, and sinus congestion."

SECOND TRIMESTER. "The placenta takes over the hormone production, and the levels of HCG drop. Along with that, the discomforts of nausea and vomiting ease up. Physical growth of the fetus crowds the abdomen, and a woman's body expands to accommodate the growth. Fetal production of thyroid stimulating hormone (TSH) begins in the fourteenth week and causes the mother's thyroid level to increase. This can lead to irritability, mood swings, mild depression, increased pulse rate, and hot flashes. Adrenal hormones become elevated and remain that way until delivery. This may cause impaired glucose tolerance and swelling. Skeletal structure becomes softer and more flexible to allow for expansion. If a woman doesn't have enough muscle flexibility in her joints, she will have some pain, as tight muscles do not allow for these adjustments. She may experience sciatic nerve pain down the lower back to the back of her legs due to the extension of the pelvis, especially at the joint of the sacrum and the pelvic bone. The growing baby puts pressure on the inferior vena cava and can cause light-headedness, nausea, drowsiness, and clamminess. Prolonged reduction of blood flow can cause backaches and hemorrhoids. Lying on the side decreases this problem.

"From the twentieth week on, the uterus expands by stretching muscle fibers. Abdominal muscles and ligaments stretch to support the uterus, and there may be abdominal pain. There is an increase in melanin production, causing darkening of the nipples and a line called linea nigra down the abdomen. If the lymph drainage system is not functioning well, an excess of melanin in the skin can cause brown spots. A well-functioning lymph drainage system is believed to keep melanin levels down so that brown spots do not occur. Increased progesterone causes sinus congestion, postnasal drip, and bleeding gums. Increased capillary permeability may cause the hands and feet to swell."

THIRD TRIMESTER. "As the baby continues to grow, the expectant mother changes her posture to shift her center of gravity. Heavier breasts can cause shoulders to slump forward. The spine is pulled out of alignment, and commonly causes backaches. The growing fetus also compresses the veins and the lymphatic system. That can cause ankle edema and varicose veins. There is increased pressure on the intestines and bladder, causing frequent urination and constipation. Pressure on the sciatic nerve can cause more lower back and leg pain. As the diaphragm starts to rise, breathing becomes more difficult. Insomnia is common."

Clinical Experience

PREGNANCY MASSAGE

Lucina tells why a pregnant woman and her unborn child benefit greatly from massage. "We tend to think of a baby in utero as being cut off from the world," she says. "In reality, the child within is a conscious being that responds to sounds, emotions, and the inner environment that its mother creates, either through her sense of well-being or lack of it."

Here Lacina describes how maternity massage promotes a comfortable and healthy pregnancy:

Relaxation and stress reduction. "This is the most important reason for a massage, and there are significant medical reasons why this is so. Research shows that prolonged stress builds up abnormal levels of toxins and chemicals in the bloodstream. These are passed through the placenta to the baby. Minimizing the buildup of toxins can be achieved by periodic deep relaxation. Relaxation increases the absorption of oxygen and nutrients by the cells of the muscles. When oxygen and nutrition increase, the woman has more energy. Some doctors also believe morning sickness and nausea are eliminated by lowering stress levels."

Improved lymphatic drainage. "Massage assists the lymphatic system in eliminating excessive toxins and hormones. Unlike the heart, the lymphatic system has no pump. It moves freely until muscles tighten up, but when muscles become too tense, either from the fetus or from stress, lymph movement decreases and the concentration of toxins rises. In the lower extremities, the growing uterus can inhibit lymph drainage, leading to swelling, varicose veins, hemorrhoids, and fluid retention. By relaxing the muscles, massage helps stimulate lymphatic drainage of toxins. It decreases the development of varicose veins by its draining effect and helps reduce swelling in the legs."

Better overall muscle tone and elasticity. "A woman's body must expand to accommodate the growing fetus. Hips widen, and abdominal, lower back, and shoulder muscles stretch. Legs must accommodate increase in weight. Massage promotes flexible muscles, joints, ligaments, and tendons. It also helps decrease muscle spasms and leg cramps by getting rid of lactic acid buildup, and can alleviate the pain caused by sciatic nerve pressure. Added flexibility helps the muscles that are needed for labor."

Hormonal balance. "Massage balances the entire glandular system. An overactive thyroid gland becomes less active, thereby decreasing irritability, mood swings, and hot flashes. An underactive thymus gland is stimulated, which increases its ability to fight infection. The alternating relaxation and stimulation that massage provides helps a woman's body function in a more balanced manner."

Maternity massage lessens symptoms associated with each stage of pregnancy. Additionally, it eases and quickens labor, and helps afterward:

First trimester. "Massage must be gentle so as not to interfere with hormonal balance. Gentle pressure with the fingers on the bridge of the nose, under the eyebrows, under the cheekbones, and under the forehead can relieve sinus congestion."

Second trimester. "Concentration is on stimulating lymph circulation, decreasing edema in the hands and feet, and working on breathing problems by massaging the chest. Massage at this time also helps increase flexibility in the muscles, joints, ligaments and tendons. Additionally, it can reduce sciatic pain and muscle spasms. To alleviate hemorrhoids, pressure can be applied to the crown of the head, for fifteen seconds three times a day."

Third trimester. "Massaging the lower hips and the area near the sacrum helps reduce back pain. Stimulation of the lymph system and blood circulation continue, especially from the thigh to the abdomen. As delivery time approaches, the massage therapist can teach the mother and her partner shiatsu and acupressure points that stimulate and speed up delivery. At about 34 weeks, peroneal massage can be learned and applied."

Peroneal massage. "This is a gentle stretch of tissues in the area between the vagina and rectum. Learning peroneal massage increases the mother's awareness of the muscles she needs to relax during the actual delivery and decreases her chances of having an episiotomy, an incision made to enlarge the vaginal opening at the time of birth. The actual procedure is as follows: Using warm vitamin E or vegetable oil, the mother places clean, oiled thumbs or index fingers an inch to an inch-and-a-half inside the vagina, and firm, gentle pressure is applied downward and outward. Stretching continues until a burning sensation is felt. This is held for a few minutes. Performing this once or twice a day, up until the time of delivery, can result in an easier birth."

During labor. "Massage during labor helps to reduce pain and anxiety by offering relief from muscle contractions. The stimulation of certain acupressure points can speed up labor."

POSTPARTUM MASSAGE

"Postpartum is the name given to the six-week recovery period after birth. During this time, hormones readjust and the uterus involutes (returns to its pre-pregnancy size). Massaging the abdomen in a circular motion helps the uterus to contract and helps to expel blood. Massage also helps to stimulate milk flow. The following techniques can be applied for this purpose: 1) The pressure point at the base of the sacrum can be held for about fifteen seconds, and then released. 2) Breast massage is another technique that can be used. Using some light oil, a woman circles her breasts with her fingertips. She places the hands flat on the breasts, starting at the nipple, and moves outward and up. That helps the glands to release milk. 3) Additionally, there is an acupressure point at the top and middle of the shoulder. If that is held for fifteen seconds, milk production is helped. 4) Pressing the point between the sixth and seventh ribs (at the nipple level on the breast bone) helps to release milk."

Lacina points out that there are instances when pregnancy massage should not be used. Contraindications include vaginal bleeding or bloody discharge, fever, abdominal pain, systemic edema (excessive swelling), sudden gush of water, severe headaches, blurry vision, excess protein in urine, diabetes, high blood pressure, heart disease, and phlebitis.

ACUPRESSURE POINTS

Thumbs can be applied to the sacrum, at the bottom of the spine, and walked up the spine to the waist. Each point is held for about five seconds.

The point in the center of the buttocks is pressed in as the mother exhales and released as she inhales.

Thumbs can be pressed along the shoulder blades between the spine and the scapula.

On the legs, pressure can be applied to spleen 6, an acupressure point located approximately three inches above the ankle, on the inside of the leg right below the tibia bone. Holding this spot for ten seconds and then releasing it helps to stimulate uterine contractions and speeds up labor.

The uterus point is on the inside of the foot, just under the ankle bone. The ovary point is on the outside of the foot, under the ankles, near the heel. Squeezing these points at the same time for about ten seconds and then releasing them, helps to speed up labor.

Breast and nipple stimulation helps to create oxytocin, the hormone that helps the uterus to contract.

ALEXANDER TECHNIQUE

The Alexander technique differs from massage in that the pregnant woman is actively engaged. Kim Jessor, senior faculty member at the American Center for Alexander Technique in New York, makes an analogy to a piano lesson: "We talk about being Alexander teachers, the people who come to us are students, and the context is a lesson. So while the results are very therapeutic, I don't think of the work as a therapy but rather as a learning process. This is significant in that it empowers students to take charge in the changing of their movement habits."

The Alexander technique is based on the concept that all of us know how to move comfortably as children, but lose that natural flexibility over time. The method teaches people how to move freely again, which is especially valuable for women undergoing the stresses of pregnancy. Jessor explains this concept with a story: "I was watching my fifteen-month-old son in the playground as he squatted down to pick something up. There was something extraordinary in watching that particular movement. It was so easy, so organic, so direct. It's the kind of movement that most of us have lost contact with.

"That made me think of a film that I saw of women in Brazil giving birth while squatting. They were working in harmony with gravity to push their baby out. While squatting is not a preferred method of delivering babies for Western doctors, it actually is one of the most efficient positions for a woman to be in to birth her baby and it is used in many cultures around the world.

"In an Alexander lesson with a woman who is pregnant, I actually work quite a bit on guiding her in and out of a squat. It's one of her movement options. Whether or not she, in fact, gives birth squatting, I think that it is a really useful way to begin to open up the pelvis.

"Young children have a certain freedom of movement that most of us lose contact with. One of the objectives of the Alexander technique is to restore that freedom of movement, which is important and wonderful for all of us, but particularly important for a pregnant woman dealing with the demands of pregnancy."

The Alexander technique is an experiential process. Real changes occur in the presence of a teacher who guides the student with hands-on training. "This is one of the special aspects of the Alexander technique," Jessor says. "You can learn a new way of moving because a teacher's hands gives a new stimulus to your nervous system. After a lesson, people tell me, 'Wow, I feel so much lighter,' or 'I can't believe how easily I am moving.' This is because they are actively participating in the lesson. But it is also a function of the Alexander teacher's hands giving that experience."

Jessor describes some of the ways the Alexander technique helps women during and after pregnancy:

Lower back pressure is relieved. "In pregnancy, women are contending with additional weight in the front of the body, which creates more pressure on the lower back. I find that most people bend over from the waist, keeping the knees straight, and pulling the head back into the spine. This creates a lot of pressure in the back. If you do that over and over, day in and day out, it starts to wear on the body. Imagine trying to do that and being pregnant at the same time; there is even more stress. I might work with a pregnant woman on a movement like bending over. I actually put my hands on her, guiding her through the movement of bending, so that she gets an experience of moving in a new way. I have had two women come to me during their second pregnancy who had a lot of back pain the first time around. Both reported little or no back pain because they learned to move in new ways that no longer put pressure on the lower back. I really feel that back pain in pregnancy is not inevitable."

Breathing improves. "Lots of pregnant women have breathing difficulties. There is a good reason for this; with the uterus growing and expanding, there is less space for the internal organs. The diaphragm has less room, so it is more difficult to breathe. The Alexander technique teaches students how to move with less downward pressure on the organs. This minimizes breathing constriction. A study on the Alexander technique and respiration, performed by a Dr. Austin at Columbia Presbyterian Hospital, here in New York, found significant improvement in breathing capacity after a course of lessons."

Rest is enhanced. "Fatigue and exhaustion is another issue in pregnancy, especially in the first and third trimesters. Women need to rest a lot, and there is an effective way to learn that in an Alexander lesson. This is not a movement component of the work, but involves lying down on the table. I have a woman lie down on her back in the beginning stages, and on her side as the pregnancy gets further along. I help her learn how to release unnecessary tension. It is easier to do this in the lying-down position because the student is not contending with gravity. The table lesson teaches the pregnant woman how to consciously release excess tension, which enables her to really rest and recuperate."

Labor is eased. "Labor is an intense situation where a woman must learn to deal with pain and fear. The Alexander technique teaches the skill of releasing muscles between contractions. By fully letting go, the woman does not remain tense in response to the pain. Rather, she is able to conserve energy. When I gave birth, I worked with another Alexander teacher for labor support. She put her hands on me and gave me verbal direction. As a result, I was able to release more effectively between contractions. Husbands of pregnant students come to me for labor support lessons where they learn to be more available to women as they give birth."

Stamina increases after delivery. "There is a lot of very challenging physical labor in being a mother. Again, there is much bending. There is also a lot of lifting. It is very important to pay attention to how you are doing this. I work with a new mother on ways of bending efficiently to pick up her baby. Recently, I taught someone how to bend over and pick up a stroller while it had a thirty-five-pound child in it. Also, the way that the baby is handled is very much affected by the way the mother is using her body. The better the use, the greater the sense of support and security for the child."

Breast-feeding is easier. "Breast-feeding also includes the component of bending. You tend to move toward the child as you are nursing, and there is the possibility of compressing your body. The Alexander technique teaches you how to maintain a sense of ease and balance while breast-feeding the baby throughout the day."

Jessor concludes by saying that there are less tangible, but equally valuable, benefits from working with the Alexander technique during pregnancy. As a woman becomes aware of different options in movement, she simultaneously opens up to greater options in her thinking: "Women begin to realize that they can make different kinds of choices about the kind of birth they want to have, where they want to have it, and who they want to use for labor support. In the same way that they begin to find freedom in movement, they find greater options in terms of the choices they make about their pregnancy."

DIET

The best insurance for a well baby is to follow a highly nutritious whole-foods diet. What you eat now will impact the health of your child later, according to nutritionist Gracia Perlstein: "When a woman is considering pregnancy, it is important that she address her diet to see how healthful it is, as many difficulties have their root in prenatal deficiencies. Scientific studies reveal that birth defects, and even problems that develop much later in life, can be prevented when the mother has excellent nutrition. I would like to include the father there too, because the quality of the sperm is also very important." Since the most crucial stage of embryonic development occurs in the first few weeks, before a women realizes that she is pregnant, good quality foods should be eaten all the time.

Eating properly means selecting unprocessed or minimally processed foods. A wide assortment of whole grains, legumes, vegetables, fruits, nuts, and seeds supplies multiple nutrients. "So many people eat the same ten or twenty foods over and over again," Perlstein says. "In traditional cultures, people have much more variety. I would like to emphasize that supplements should only enhance an excellent diet. Make the effort to eat high-quality, nutrient-dense foods. That means whole foods, the way nature produced them."

The body intuitively knows what it needs to support new life, and paying attention to its messages can be a helpful guide. "A woman's body is very wise when she is pregnant. Many women can't stand the look or smell of coffee or cigarettes, even when they used to smoke or drink coffee several times a day," states Perlstein. She adds that worrying about eating the right foods all the time is stressful and can produce more harm than good. But nutrition education can benefit women with highly processed diets, who need to learn about better food choices. "Vegetarian women may crave animal foods or be drawn to dairy when they are pregnant. Usually it is good to pay attention to these cravings, but to respond in the most wholesome way possible."

Wholesome means organically grown. Pesticide-free fare is better for everyone, of course, but vitally important for young children and developing fetuses, according to recent research. Dairy and animal products should be from creatures naturally raised. One reason for this is that pesticides and other contaminants tend to concentrate in an animal's tissues. The higher up the food chain, the higher the concentration of toxins. Fortunately, many health food stores, and more and more supermarkets sell the healthful varieties.

Animal products, when a part of the diet, should be eaten in moderation. Although protein needs increase, they can be abundantly obtained from vegetarian sources, which are less toxic than their animal counterparts. Excellent vegetarian protein sources include fortified soy milk, tofu, tempeh, beans, nuts, and seeds, for example.

The increased need for calcium is similarly fulfilled in such a diet: "Many women do not realize that there are excellent sources of calcium other than milk and dairy. There are green leafy vegetables, fortified soy milk, tofu, almonds, and many other calcium-containing foods. If you eat a diet rich in fresh vegetables and fruits, you tend to get quite a bit of calcium. If you want a supplement, calcium citrate is easiest on the stomach. Other forms sometimes cause digestive upsets or constipation. Definitely avoid calcium-depleting foods—coffee, chocolate, and sodium."

Perlstein adds that eating several small meals throughout the day offsets common complications: "Hunger, not calorie counting, is the most reliable guide to eating during pregnancy. Five to six small, nutrient-dense meals per day is a sensible ideal. This is a good habit to develop in the last trimester of pregnancy, when the organs in your stomach are somewhat constricted, and good in the early stages to prevent nausea. It keeps the blood sugar from falling, and nausea has a lot to do with low blood sugar."

Water should be pure and taken in adequate amounts. Eight to twelve glasses are recommended to help flush out toxins from the liver and kidneys: "Many people do not drink enough fluids," notes Perlstein. "This is especially important during pregnancy because the woman is filtering the waste for two bodies."

WHAT TO AVOID. Equally important is knowing what not to take in. Perlstein lists substances that can harm a growing fetus:

Harmful household chemicals. "First on the list of what to avoid is chemical exposure to toxic household cleansers. Natural food stores are a good source for environmentally harmless cleansers of various kinds. You want to avoid fumes from paints, thinners, solvents, wood preservatives, varnishes, glues, spray adhesives, benzene, dry cleaning fluid, anything chemically based and questionable. Stay away from household pesticides. I want to emphasize again that you don't want to go spraying for fleas, roaches, or ants with commercially available pesticides when you are pregnant or looking to become pregnant."

Radiation. "Avoid radiation and x-rays, especially during the first three months. If a doctor feels an x-ray is required, be sure to mention that you may be pregnant. Ask if it can be put off until after the first trimester, if possible."

Certain herbs. "Basic rule of thumb is not to have bitter herbs, such as goldenseal and pennyroyal. Many books list these herbs specifically."

Antihistamines. "You want to avoid antihistamines. That includes some from the natural food stores such as ma huang and osha root."

Laxatives. "If you are having problem with constipation, adequate fluids, whole grains, and fresh vegetables should correct that problem quite easily. You want to avoid senna, castor oil, and *cascara sagrada* as well as diuretics, including the herbs buchu, horsetail, and juniper berries. If you drink adequate fluids and don't consume excess sodium or animal protein, your kidneys should be able to filter without water retention."

Hair dyes. "Avoid dying your hair with chemicals. Nonchemical hair dyes are available, which usually do the trick."

Hormones. "Hormones are another reason to stay away from commercial meats."

Substance abuse. "Of course, you need to stay away from intoxicants and strong substances, including cigarettes, alcohol and recreational drugs."

High temperatures. "Avoid very high temperatures for a prolonged period—for example, hot tubs or saunas."

Toxic surroundings. "As much as possible, avoid stress, negative people, and aggravating situations. Instead, try to spend quality time alone and with loved ones, people who are supportive. Spend time in nature. Read inspiring literature. Listen to beautiful music. This has a beneficial effect on your mental and emotional state. That, in turn, affects your baby's biochemistry."

SUPPLEMENTS. Beyond an excellent diet, Perlstein recommends the following daily nutrients for pregnant women:

>Multiple vitamin/mineral supplement
>Vitamin C
>B12
>Zinc
>Vitamin E—400 units
>Folic acid

Folic acid, which is also contained in green leafy vegetable and whole grains, is especially important in pregnancy because science has shown it to prevent neural tube defects. Even when included in the diet, extra folic acid should be taken in supplement form as it is fragile and easily damaged by heat. Additionally, acidophilus helps prevent constipation and other types of colon problems.

Extra iron may be needed, but a woman should have her hemoglobin tested first, just to be sure. Research shows that excess iron in the system can have damaging effects.

EXERCISE

The American College of Gynecologists and Obstetricians (ACOG) endorses physical activity during pregnancy and has created specific guidelines for the dos and don'ts of exercise:

Pregnant women derive health benefits from a mild to moderate exercise routine. Exercising 60 minutes, three times per week, is preferable to intermittent activity, but some benefit can be derived from shorter durations as well. Sometimes little oxygen is available for aerobic exercise due to the body's increased oxygen demands. Therefore, a woman should begin an aerobic activity slowly, and gradually build to capacity. She should not push too hard, and certainly not to the point of breathlessness. Pregnant women should not exercise in the face-up position after the first trimester. This position limits blood supply to the baby.

Standing for prolonged periods of time, doing heavy work in the standing position, and exercising at high intensities are to be avoided. These activities are associated with diminished birth weight in newborns. It's better for women to engage in non-weight-bearing activities such as cycling and swimming, rather than exercises like running. Non-weight-bearing exercise minimizes risk of injury and allows activity levels to remain closer to prepregnancy levels, right up to delivery. A woman should be aware that her center of gravity is different, and that she might lose her balance when exercising. Anything that could involve falling over, or even mild abdominal trauma, should be avoided.

Pregnant women require an extra 300 calories per day in order to maintain their normal metabolic rate. Exercise increases the need for more calories.

A pregnant woman must be careful not to raise body temperature with vigorous workouts, especially in the first trimester. Excessive body heat in the mother can adversely affect the development of brain tissue in the baby. The threshold for this is a body temperature of about 39.2 degrees C, which is 100 or 101 degrees F. The conclusion here is to exercise, but never to the point of raising body temperature. Pool exercises help to dissipate heat.

After delivery, gradually build up to prepregnancy exercise levels.

Chiropractor Richard Statler of Long Island, New York, answers some commonly asked questions on the subject of pregnancy and exercise:

WHEN SHOULD A PREGNANT WOMEN NOT EXERCISE?

"Basically, every pregnant woman can benefit from starting an exercise program at any point in pregnancy. However, there are certain exceptions to this rule. In these situations, an expectant woman should avoid or limit exercise:

Pregnancy-induced hypertension

Premature rupture of membranes

Incompetent cervix

Persistent second or third trimester bleeding

Premature labor during the prior or current pregnancy

Intrauterine growth retardation

Other medical contraindications include thyroid, heart, vascular or pulmonary conditions. Women with medical problems need a physician's evaluation to determine whether an exercise program is appropriate."

HOW MUCH EXERCISE SHOULD A PREGNANT WOMAN GET?

"How much exercise a woman is capable of largely depends on her fitness level before pregnancy. Someone who has never exercised should not begin a heavy program. Nor should someone who was an avid exerciser completely give it up. For a marathon runner to suddenly stop because she is pregnant can be as problematic as a nonrunner deciding to run marathons during her pregnancy."

WHAT ARE THE BENEFITS OF EXERCISING DURING PREGNANCY?

"Statistics show that women who exercise during pregnancy usually have an easier, shorter labor and safer delivery. There are fewer premature births. During pregnancy the woman feels more energetic and vital, and less stressed. Exercise alleviates a good portion of discomfort from back pain or sciatica. By stabilizing the blood sugar, exercise can even help women who are diabetic. Mothers who exercise see quicker recovery times after delivery.

"One benefit to exercising in a group program is the social aspect. An exercise group can provide informal support. First-timers speak to women who have been there, and get real-life input and suggestions. That's important in this day and age, when people no longer live with extended families who traditionally passed down such wisdom."

HOW DOES EXERCISING AFFECT THE BABY?

"When a mother exercises, she gets more oxygen and is able to pass that to her baby. Better nutritional delivery, better oxygen, and better blood flow can only be helpful. There is also less complication with labor and birth, and that can mean a healthier baby."

Dr. Statler says that exercises geared toward opening up the pelvis are particularly important in preparing women for delivery: "The pelvic area is where the baby sits. It must expand so that the baby can pass through. The pelvis has three contact points. In the front is the pubic bone area; in the back are two sacroiliac joints, one to the left and one to the right. Those joints can stretch and open up to allow the pelvis to expand. Although hormones secreted during this time allow the pelvis to open up tremendously, placing the woman in the typical birth position of lying on her back compresses the sacroiliac joints. We can potentially lock up two-thirds of her ability to stretch."

Stretching exercises are key for opening up this area. Here are three that Dr. Statler recommends:

Hip stretch. Stand with feet shoulder-width apart. Rotate on the balls of the feet until the heels are turned out. In this position, do a half squat, keeping the back straight. It may help to do this while leaning against a wall. It can also be done on a supermarket line, while holding onto a shopping cart. An alternate way of doing the exercise is seated. Once again, feet are shoulder-width apart, and feet are flat on the floor. Shimmy forward slightly to keep from sitting back in the chair. Lean back a little bit to take the weight of the body off the hip joint. That allows for better movement. Place a child's volleyball or play ball between the knees and hold it there. Pivot on the balls of the feet to turn the heels out, keeping the heels flat on the floor. Now gently squeeze the ball while pushing the legs together and internally rotating the thighs toward the midline. Hold for ten seconds and relax.

Either of these exercises is great for opening up the hip and sacroiliac joints. They prepare the mother for delivery by developing more stable joints throughout pregnancy.

Pubic stretch. This exercise helps the front of the pelvis by using motions that are opposite to those used in the previous exercise. Standing, with feet one shoulder-width apart, turn toes and thighs out. Bend knees slightly. As before, this can be done in a supermarket while holding on to a shopping cart. In the seated position, sit on the floor with soles of the feet together and knees apart. Use the back against the wall for support. Pull the feet as close to the body as is comfortable. Place the hands on the knees, and gently press the knees down and apart from each other toward the floor. Hold that for thirty seconds while breathing deeply. Repeat two or more times. Never do any bouncing or jerky motions. These are slow stretches.

Cat arch. Lie on all fours so that hands and knees are touching the floor. Arch the back like a cat, while slowly inhaling. Allow the back to return to the flat back position while exhaling. Do not curve the back in. Hold for a few seconds and relax. Repeat ten to fifteen times.

AROMATHERAPY

Ann Berwick reports that in Europe, where aromatherapy is scientifically studied and widely prescribed, hospital maternity wings utilize essential oils for their soothing and uplifting mind/body effects: "There is a report of one woman who had severe anxiety throughout her pregnancy. They gave her neroli oil, which helped to keep her blood pressure down and allowed her to go into delivery in a more relaxed state. During delivery, she was given lavender and clary sage to relax her uterus. Clary sage is also slightly euphoric, so it helped her to cope mentally with the birth." Here are some formulas to try before, during, and after birth:

As an antidote for nausea and vomiting, peppermint is effective when a very dilute amount is rubbed into the stomach or inhaled.

For relaxation, 8 ounces vegetable oil, 13 drops lavender, 2 drops geranium, and 10 drops sandalwood can be massaged into the skin or used as a compress.

To clear nasal congestion, a teaspoon of eucalyptus oil can be added to a cold air humidifier or pan of hot water. The steam inhaled lessens congestion.

To help heartburn, place 2 to 3 drops of diluted peppermint oil on the back of the tongue.

Five drops rose oil, 12 drops clary sage, and 5 drops ylang-ylang in 2 to 3 ounces vegetable oil can be used as a massage oil during labor.

To prevent stretch marks, massage 2 ounces wheat germ oil, 20 drops lavender, and 5 drops neroli oil into thighs.

To soothe sore nipples, mix one pint cold water, one drop geranium oil, one drop lavender oil, and one drop rose oil.

After an episiotomy a sitz (shallow) bath is helpful, especially when 2 drops of cyprus oil and 4 drops of lavender oil are added. Soak for fifteen to twenty minutes.

To promote milk production, take two drops fennel oil with some honey water, every two hours.

Hemorrhoids will be helped by 5 drops of cyprus oil, added to the bath.

The astringent action of cyprus and lemon oil constricts varicose veins. A few drops can be added to a body lotion and applied to the veins morning and evening.

HERBS

Raspberry tea throughout the pregnancy strengthens uterine muscle. It contains fragine, a smooth-muscle relaxer. In the final stages of pregnancy, it can be combined with black cohosh, squaw vine, and peppermint to relax the pelvis, speed up delivery, and make delivery less bloody.

Ginger is one of the best natural remedies for nausea, especially when accompanied by small, frequent, meals, fresh air, and plenty of rest. Ginger can be taken as a capsule or tea.

A washcloth soaked in ginger or comfrey tea and applied to the area promotes healing of an episiotomy.

Rosemary added to bath water relieves tension and back pain.

Adding jasmine and clary sage to a bath has an uplifting effect, and prevents postpartum depression.

HOMEOPATHIC REMEDIES

Homeopathic physician Stephanie Odinov Pukit lists a variety of remedies for all stages of pregnancy. She begins with treatments for morning sickness, noting, "Along with the dry biscuit in bed with a hot beverage, homeopathic remedies can be extremely important at this time."

Sepia. Ambivalence is the key word here. There is a conflict between self-preservation and the urge to procreate, which makes wanting a child questionable. The woman becomes angry and irritable and feels as if a black cloud hovers over her. Although her appetite is insatiable, heavy pains worsen with smells or thoughts of food.

Pulsatilla. This is the opposite scenario. Pulsatilla is an excellent remedy for the woman who is cheerful, sweet, somewhat helpless. The person is warm and may throw the covers off at night. She becomes worse with emotional excitement. Nausea comes and goes and is characteristically worse in early evening.

Nux vomica. This is a wonderful remedy for soothing the nerves after a woman has abused her body with alcohol, drugs or coffee. She tends to be constipated. She tends to wake up at night to think about business because she is ambitious and driven.

Arsenicum. The picture here is a person constantly anxious about her state of health. She always runs to the doctor fearing that something is wrong. The woman tends to have burning pains. She has great thirst and takes little sips. Symptoms are usually exacerbated at midnight.

Cocculus indicus. This remedy specifically helps motion sickness. The woman tends to lose sleep and to be constantly exhausted. She may be nursing children, or caring for someone. The woman feels dizzy standing and better when lying down. She is worse in fresh air.

Petroleum may be needed if there is a voracious appetite followed by persistent vomiting.

Bryonia. The person has strong sensitivity to smells and may have connective tissue and arthritic problems. Nausea becomes worse with motion.

Dr. Odinov Pukit suggests these remedies for problems that occur in the latter stages of pregnancy:

Sepia or pulsatilla. In the third to sixth month, the fetus presses high up in the abdomen, causing heartburn, shortness of breath, and indigestion. These remedies also help hemorrhoid problems. The one chosen depends on the other symptoms manifested. Sepia is for a gloomy disposition, while pulsatilla is for a sweet nature.

Carbo vegetabilis. The woman is slightly heavy and tends to have indigestion and shortness of breath due to poor oxygenation. Although she tends to be chilly, she prefers open windows with the air directly on her.

Bellis perennis. As the baby drops into the pelvis, pressure is felt on the organs in the lower part of the bladder. Pain and arthritis may occur as a result. Bellis perennis is specific for pain in the uterine area or groin. The woman might be walking when all of a sudden her legs weaken from a sharp nerve pain. After childbirth, when arnica has done its job and there are still some lumps remaining in the tissues, bellis perennis is also excellent.

Kali carb is for women with back pain, especially those who tend to wake up between 2 and 4 in the morning. This individual's personality is somewhat crabby and closed. She is vague and evasive about answering questions. Pains are better with pressure and rubbing. The person tends to be anxious and chilly.

Aconite. High-potency aconite is wonderful to use at any point in pregnancy when there has been shock or fright. Arnica and calendula may be useful for this purpose as well.

In addition, Dr. Odinov Pukit works with abnormal presentation. She finds that homeopathic remedies can help turn the baby over when used between 32 and 36 weeks: "Pulsatilla works in 40 percent of the cases, and other remedies are used when they match the woman's constitution. A wonderful remedy for that woman in general may help in that specific area as well."

Midwife Jeannette Breen finds homeopathy useful during labor, and after birth. "I seem to be using more and more homeopathic remedies since I've been seeing the advantages." These are a few she recommends:

Arnica. Starting a month before delivery, regular application of arnica directly to the nipples prevents their later tearing and cracking with breast-feeding. After birth, arnica quickens recuperation. Calendula can be used in the same way.

Califilum. May help a stalled labor. This is specific for a weak uterus or a uterus running out of steam. The woman often experiences weakness, exhaustion, trembling, and shivering. Sharp, brief, unstable, and painful lower uterine contractions fail to completely dilate the cervix and push the baby.

Gelsemium. May be indicated as a follow-up to califilum. Also good for neuralgia, rheumatic discomfort, and pains in the bladder and vaginal area. The person tends to be thirsty and chilly.

Cimicifuga. Also good for stalled labor, especially when woman is becoming fearful, hysterical, and exhausted, and the pains are becoming erratic. This tones the uterus, calms it down, and helps it to become more coordinated.

Breen cautions that homeopathic remedies should not be used as a quick fix. "There is not always a pill to take care of every problem in labor and birth. Sometimes you have to be patient. That's what midwives are good at. They try to be as patient and supportive as possible during this time."

Odinov Pukit adds that after birth homeopathic remedies can help newborns as well: "If the baby is distressed, we might need arnica rescue remedy. Carbo veg is wonderful if there is cyanosis with some respiratory effect. And arsenicum if the baby is born lifeless."

WATER BIRTH

Jeannette Breen is a great enthusiast for using water during labor: "It has a wonderful analgesic quality, which is much better than an epidural. Being immersed in water provides tremendous relaxation. It does not take the pain away, but women do report feeling less pain in the water. They feel less effect from the pull of gravity. Their movements are very easy, and there is much better tissue relaxation, which means there is almost no tearing in a water birth. It is also easier for the baby because the mother is more relaxed and moving freely. She is not stuck in one position. It is easier for the baby to negotiate the pelvis and to slip out in a warm, moist environment that is quite familiar."

SOCIAL SUPPORT

"Two keys to a normal healthy pregnancy and birth are a healthy diet and good social support," says Breen. "Those seem to be overlooked, especially in traditional maternity care in this country. The focus is on diagnostic testing, but not a lot of emphasis is placed on healthy diets, other than prescribing women prenatal vitamins and iron. There is no question that a high quality diet rich in all the nutrients can make a woman's whole body work more efficiently and effectively.

"Social support creates an environment of love that is all-important but too often overlooked in hospitalized birthing environments that focus solely on technology. No one can have the baby for the pregnant woman; she has to do it herself. But if she is surrounded by love and support, rather than fear and technology, she is able to give birth in a very intuitive, instinctual way which is satisfying and safe."

CORRECTIVE VAGINAL SURGERY

In the United States, about 80 percent of women give birth by episiotomy. Of those operations, approximately 90 percent are improperly performed. "Doctors are just not instructed in how to do this surgery," says Dr. Vicki Hufnagel. "All you have to do is go to your local medical school, get out the textbook on obstetrics, and look at what an episiotomy is. It will have a drawing, and a discussion that says to put one or two sutures here, and one or two there. They are teaching physicians to close an entire organ system in just one or two layers. If you were to close a laceration on your face in one or two layers, your muscles wouldn't work, your face wouldn't work. You'd be a real mess. We are teaching students how to close the vaginal vault area in a manner that is not allowable in other places. That is the standard of care that we have, and it is completely unacceptable."

Incorrectly performed episiotomies result in problems down the road. Without support of the vaginal muscles, the cervix pushes through the vagina. It appears that the uterus is being forced out, when really it is not. Doctors mistakenly diagnose a prolapsed uterus and commonly recommend a hysterectomy. Tragically, 100,000 to 200,000 women with this misdiagnosis receive this operation each year.

Corrective surgery easily ameliorates the problem. Repairing the vagina is a simple procedure that can be performed in a doctor's office. It takes all of 45 minutes, and patients can go home the same day.

Postpartum Depression

Depression after childbirth affects thousands of women each year. Although the exact cause is unknown, hormonal shifts after birth, particularly drops in progesterone, may play a large role. Research also links the condition to low levels of the neurotransmitter serotonin. Emotionally, it is often connected to difficult labor and disappointments after birth.

Symptoms range in degree, but are generally worse than a temporary feeling of the blues immediately following childbirth, according to Dr. Marjorie Ordene, a complementary gynecologist from Brooklyn, New York: "Postpartum depression is defined as a gradually increasingly sullen mood and a loss of interest and enthusiasm starting around the third postpartum week. This is different from the baby blues, which is a frequent and common occurrence in the normal population. The blues happens the first week postpartum, and basically goes away by itself. We are talking about something much more severe." In the worst-case scenario, women can become sick for years, and lose touch with reality.

HOMEOPATHY

Homeopathic physician Dr. Jane Cicchetti recommends that women try the 30c potency of the remedy that best addresses their symptoms. If this does not help, a visit to a homeopathic physician can provide more individual support:

Sepia. Sepia may be needed after an exhausting delivery, after giving birth to two or more children at once, or after having several children. The woman feels completely worn out and depressed. Physically, she feels as if her uterus might fall out, and finds herself crossing her legs a lot. Often there is an actual prolapse of the uterus. Emotionally, a woman who loved her husband and children suddenly has an aversion to them. In fact, she has an aversion to everyone and wants to be alone. She becomes irritable and angry if anyone bothers her, and has an aversion to sex. The woman cries often but cannot understand what is wrong; in fact this problem is caused by a hormonal disturbance rather than an emotional one.

Natmur. Natmur is for chronic grief. The woman is introverted and dwells on past, unpleasant memories but keeps them to herself. She tries to put on the appearance that everything is fine, and becomes aggravated if someone tries to comfort her.

Ignatia. Ignatia is for postpartum depression brought on by emotions. It is needed when disappointment follows childbirth. A woman imagines an ideal pregnancy and birthing situation. When that does not work out, she feels extremely let down and depressed. These feelings may occur after a stillbirth or a miscarriage. There is uncontrollable sobbing and sighing, and a rapid change of emotions, which are often contradictory. Depression is acute, while natmur depression is chronic.

Arnica. This commonly needed remedy is useful for depression, upset, and malaise brought on by bruising, soreness, and pain that lasts a long time. Arnica helps heal the physical trauma, and improves the mother's energy and emotional state.

Pulsatilla. Pulsatilla is given when a woman cries a lot and wants to be taken care of. She needs to attend to her newborn baby, but feels as if someone should be attending to her. This individual will eat sweets and other goodies to alleviate overwhelming feelings of sadness and loneliness. The woman often is warm-blooded and enjoys the fresh air. She is happier walking around outside, and much happier if she can be with people.

Cimicifuga. This remedy is used less often, but is very important for those who need it. Cimicifuga is derived from black cohosh, a powerful herb for treating hysteria and female complaints. It is needed when a woman feels as if a dark cloud of gloom has settled over her. She fears losing her mind. Often this stems from a very difficult delivery where the woman had a mini nervous breakdown, feeling at one point as if she was going insane. This leaves her with a great fear of ever having a baby again. Often she has alternating states. When she is not under this dark cloud of gloom, she becomes excitable and talkative, jumping from one subject to another in an almost hysterical fashion. Cimicifuga heals the nervous system.

Kali carbonicum. This deep mineral remedy is indicated for women who become anxious and irritable after a delivery that leaves them feeling weak. Easily startled, they want to be left alone and have an aversion to being touched. They tend to be chilly and to have insomnia from 2 to 4 A.M. Further, they are regimented and have trouble going with the flow of caring for a new baby. Often these symptoms follow a delivery that primarily consists of back labor. Sciatica develops to some degree, which then leads to this emotional state.

Phosphoric acid. Here a woman is extremely disappointed from physical or emotional shock. She may have lost the baby, or something might be wrong with it. A loved one may have died at the time of birth, or she may be affected from the loss of much bodily fluid during delivery. Indifferent to everything, the woman lies in bed with her face to the wall. It is as if her emotions have completely disappeared. She doesn't want to talk, think, or answer questions.

Cocculus. This is a remedy for fatigue and emotional depression brought on by loss of sleep. The woman feels drunk and may go through the day feeling dizzy and staggering. These feelings are brought on by sleep deprivation.

Aurum metallicum. For profound depression characterized by total hopelessness, self-destructive behavior, and a longing for death.

These remedies can make a difference because they get to the root of the problem. Regarding conventional treatment methods that use antidepressants, Dr. Cicchetti says, "Women just suppress their symptoms, and their health does not really get any better."

NATURAL PROGESTERONE

"Studies show that postpartum depression can be prevented by treating women with progesterone," reports Dr. Ordene. "Companies that make natural progesterone recommend taking a half teaspoon twice daily, starting a month after delivery. Since postpartum depression is supposed to start three weeks after giving birth, it makes sense to begin using the natural progesterone cream at that time."

VITAMIN B6

According to research, vitamin B6 raises serotonin levels. Patients given B6 for 28 days after delivery did not have a recurrence of postpartum depression.

Miscarriage

Surprisingly, two-thirds of all pregnancies end up as miscarriages. One reason for this phenomenon is that many women miscarry before they even know that they are pregnant. Most commonly, genetic abnormalities precipitate the problem. Embryos develop wrongly, and a woman's body naturally aborts the fetus. Endocrine system imbalances are also associated with miscarriages. Women in their late forties have an especially difficult time carrying full-term, due to hormonal changes that accompany aging. Poor thyroid gland functioning can also interfere with pregnancy, as can intercourse during pregnancy. Another cause of miscarriages is low-grade infections, which are often the result of sexually transmitted diseases. Women do not consciously realize a problem exists, but the body knows, and rejects the fetus. Bladder infections are also common; as the uterus enlarges, it places great pressure on this organ. Miscarriages may also occur when women are hard on their bodies. These women push themselves to the limit by overexercising and undereating to the point of anorexia. Their unhealthy state doesn't provide enough nutrition for themselves or their fetus.

PREVENTING MISCARRIAGES

When a miscarriage occurs more than once, a woman needs to have a thorough medical workup. Once the problem is understood, it is often correctable. If a woman is having intercourse during pregnancy, for example, she may simply need to take precautions. Using a condom during intercourse can prevent a miscarriage because it keeps male prostaglandins out of the female system, which, in turn, prevents premature uterine contractions. Low-grade infections must be cleared up, and increasing the intake of liquids and vitamin C can sometimes do the trick. Mixing four ounces of strawberry juice with four ounces of water is an especially good source of vitamin C, which acidifies the urine and helps prevent bladder infections. More serious infections should be cultured, and treated appropriately. Sometimes, this means antibiotics. Older women, who are having a difficult time holding on to a pregnancy due to hormonal changes, may need low doses of progesterone, about 25 mg, in suppository form.

Breast-Feeding Fallacies

The following section lists corrections to common fallacies related to lactation and breast-feeding:

Nipple soreness is not related to skin color.
The lactating breast is never empty.
All women do not experience pain during each breast-feeding.
Nipples do not get tougher with nursing.
Creams and oils on the breast are not encouraged for nipple soreness; vitamin E toxicity could be a concern because of liberal applications, and pesticide residues are a concern in sheep-fat-derived lanolin.
Engorgement may be experienced by newly breast-feeding mothers but is almost always indicative of inappropriate or infrequent suckling.
The let-down process is not a singular event, but occurs continually during suckling.
The human nipple is different from artificial nipples: it can stretch two to three times its non-suckled length. It contains fifteen to twenty pores, which spurt a fine stream of milk. The

milk ejection occurs in a rhythmic fashion. The nipple remains elongated only with active suckling. It does not drip continuously.

Noninfectious mastitis rarely requires antibiotic therapy; infectious mastitis includes temperature elevation and flulike systems as well.

Extra fluid intake is not needed for breast-feeding; drinking to quench one's thirst is sufficient.

The lactating mother's breasts become full usually between one to three days after the infant starts suckling.

Colostrum, which is a highly concentrated source of protein and antibodies, is produced as early as the third month of pregnancy.

Women with inverted nipples can breast-feed.

Healthy babies do not need supplemental feedings before the mother's milk comes in.

Breast milk helps reduce bilirubin concentrations by coating the small intestines, reducing bilirubin recirculation.

Additional water or glucose given to the infant reduces total caloric intake and reduces the coating action of milk feedings.

Human milk is far superior in all aspects to artificial formula.

Source: K. G. Auerbach, "Breast-Feeding Fallacies: Their Relationship to Understanding Lactation," *Birth* 17, no. 1 (March 1990): 44–49.

Herbal Pharmacy

Plants containing phytochemicals with anti-morning-sickness properties, in order of potency:

> *Persea americana* (avocado)
> *Triticum aestivum* (wheat)
> *Hordeum vulgare* (barley)
> *Oryza sativa* (rice)
> *Sesamum indicum* (sesame)
> *Glycine max* (soybean)
> *Lens culinaris* (lentil)
> *Avena sativa* (oats plant)
> *Zea mays* (corn)
> *Avena sativa* (oats seed)
> *Tamarindus indica* (tamarind)
> *Pisum sativum* (pea)
> *Theobroma cacao* (cacao)
> *Gossypium* sp. (cotton)

Patient Stories

LAURIE

I started massage about three years ago. I'm a nurse and I was working a twelve-hour shift in an intensive care unit, which really turned out to be thirteen- or fourteen-hour shifts. I was pregnant with my third child and having a great deal of back discomfort. A friend of mine, who had hurt her shoulder, recommended a massage therapist. I started to go and it helped tremendously. I felt wonderful.

After having the baby, I stopped going for a while because of finances. But then I started going again because I was having trouble with carpal tunnel where part of my fingers would get numb. And it helped tremendously with that.

To be honest, I had seen an orthopedic doctor about the carpal tunnel, and I didn't want surgery. I wanted to try to avoid that. I have to say, I feel perfect now just from going to the massage therapist for that problem.

Working in intensive care is very stressful, and I'm a wired type of person. The only time I sit down is to drive a car or go to the bathroom. This relaxes me and gets my whole mind clear for the week. It's really fantastic.

DARLENE

I had severe back pain. When I became pregnant, I became quite worried about it. My chiropractor helped me to feel much better. He made the whole pregnancy easier.

My baby was colicky from birth, and my chiropractor suggested that I bring her in when she was seven days old for an adjustment. Every time she was a little gassy, I would bring her in, and he would adjust her. After that, she was a satisfied child who slept through the night. He really helped her.

As far as chiropractic treatment goes, I swear by it.

Hot News

Morning sickness has been the subject of much recent research; among treatments found effective by studies are acupressure on the pericardium 6 point, or the use of a wristband that puts pressure on this point; vitamin B6 supplementation; and powdered ginger capsules. One study concludes, however, that morning sickness may not be an unmitigated evil; it is connected with a lower miscarriage rate and may serve to protect the fetus from food poisoning.

Research has indicated that cesarean sections, as well as being associated with greater risks to mother and infant, are often unnecessary. Women who have had one cesarean section may later give birth vaginally, however; in the United States, the number of women giving birth vaginally after an earlier C-section has risen in recent years. Another encouraging statistic is that, according to one study, women over thirty-five years old generally have no more complications and bear children with less infant mortality and fewer congenital anomalies than younger women, although they do more often require surgical intervention to give birth.

Another subject of studies has been birthing positions; several studies have concluded that use of upright posture in a birthing chair is as safe as the traditional semirecumbent posture, and may allow less pain during labor. Water birth is another method that has received recent attention. Other strategies that reduce labor pain include biofeedback during labor, acupuncture, transcutaneous electrical nerve stimulation (TENS), Lamaze training, and hypnosis. Many studies have pointed to the advantages of birthing centers or midwife-attended home births over hospitals, and demonstrated their equal safety. *(See below.)*

FROM THE MEDICAL LITERATURE ON PREGNANCY

NAUSEA/MORNING SICKNESS

A double-blind, cross-over study examined the effects of acupressure on morning sickness. Results showed that acupressure (on the pericardium 6 point) significantly reduced nausea, and that two-thirds of the women in the study favored it over sham acupressure.

J. Bayreuther et al., "A Double-Blind, Cross-Over Study to Evaluate the Effectiveness of Acupressure at Pericardium 6 (P6) in the Treatment of Early Morning Sickness (EMS)," *Complementary Therapies in Medicine* 2 (1994): 70–76.

A placebo-controlled study examined the efficacy of acupressure on the P6 point in preventing morning sickness in women during early pregnancy. Both treatment and placebo groups showed significant improvements relative to women who received no treatment at all.

J. W. Dundee et al., "P6 Acupressure Reduces Morning Sickness," *J-R-Soc.-Med.*81, no. 8 (August 1988): 456–57.

Results of a placebo-controlled study showed that 60 percent of pregnant women in their first trimester who wore a wristband, putting pressure underneath the wrist, reported reductions in nausea (compared to 30 percent of controls, who wore placebo bands).

"Band Said to Ease Morning Sickness," *Medical Tribune* (December 24, 1992): 4.

The use of SeaBands reduced nausea and vomiting by 50 percent in pregnant women between 5 and 22 weeks gestation. The sooner the bands were applied, the more effective they proved to be.

M. C. Stainton and E. J. Neff, "The Efficacy of SeaBands for the Control of Nausea and Vomiting in Pregnancy," *Health Care Women International* 15, no. 6 (November–December 1994): 563–75.

Morning sickness may have evolved as a means of protecting embryos from food toxicity. Several studies have associated morning sickness with lower rates of miscarriage.

M. Profet, "Mother Nature Knows Best," *Nutrition Week* 22, no. 32 (August 21, 1992): 1.

In a double-blind, placebo-controlled study, 31 pregnant women were given 25 mg of vitamin B6 every 8 hours over a 72-hour period. Results: The vitamin treatment significantly reduced the incidence of nausea and vomiting.

V. Sahakian et al., "Vitamin B6 is Effective Therapy for Nausea and Vomiting of Pregnancy: A Randomized, Double-Blind Placebo-Controlled Study," *Obstetrics and Gynecology* 78, no. 1 (July 1991): 33–36.

Preliminary results from an ongoing Hungarian placebo-controlled study on the effects of multivitamin/mineral supplements in pregnant women have shown that women taking the supplements had significantly lower rates of vertigo, nausea, and vomiting during the first trimester than did controls.

A. E. Czeizel et al., "The Effect of Periconceptional Multivitamin-Mineral Supplementation on Vertigo, Nausea and Vomiting in the First Trimester of Pregnancy," *Archives Gynecology and Obstetrics* 251, no. 4 (1992): 181–85.

A placebo-controlled study gave 250 mg of powdered ginger root to women with nausea and vomiting 4 times a day for a total of 4 days. Seventy percent of the women taking the ginger root experienced relief.

W. Fischer-Rasmussen et al., "Ginger Treatment of Hyperemesis Gravidarum," *European Journal of Obstet. Gynaecol. Reprod. Biology* 38 (1990): 19–24.

It was demonstrated that taking 3–8 capsules of ginger root before arising, and 3–5 more upon experiencing the first signs of pregnancy-related nausea, eliminated or reduced the nausea in 75 percent of the women studied.

D. B. Mowrey, *The Scientific Validation of Herbal Medicine* (New Canaan, Conn.: Keats Publishing, 1986).

A case study of a woman with severe nausea through her entire first pregnancy reports that when the same trouble plagued her halfway through her second, she started taking 500 mg capsules of ginger 20 times a day. The treatment brought symptoms under control and allowed her to complete two additional pregnancies without suffering again from the same disorder.

B. Roach, *Townsend Letter for Doctors* (July 1983, September 1984, and June 1986).

CESAREAN SECTIONS

Noting the danger associated with cesarean section relative to giving birth vaginally, a retrospective study of 194 pregnant women who had previously undergone cesarean sections showed that 79 percent were able to deliver vaginally when they did so under careful surveillance.

N. P. Veridiano et al., "Vaginal Delivery After Cesarean Section," *International Journal of Gynecology and Obstetrics* 29 (1989): 307–11.

A review article examines the prospects of giving birth vaginally for women who have had previous cesarean sections. In 1985, the vaginal birth rate after cesarean section was 7 percent. By 1990 it had risen to 20 percent, while the number of cesarean sections had leveled off. Advantages of vaginal birth include shorter hospital stays, quicker maternal recovery, lower cost, and lower risk of infection. While the authors argue that safe vaginal births can be achieved, they do note the following contraindications: previous classical vertical uterine incisions, previous low vertical uterine incisions, unknown type of uterine incision, multiple gestation, breech presentation, and an unusually large baby.

Neal Clemenson, "Promoting Vaginal Birth after Cesarean Section," *American Family Physician* 47, no. 1 (January 1993): 139–44.

More than 6,000 women who had undergone cesarean sections were compared to age-matched controls. It was found that among women who had had the cesarean sections, there were a greater number of visits to both general and mental hospitals, and more operations performed. Cesarean-section women also had a higher risk of sterilization and pregnancies relative to the controls.

E. Hemminki, "Long-Term Maternal Health Effects of Cesarean Section," *Journal of Epidemiology and Community Health* 45 (1991): 24–28.

Researchers showed that, independent of other factors, advanced maternal age may influence a doctor's decision whether or not to perform a cesarean section.

D. Gordon et al., "Advanced Maternal Age as a Risk Factor for Cesarean Delivery," *Obstetrics and Gynecology* 77, no. 4 (April 1991): 493–97.

A study found that rates of cesarean sections increased from 9 percent in 1974 to 15 percent in 1978, and then up to 21 percent in 1984. One-third of the rise in the cesarean rate from 1974 to 1978 was due to repeat cesareans, and 9 percent was due to fetal distress. From 1978 to 1984, 47 percent of the rise in the cesarean rate was attributed to repeat cesareans, and 16 percent to fetal distress. Ninety-six percent of women giving birth after a previous cesarean section had a cesarean delivery again.

P. H. Shionoet al., "Reasons for the Rising Cesarean Delivery Rates: 1978–1984," *Obstetrics and Gynecology* 69, no. 5 (May 1987): 696–700.

Women receiving transcutaneous electrical nerve stimulation to control pain following cesarean section had a decreased need for medication and therefore less risk of side effects than women who did not receive TENS.

J. L. Hollinger et al., "Transcutaneous Electrical Nerve Stimulation After Cesarean Birth," *Physical Therapy* 66, no. 1 (January 1986): 36–38.

A study found that mothers who gave birth by cesarean section tended to have a bout of amnesia after birth, and thus their earliest recognitions of first contact with the infant were later than those of mothers giving birth vaginally. It was also shown that cesarean-section mothers had lower levels of eye-to-eye contact with their babies compared to controls a month after birth. Cesarean-section mothers suffered more depression, had more doubts about their abilities to adequately care for their babies, and began viewing their babies as persons later than controls did.

J. Trowell et al., "Possible Effects of Emergency Cesarean Section on the Mother-Child Relationship," *Early Human Development* 7, no. 1 (October 1982): 41–51.

Compared to women who delivered vaginally, a study reports, women who gave birth via cesarean section were found to suffer from higher rates of maternal depression, more obstetrical complications, and more difficult convalescence.

S. E. Gottlieb and D. E. Barrett, "Effects of Unanticipated Cesarean Section on Mothers, Infants, and their Interaction in the First Month of Life," *Journal of Dev. Behav. Pediatrics* 7, no. 3 (June 1986): 180–85.

Black women have a 24 percent higher risk of cesarean section birth than do white women, and the rate climbs to over 40 percent for black non-English-speaking women giving birth in for-profit hospitals to large babies. Latinas born in the United States have the second highest risk. Biological differences or sociological factors do not seem to account for such discrepancies.

P. Braveman et al., "Racial/Ethnic Differences in the Likelihood of Cesarean Delivery, California," *American Journal of Public Health* 85, no. 5 (May 1995): 625.

The highest cesarean-section rates in the country tend to be in the South, at large for-profit hospitals. The national average is about 23 percent, which makes cesarean section the most common major operation in the United States. States with rates above 24 percent include: Arkansas, Louisiana, Mississippi, Texas, West Virginia, Washington, D.C., Alabama, Florida, New Jersey, and Kentucky. Colorado had the nation's lowest C-section rate, at 16 percent. The Public Citizen group argues that the rate should be no higher than 12 percent and that, using this standard, 420,000 unnecessary C-sections were performed in 1992, at a cost of $1.3 billion.

"Consumer Group Challenges C-section Rate," *Special Delivery* 17, no. 3 (Summer 1994): 4.

An article on the relationship between cesarean sections and malpractice suits in the United States notes that the rate of cesarean delivery has increased from 4.5 per 100 births in 1964 to 24.1 per 100 births in 1986. One study of hospitals in New York state covering approximately 60,000 cesarean deliveries showed a clear relation to physician malpractice insurance premiums, the number of claims against obstetric staff per 100 doctors, and the number of claims against a hospital per 1000 patients discharged.

A. Localio et al., "Relationship Between Malpractice Claims and Cesarean Delivery," *JAMA* 269, no. 3 (January 20, 1993): 366.

CIRCUMCISION

Many third-party payers have started refusing to cover the cost for male circumcision, which may lead to a reduction in the number performed, an article notes. The author argues that since many doctors believe there to be little medical need for the practice, parents' decisions on whether or not to circumcise are not based on adequate medical information.

R. Rockney, "Newborn Circumcision," *American Family Physician* 38, no. 4 (October 1988): 151–55.

The American Academy of Pediatrics stated, in 1975, that there is "no medical indication for routine circumcision of the newborn." However, physician surveys showed that 41 percent of doctors were still recommending circumcision. Factors influencing the physicians' views included concerns about hygiene, the physician's age and medical specialty, and religious customs. The AAP statement did not seem to have an impact on the rate of male circumcision in the United States.

D. A. Patel et al., "Factors Affecting the Practice of Circumcision," *American Journal Dis. Child* 136, no. 7 (July 1982): 634–36.

A study surveyed new parents soon after they made their decision on whether or not to circumcise. Results showed that the factor most significantly associated with the decision was the status of the father. Concerns over the son's self-concept in the future, and treatment by his future peers, played an important part in the decision as well.

M. S. Brown and C. A. Brown, "Circumcision Decision: Prominence of Social Concerns," *Pediatrics* 80, no. 2 (August 1987): 215–19.

The majority of doctors performing circumcisions do not use analgesia, despite evidence that newborns can perceive pain and experience physiological stress from the procedure.

N. Wellington and M. J. Rieder, "Attitudes and Practices Regarding Analgesia for Newborn Circumcision," *Pediatrics* 92, no. 4 (October 1993): 541–43.

A study found that counseling parents with a videotape version of informed consent prior to the decision on whether or not to circumcise significantly reduced the incidence of circumcision (compared to when parents received oral counseling only).

R. W. Enzenauer et al., "Decreased Circumcision Rate with Videotaped Counseling," *Southern Medical Journal* 79, no. 6 (June 1986): 717–20.

A review article comments on the fact that while ritual circumcision of males has been practiced for millennia, the United States is the only English-speaking country not to have abandoned the practice.

E. Wallerstein, "Circumcision: The Uniquely American Medical Enigma," *Urol. Clin. North America* 12, no. 1 (February 1985): 123–32.

A study suggests that the circumcision of male infants may result in a greater pain response during later vaccination. Results showed that 30 boys who had been circumcised at birth out of a total of 42 who received various vaccinations at 46 months cried longer, and were deemed to be experiencing more pain, than uncircumcised boys.

Taddio et al., "Effect of Neonatal Circumcision on Pain Responses During Vaccination in Boys," *Lancet* 345, no. 8945 (February 4, 1995): 291.

BIRTHING POSITIONS

A study assessed the advantages and disadvantages of upright posture during the second stage of labor in women giving birth for the first time. Results showed that there were no significant differences between giving birth in a birthing chair and doing so in a recumbent position in bed. The authors thus argue that the upright posture is a safe and acceptable means of giving birth.

H. S. Liddell and P. R. Fisher, "The Birthing Chair in the Second Stage of Labour," *Australian and New Zealand Journal of Obstetrics and Gynaecology* 25, no. 1 (February 1985): 65–68.

Delivery using a birthing stool was compared to delivery in a conventional semirecumbent position. No significant differences were found between the two methods with respect to mode of delivery, length of second stage of labor, oxytocin augmentation, perineal trauma, labial lacerations, or vulvar edema. Women in the birthing chair group reported an overall satisfaction with their birth position and experienced less pain during the second stage of labor than did women in the semirecumbent position.

U. Waldenstrom and K. Gottvall, "A Randomized Trial of Birthing Stool or Conventional Semirecumbent Position for Second-Stage Labor," *Birth* 18, no. 1 (March 1991): 5–10.

POSTPARTUM RELAXATION

A study examined the effects of a protocol involving relaxation with guided imagery on various behavioral measures during the first 4 weeks of the postpartum period. Women on the protocol reported significantly higher levels of self-esteem and significantly lower levels of depression and anxiety than did controls after the 4 weeks.

B. L. Rees et al., "Effect of Relaxation with Guided Imagery on Anxiety, Depression, and Self-Esteem in Primiparas," *Journal of Holistic Nursing* 13, no. 3 (September 1995): 255–67.

BREAST-FEEDING

Exercise increases sour-tasting concentrations of lactic acid in breast milk. A study examined 26 2- to 6-month-old babies and found that they were less likely to accept breast milk 10-30 minutes following the mother's exercise compared to breast milk prior to exercise.

"Post-Exercise Lactic Acid Taints Breast Milk," *Medical Tribune* (January 29, 1992): 40.

In a survey of approximately 5,000 medical residents and physicians, less than 50 percent of the residents knew the correct answers to questions concerning the ideal treatment for a breast abscess or breast-fed jaundiced baby. Physicians did not do much better, with over 30 percent incapable of correctly advising mothers how to handle low milk supply. When residents were questioned about their medical training, just 55 percent reported even a single incident of precepting related to breast-feeding. The number of residents shown breast-feeding techniques at least five times was under 20 percent. Over half of the physicians believed their residency training with respect to breast-feeding was inadequate, yet more than 90 percent of them endorsed physician involvement in the promotion of breast-feeding. Based on these findings, the authors argue that physicians are not prepared to counsel women on breast-feeding.

G. L. Freed et al., "National Assessment of Physicians' Breast-Feeding Knowledge, Attitudes, Training and Experience," *JAMA* 273, no. 6 (February 8, 1995): 472–76.

The rate of new mothers breast-feeding in hospitals peaked in 1982 at approximately 62 percent, after bottoming out in 1972, an article reports. In the mid-1990s, 50 percent of women are breast-feeding at the time of hospital discharge. Reduced hospital time following birth has resulted in less opportunity to educate mothers about breast-feeding. The author argues that breast-feeding promotion is 30 years behind the knowledge about its nutritional and infection-fighting benefits, and that it is a cost-effective preventive medicine.

Calvin Pierce, "Breast-Feeding is Failing to Thrive," *Family Practice News* (April 15, 1994): 5.

All of the essential vitamins, minerals, and trace elements required by an infant are provided in breast milk, and neither moderate deficiencies nor excessive micronutrients in the mother should affect the levels available to the infant.

C. J. Bates and Ann Prentice, "Mother's Milk is a Source of Vitamins, Essential Minerals and Trace Elements," *Pharmac. Therapy* 62 (1994): 193–220.

Despite an officially stated goal of increasing the percentage of mothers breast-feeding in the United States to 75 by the year 2000, rates declined from 60 percent in 1984 to 52 percent in 1989 for newborns and from 24 percent to 18 percent for infants 5–6 months old.

G. L. Freed, "Breast-Feeding: Time to Teach What We Preach," *JAMA* 269, no. 2 (January 13, 1993): 243–45.

A study found that the consumption of 1.5 g of garlic 2 hours prior to breast-feeding made the milk more appetizing to infants and thus resulted in their consuming more.

"Breast-Feeding Moms: Shun Alcohol, but Eat Garlic?" *Human Sexuality* 26, no. 1 (January 1992): 16.

The short-term consumption of alcohol by breast-feeding mothers, it was found, affects the odor of breast milk and thus reduces its intake by the infant.

J. A. Mennella and G. K. Beauchamp, "Transfer of Alcohol to Human Milk: Effects on Flavor and the Infant's Behavior," *New England Journal of Medicine* 325, no. 14 (October 3, 1991): 981–85.

An editorial argues that breast-feeding during the first 3–6 months of life is nutritious, economical, hard to contaminate, helpful in disease prevention, and beneficial to mother/child bonding.

J. Janine, "Breast-Feeding in 1991," *New England Journal of Medicine* 325, no. 14 (October 3, 1991): 1036–38.

The position of the World Health Organization on breast-feeding is that in all populations, irrespective of HIV infection rates, breast-feeding should continue to be protected, promoted, and supported.

L. D. Arnold and E. Larson, "Immunologic Benefits of Breast Milk in Relation to Human Milk Banking," *American Journal of Infection Control* 21, no. 5 (October 1993): 235–42.

PREGNANCY AFTER 35

Women over 35 giving birth in a modern tertiary care facility are at no significantly higher risk of difficulties than are younger women, a case-control study found.

D. S. Kirz et al., "Advanced Maternal Age: The Mature Gravida," *American Journal of Obstetrics and Gynecology* 152, no. 1 (May 1, 1985): 7–12.

Women 35 or older have twice as many cesarean sections as those in the 20-to-29-year age range.

V. Edge and R. K. Laros, Jr., "Pregnancy Outcome in Nulliparous Women Aged 35 or Older," *American Journal of Obstetrics and Gynecology* 168, no. 6, pt. 1 (June 1993): 1881–85.

A study of over 26,000 children with birth defects of unknown cause in British Columbia found no association between maternal age and the incidence of such birth defects.

P. A. Baird et al., "Maternal Age and Birth Defects: A Population Study," *Lancet* 337, no. 8740 (March 2, 1991): 527–30.

A study compared the outcomes of singleton pregnancies in women having their first child at 35 or older with those having their first child between 20 and 29. Results showed that breech presentations and cesarean sections were nearly twice as prevalent in the older group and that only 27 percent of the older women experienced spontaneous vaginal delivery. Older women had longer hospital stays for both cesarean and vaginal deliveries.

O. Jonas et al., "Pregnancy Outcomes in Primigravid Women Aged 35 Years and Over in South Australia, 1986–1988," *Medical Journal of Australia* 154, no. 4 (February 18, 1991): 246–49.

When researchers looked at the effects of maternal age on first-birth pregnancies, they found that low-birth-rate risk was slightly increased in women 35 or older compared to women between 20 and 29. Women 30 or older showed an increased risk of cesarean delivery, and those over 35 were significantly more likely to experience pregnancy and birth complications.

G. S. Berkowitz et al., "Delayed Childbearing and the Outcome of Pregnancy," *New England Journal of Medicine* 322, no. 10 (March 8, 1990): 659–64.

A study comparing outcome of pregnancies in women 35 and older to pregnancy outcome in younger women found that maternal complications were no more prevalent in the older group than in those 34 and younger. Older women gave birth to fewer infants with congenital anomalies, although they did have births requiring significantly more operative delivery. Infant mortality was also lower for the group of infants born to older women.

K. L. Ales et al., "Impact of Advanced Maternal Age on the Outcome of Pregnancy," *Surg. Gynecol. Obstet.* 171, no. 3 (September 1990): 209–16.

ULTRASOUND

The author of a review article on ultrasound argues that using it in the screening of low-risk women provides no clinical benefits for either mother or child and adds millions to the cost of health care. Results of the Routine Antenatal Diagnostic Imaging with Ultrasound (RADIUS) trial, which compared over 15,000 low-risk pregnant women who were routinely screened with ultrasound to a group who received ultrasound examinations only when these were specifically indicated, appear to support the author's conclusions in that death or morbidity occurred in 4.98 percent of the babies in the screened groups versus 4.91 percent in the controls. Experts have estimated the cost of routinely screening 4 million pregnant women annually in the United States at approximately $1 billion.

S. Boschert, "Routine Prenatal Ultrasound Has 'No Benefit' in Low-Risk Women," *Family Practice News* 23, no. 14 (July 15, 1993): 1, 15.

DELIVERY

A study found that women using biofeedback during labor experienced significantly less pain compared to controls, and that those receiving biofeedback had a mean labor time of 2 hours less and required 30 percent less medication than did controls.

P. Duchene, "Effects of Biofeedback on Childbirth Pain," *Journal of Pain and Symptom Management* 4, no. 3 (1989): 117–23.

Conventional analgesics and acupuncture were compared in how well they controlled labor pains. Women who received acupuncture reported feelings of well-being, calmness, and being in control of labor and delivery. Acupuncture was also associated with a shorter first stage of labor.

I. F. Skelton and M. W. Flowerdew, "Acupuncture and Labour—A Summary of Results," *Midwives Chron.* 101, no. 1204 (May 1988): 134–38.

Results of a case-control study indicated that the application of fresh ginger paste at the Zhihying acupoint before retiring proved to be a significantly effective treatment for correcting breech positions in pregnant women.

R. Cai et al., [Study on Correction of Abnormal Fetal Position by Applying Ginger Paste at Zhihying Acupoint: A Report of 133 Cases], *Chen Tzu Yen Chiu Acupuncture Research* 15, no. 2 (1990): 89–91.

Transcutaneous electrical nerve stimulation (TENS) was shown to be an effective means of pain relief during labor, according to a study. Results showed that 23 percent of patients receiving the treatment reported considerable pain relief, 60 percent judged it to be of help, and 7 percent did not require any additional analgesia. Another study looking at TENS and labor pains found that 20 percent reported it to be of great benefit and 82 percent said it was of some benefit.

P. Stewart et al., "Transcutaneous Nerve Stimulation as a Method of Analgesia in Labour," *Anesthesia* 34, no. 4 (April 1979): 361–64.

In a study assessing the effects of acupuncture on normal delivery, of those women who were giving birth for the first time, 60 percent experienced definite objective and subjective relief, as did about 90 percent of the women having their second or subsequent childbirth experience. Duration of the delivery was reduced, and no side effects were reported in mother or child.

M. Hyodo and O. Gega, "Use of Acupuncture Anesthesia for Normal Delivery," *American Journal of Chinese Medicine* 5, no. 1 (Spring 1977): 63–69.

Clinical evidence suggests that black cohosh relieves the pain and distress of pregnancy, contributes to easy, quick, and uncomplicated deliveries, and promotes uterine involution and recovery.

D. B. Mowrey, *The Scientific Validation of Herbal Medicine* (New Canaan, Conn.: Keats Publishing, 1986): 108.

BIRTHING CENTERS

A review of the cases of over 11,000 women with low-risk pregnancies admitted for labor to free-standing birth centers found that there were fewer cesarean sections than would have been the case had the women gone to the hospital, and that the rates of infant mortality, as well as Apgar scores, were in line with what would have been expected in low-risk hospital birth.

J. Rooks et al., "Outcomes of Care in Birth Centers: The National Birth Center Study," *New England Journal of Medicine* 321, no. 26 (December28, 1989): 1804–11.

An article comments on a study of midwife-staffed health centers that showed that the total cost per patient was $3,200, compared to $4,600 for similar care at a community hospital. Researchers calculated that the cost of prenatal care and delivery could be reduced by 40 percent if such birthing centers existed in all communities.

C. Laino, "Birthing Centers Present Option," *Medical Tribune* (June 2, 1994): 12.

Researchers contrasted numerous aspects of the childbirth experience at an in-hospital birth center with more conventional maternity practices. They reported that women delivering in the birthing center felt more satisfaction with their own achievement and more involved in the birthing process than women receiving the more standard care. Differences were also noted between the level of support women experienced, the freedom of expression of feelings, and pain relief. All favored the birthing center approach.

U. Waldenstrom and C.A. Nilsson, "Experience of Childbirth in Birth Center Care: A Randomized Controlled Study," *Acta Obstet. Gynecol. Scand.* 73, no. 7 (August 1994): 547–54.

A Swedish study compared low-risk women's satisfaction with care at an in-hospital birth center with standard obstetric care. Results: Women in the birth center group were more satisfied with their care before, during, and after the births of their babies.

U. Waldenstrom and C. A. Nilsson, "Women's Satisfaction with Birth Center Care: A Randomized, Controlled Study," *Birth* 20, no. 1 (March 1993): 3–13.

The advantages of nontraditional settings for childbirth over traditional hospital settings include lower cost and decreased use of medical childbirth procedures.

L. L. Albers and V. L. Katz, "Birth Setting for Low-Risk Pregnancies: An Analysis of the Current Literature," *Journal of Nurse Midwifery* 36, no. 4 (July–August 1991): 215–20.

Data have shown birth centers to be as safe as hospitals for low-risk women. Also, such centers are less expensive, do fewer cesarean deliveries and invasive procedures, and rate higher in patient satisfaction.

M. C. Spitzer, "Birth Centers: Economy, Safety, and Empowerment," *Journal of Nurse Midwifery* 40, no. 4 (July–August, 1995): 371–75.

The 1989 National Birth Center Study concluded birth centers are safe and provide an acceptable alternative for women at low risk for birth complications.

J. T. Fullerton and R. Severino, "In-Hospital Care for Low-Risk Childbirth: Comparison with Results from the National Birth Center Study," *Journal of Nurse Midwifery* 37, no. 5 (September–October 1992): 331–40.

HOME BIRTHS

A study compared the outcome of women who gave birth using a home birth service with physician-attended hospital deliveries. Conclusions: Home births attended by lay midwives can be done with less intervention as safely as deliveries performed in the hospital.

A. M. Duran et al., "The Safety of Home Birth: The Farm Study," *American Journal of Public Health* 82, no. 3 (March 1992): 450-53.

A European review article argues that it is at least as safe—if not safer—for healthy women to give birth at home as it is in the hospital. Studies are cited.

O. Olsen, "Hjemmefodsler og Videnskabelig Tankegang" [Home Delivery and Scientific Reasoning], *Tidsskr. Nor. Laegeforen*, 114, no. 30 (December 10, 1994): 3655–57.

Results of an Australian survey-based study found that women giving birth in the home were older, more educated, more feminist, more willing to accept responsibility for maintaining their own health, more well read on childbirth, and more likely to have had previous children. Also, they gave higher ratings of their midwives than did labor-ward mothers.

J. D. Cunningham, "Experiences of Australian Mothers Who Gave Birth Either at Home, at a Birth Centre, or in Hospital Labour Wards," *Soc. Sci. Med.* 36, no. 4 (February 1993): 475–83.

MIDWIFERY

A look at the differences between nurse midwives and family practitioners in rural hospitals found that family physicians used episiotomy for delivery more frequently and were more likely to perform cesarean sections due to a diagnosis of dystocia (difficult labor).

W. J. Hueston and Mary Rudy, "A Comparison of Labor and Delivery Management Between Nurse Midwives and Family Physicians," *Journal of Family Practice* 37, no. 5 (1993): 449–54.

A Washington State study compared the outcomes of births attended by licensed midwives out of the hospital to those attended by physicians or certified nurse-midwives in hospitals and certified nurse-midwives out of hospitals. Results showed the only difference was a lower risk for low birthweight in births attended out of the hospital by licensed midwives versus those attended in hospitals by certified nurse-midwives.

P. A. Janssen et al., "Licensed Midwife-Attended, Out-of-Hospital Births in Washington State: Are They Safe?" *Birth* 21, no. 3 (September 1994): 141–48.

U.S. women assisted by midwives either in or out of hospital settings have experienced cesarean section rates much lower than those of women with similar circumstances receiving assistance from physicians in hospitals. Studies have also shown that excellent outcomes have been achieved by women at an elevated risk for adverse perinatal outcomes under the care of midwives.

C. Sakala, "Midwifery Care and Out-of-Hospital Birth Settings: How Do they Reduce Unnecessary Cesarean Section Births?" *Social Scien. Med.* 37, no. 10 (November 1993): 1233–50.

WATER BIRTH

A recent conference on the prevention of prematurity and neonatal mortality asserted that immersion in warm water is a safe and effective way of decreasing labor pain during birth.

"Warm Bath Can Ease Birth Pain," *Family Practice News* (May 15–31, 1991): 61.

Noting the many drawbacks of institutionalized obstetrics in the United States, an article argues for the acceptance of water birth as a safe and effective alternative to mainstream birthing.

K. Daniels, "Water Birth: The Newest Form of Safe, Gentle, Joyous Birth," *Journal of Nurse Midwifery* 34, no. 4 (July–August 1989): 198–205.

An article notes that of 831 women using the water birth approach at a family birthing clinic in California, 483 gave birth in the water with good Apgar scores and only one woman experienced a minor infection. The author argues that such results lend support to the efficacy of water birth an alternative means of delivery for many women.

L. K. Church, "Water Birth: One Birthing Center's Observations," *Journal of Nurse Midwifery* 34, no. 4 (July–August 1989): 165–70.

ACUPUNCTURE

In a study, 80 pregnant women at risk for difficult labor received acupuncture for 3–6 days prior to delivery. Results showed that spontaneous labor was without difficulty and there was significantly less blood loss compared to that for mothers not given the treatment.

E. V. Aleksandrina et al., [The Acupuncture Prevention of Anomalies in Labor Strength in Pregnant Women of a Risk Group], *Akusherstvo i Ginekologia* 8, no. 12 (1992): 22–24.

LAMAZE/PSYCHOPROPHYLAXIS

Results of a study showed that women who received Lamaze training had significantly shorter first stages of labor than a similar group of women who did not undergo Lamaze training.

I. Delke et al., "Effect of Lamaze Childbirth Preparation on Maternal Plasma Beta-Endorphin Immunoreactivity in Active Labor," *American Journal Perinatol.* 2, no. 4 (October 1985): 317–19.

Women giving birth for the first time who completed Lamaze training were compared with matched controls who didn't. The Lamaze group received less conduction anesthesia, had a higher rate of spontaneous vaginal deliveries, and were given narcotics less frequently during labor than were controls.

J. R. Scott and N. B. Rose et al., "Effect of Psychoprophylaxis (Lamaze Preparation) on Labor and Delivery in Primiparas," *New England Journal of Medicine* 294, no. 22 (May 27, 1976): 1205–7.

A study on childbirth-related factors compared 500 Lamaze-prepared patients to 500 age-, race-, parity- (number of children), and education-matched controls. Results found Lamaze to significantly benefit almost every measure examined. For example, Lamaze subjects had one-fifth the amount of fetal distress of controls and a fourth as many cesarean sections. They had a third fewer postpartum infections and fewer perineal lacerations. And cases of pregnancy toxemia were three times higher in controls, with the incidence of prematurity being double that of the Lamaze group.

M. J. Hughey et al., "Maternal and Fetal Outcome of Lamaze-Prepared Patients," *Obstetrics and Gynecology* 51, no. 16 (June 1978): 643–47.

HYPNOSIS

Hypnosis can help normalize fetal position. A case-control study of pregnant women with fetuses in the breech position showed that hypnotism resulted in an 81 percent conversion rate to a normal fetal position, compared to 48 percent in controls.

L. E. Mehl, "Hypnosis and Conversion of the Breech to the Vertex Presentation," *Archives of Family Medicine* 3, no. 10 (1994): 881–87.

In a study, hypnosis reduced first-stage labor time by 98 minutes for primiparas (women having their first baby) and 40 minutes for multiparas, relative to women receiving psychoprophylaxis. Women receiving hypnosis also reported more satisfaction with labor than those receiving psychoprophylaxis, as well as a reduction in anxiety and problems falling asleep.

L. R. Brann and S. A. Guzvica, "Comparison of Hypnosis with Conventional Relaxation for Antenatal and Intrapartum Use: A Feasibility Study in General Practice," *Journal of the Royal College of General Practitioners* 37, no. 303 (October 1987): 437–40.

The effects of hypnotherapy on labor in pregnant women were measured. First-stage mean labor time in women having their first babies receiving hypnosis was 6.4 hours, compared to 9.3 hours for controls. For other women, the hypnosis group mean time was 5.3 hours, versus 6.2 for controls. Both groups receiving hypnosis experienced a significant reduction in the need for analgesic agents.

M. W. Jenkins and M. H. Pritchard, "Hypnosis: Practical Applications and Theoretical Considerations in Normal Labour," *British Journal of Obstetrics and Gynaecology* 100, no. 3 (March 1993): 221–26.

EXERCISE

Exercise during pregnancy can be beneficial in a variety of ways. A study showed that women who exercised began labor significantly earlier than controls and had a lower incidence of vaginal and abdominal operative delivery. In those delivering vaginally, active labor time was reduced relative to controls. Acute fetal stress was also found to be less common among women who exercised during pregnancy than in those who did not.

J. F. Clapp, III, "The Course of Labor after Endurance Exercise during Pregnancy," *American Journal of Obstet. Gynecol.* 163, no. 6, pt. 1 (December 1990): 1799–1805.

According to a Dutch study, strenuous exercise of limited duration during pregnancy is not harmful to either the fetus or the mother.

"Experts Differ on Prenatal Exercise: Some Say Women Can Exercise Strenuously for More Than Fifteen Minutes," *Medical Tribune* (April 23, 1992).

Healthy women who exercise regularly during pregnancy have no higher levels of abortion, infertility, abnormal presentation, premature rupture of membranes, congenital abnormalities, or preterm labor than do nonexercisers. Babies born to exercising mothers have less body fat, and there is significantly less incidence of fetal distress during labor in these women as well.

J. F. Clapp, III, "Exercise and Fetal Health," *Journal of Developmental Physiology* 15 (1991): 9–14.

Results of a study showed that the level of exercise during pregnancy was inversely associated with the number of pregnancy symptoms.

B. Sternfeld et al., "Exercise During Pregnancy and Pregnancy Outcome," *Med. Science Sports Exercise* 27, no. 5 (May 1995): 634–640.

HOMEOPATHY

The effectiveness of homeopathic remedies on uterine contraction has been documented by studies. A study comparing conventional and homeopathic therapies in women at risk for contraction abnormalities showed that the only notable differences between the two were that fewer hemorrhages and a reduced number of abnormal contractions were associated with homeopathic treatments.

B. Hochstrasser and P. Mattmann, "Homeopathy and Conventional Medicine and Obstetrics," *Schwitz. Med. Wochenschr.* 124, suppl. 62 (1994).

ECTOPIC PREGNANCY

In the United States, the leading cause of maternal death in the first trimester of pregnancy is ectopic pregnancy.

A. Kalandidi et al., "Induced Abortions, Contraceptive Practices, and Tobacco Smoking as Risk Factors for Ectopic Pregnancy in Athens, Greece," *British Journal of Obstetrics and Gynecology* 98, no. 2 (February 1991): 207.

From 1970 to 1989, the rate of ectopic pregnancy per 1,000 pregnancies increased almost fourfold; per 1,000 live births, the increase was fivefold.

"Ectopic Pregnancy—United States, 1988–1989," *MMWR* 41, no. 32 (August 14, 1992): 591.

Vaginal douching has been found to be a risk factor for both eptopic pregnancy and pelvic inflammatory disease. Smoking is also a risk factor for both of these conditions, as is sexually transmitted disease.

J. Schachter and J. M. Chow, "Vaginal Douching as It Relates to Reproductive Health Complications," *Current Opinion in Infectious Diseases* 6 (1993): 27–30.

Smoking at the time of conception is a significant dose-related risk factor for ectopic pregnancy, a case-control study revealed.

J. Coste et al., "Risk Factors for Ectopic Pregnancy: A Case Controlled Study in France with Special Focus on Infectious Factors," *American Journal of Epidemiology* 133, no. 9 (May 1, 1991): 839–49.

Smoking at the time of conception increases ectopic pregnancy risk by 40 percent.

A. Stergachis et al., "Maternal Cigarette Smoking and the Risk of Tubal Pregnancy," *American Journal of Epidemiology* 133, no. 4 (1991): 332–37.

Smoking increases the odds of having an ectopic pregnancy. For those women smoking fewer than 10 cigarettes per day, the odds are raised to 1.4. The odds ratio for those smoking 1.5 packs or more per day go up to 5.0.

A. Handler et al., "The Relationship of Smoking and Ectopic Pregnancy," *American Journal of Public Health* 79, no. 9 (September 1989): 1239–42.

A study of 70 women links smoking to a twofold increase in ectopic pregnancy.

A. Kalandidi et al., "Induced Abortions, Contraceptive Practices, and Tobacco Smoking as Risk Factors for Ectopic Pregnancy in Athens, Greece," *British Journal of Obstetrics and Gynecology* 98, no. 2 (February 1991): 207.

According to the results of a study of over 700 pregnancies, risk factors for ectopic pregnancy include age, number of previous pregnancies, and antineoplastic drugs. During the past two decades, the incidence of ectopic pregnancy has increased.

M. J. Saurel-Cubizolles et al., "Ectopic Pregnancy and Occupational Exposure to Antineoplastic Drugs," *Lancet* 341 (May 8, 1993): 1169–71.

A case-controlled study determined the following as risk factors for ectopic pregnancy: having had an appendectomy or prior tubal surgery, prior ectopic pregnancy, and induced conception cycle.

J. Coste et al., "Risk Factors for Ectopic Pregnancy: A Case Controlled Study in France with Special Focus on Infectious Factors," *American Journal of Epidemiology* 133, no. 9 (May 1, 1991): 839–49.

Illegal abortion produces a tenfold increase in ectopic pregnancy risk, according to a study performed in Greece when abortion was illegal. Legal abortion, by contrast, carries with it much less risk of a later ectopic pregnancy.

A. Kalandidi et al., "Induced Abortions, Contraceptive Practices, and Tobacco Smoking as Risk Factors for Ectopic Pregnancy in Athens, Greece," *British Journal of Obstetrics and Gynecology* 98, no. 2 (February 1991): 207.

Intrauterine devices are more effective at preventing intrauterine pregnancy than ectopic pregnancy, a study confirmed.

J. Coste et al., "Risk Factors for Ectopic Pregnancy: A Case Controlled Study in France with Special Focus on Infectious Factors," *American Journal of Epidemiology* 133, no. 9 (May 1, 1991): 839–49.

A fourfold increase in ectopic pregnancy risk is associated with the use of an intrauterine device, and risk increases with duration of use, a study determined. Factors not associated with increased risk of ectopic pregnancy, according to the study, are oral contraceptive use and miscarriages.

A. Kalandidi et al., "Induced Abortions, Contraceptive Practices, and Tobacco Smoking as Risk Factors for Ectopic Pregnancy in Athens, Greece," *British Journal of Obstetrics and Gynecology*, 98, no. 2 (February 1991): 207.

A case-controlled study found that postpartum or interval tubal sterilization increases ectopic pregnancy risk 2.8 times compared to the barrier method, and 3.7 times compared to oral contraceptives. The risk from interval sterilization is similar to that from intrauterine devices. However, in comparison to using no contraceptives, interval sterilization reduces ectopic pregnancy risk.

V. Holt et al., "Tubal Sterilization and Subsequent Ectopic Pregnancy: A Case Controlled Study," *JAMA* 266, no. 2 (July 10, 1991): 242–46.

Laparoscopy and traditional Chinese medicine have been used to successfully treat cases of ectopic pregnancy.

Y. N. Wu et al., [Conservative Therapy of Combining Laparoscopy and Chinese Medicine for Ectopic Pregnancy], *Chung Kuo Chung Hsi I Chieh Ho Tsa Chih* 14, no. 10 (October 1994): 583–85.

22. PRE-MENSTRUAL SYNDROME (PMS)

PMS is more widespread in Western societies than in primitive cultures, because of diet and lifestyle. Dr. Michael Janson, an orthomolecular physician from Cambridge, Massachusetts and author of *The Vitamin Revolution*, says, "Sugar, caffeine, and alcohol precipitate or worsen symptoms and should be avoided. This is because a lot of patients with PMS have frank hypoglycemia. Their sugar levels fluctuate up and down. Eating sugar sends blood sugar levels way up, and the body responds by dropping sugar levels way down. Additionally, caffeine, even when taken in small amounts in the morning, can aggravate symptoms, such as breast tenderness, and sleep disturbances."

Symptoms

The effects of PMS can range from mild to severe and vary from person to person. They may include bloating, cramps, headaches, swelling, fluid retention, low back pain, depression, abdominal pressure, insomnia, sugar cravings, anxiety, irritability, breast tenderness, mood swings, and acne.

Clinical Experience

DIET
According to Dr. Janson, the best diet to lessen the symptoms of PMS is high in fiber and complex carbohydrates, with small meals and snacks in between. This helps to regulate blood sugar, and in many cases is enough to reduce or eliminate PMS symptoms. Herbalist Letha Hadady recommends cool green foods such as salads and the avoidance of hot, spicy, and acidic foods as well as the elimination of coffee. Some people, however, need more help and can benefit from vitamin therapy, exercise, and a stress management program.

NUTRITIONAL SUPPLEMENTS
When symptoms are severe, diet alone may not be enough. These nutrients may prove useful:

Vitamin B6 (pyridoxine). This has a number of helpful properties for alleviating PMS. As a smooth muscle relaxant, it can decrease cramps. As a diuretic, it reduces fluid retention, swelling, and breast tenderness. Between 200 and 400 mg should be taken daily. Vitamin B6 can be taken throughout the month, rather than just pre-menstrually. One hundred mg in a B-complex vitamin can be taken the first two weeks of the period, and an additional 250 the last two weeks of the cycle. More B6 increases the need for magnesium.

Magnesium. Magnesium calms the nervous system and relieves anxiety, depression, irritability, nervousness, and insomnia. As an antispasmodic, it alleviates cramps and back pain. Magnesium also helps reduce cravings for sweets. Between 500 and 1,000 mg may be needed.

Gammalinolenic acid (GLA). GLA is a precursor to prostaglandin-E1, a hormonelike substance that helps to regulate neurological and hormonal functions. Prostaglandin-E1 helps reduce muscle spasms, cramping, sugar cravings, mood swings, depression, anxiety, irritability, acne, and to some extent breast tenderness. It also reduces inflammation and decreases the stickiness of the platelets, which prevents blood clotting. GLA is found in evening primrose oil, borage oil, and black currant oil. Borage oil is the most concentrated source of GLA, containing 24 percent GLA, the equivalent of six capsules of evening primrose oil. One 1,000 mg capsule of borage oil provides a daily dose of 240 mg GLA.

Eicosapentaenoic acid (EPA). This oil found in fish and flaxseed oil produces prostaglandin-E3, which helps to alleviate breast tenderness. Flaxseed oil is fragile and should not be used in cooking. It can be used in salad dressings or over cooked foods.

Vitamin E. 400–800 IU can reduce cramps, breast tenderness, and fibrocystic breasts, which often swell up before the period.

Multiple vitamin/mineral supplement. A balanced multivitamin/mineral supplement can help to balance the system.

EXERCISE

Exercise helps to improve mood, reduce cramps, eliminate excess fluid, and control sugar cravings. Aerobic exercises should be performed three to four times per week.

HERBS

Herbalist Letha Hadady finds these Chinese herbs useful for alleviating symptoms of PMS:

Lungtanxieganwan. A Chinese remedy that alleviates anger associated with PMS.

Xiao Yao Wan. Helps relieve PMS symptoms of depression, poor circulation, indigestion, and bloating.

Women's Harmony. Increases circulation.

These remedies can be ordered from a mail order source in Oakland, California called Health Concerns (800-233-9355).

HOMEOPATHY

The homeopathic remedy chosen should correspond to the symptoms described; only one should be used for best results. Sometimes it's a matter of trial and error; if one does not work, try another. Dr. Ken Korins, a classically trained homeopathic physician in New York City, recommends these remedies for PMS.

Lachasis helps most physical and emotional symptoms that accompany PMS, such as headaches, right ovarian pain, breast tenderness. It may be indicated if PMS symptoms stop once menstrual flow stops. Also, symptoms get worse with heat and with constricted clothing around the abdomen. Emotional indications are restlessness, paranoia, and a tendency to be talkative.

Laccaninum. Think of this remedy when the only symptom is a painful, swollen breast. Pain leaves once the menstrual flow begins. There is a tendency to be irritable.

Bovista. Gastrointestinal symptoms occur before the period, such as diarrhea. There may also be traces of blood before the actual flow begins. Subjective and objective feelings of swelling occur throughout the body, even through the hands, causing a tendency to feel clumsy.

Pulsatilla. Emotional symptoms of PMS, such as a weepy, mild disposition. There is a need for consolation from others. Strong craving for sweets.

Natmur. Emotional state is melancholy and sad, and worsens with attempts to console by others. Headaches occur before, during, or after period. Craving for salty foods and an aversion toward sex at the time of the period.

Sepia. For sadness, depression, indifference, and feelings of discontent and discouragement about life. Often a colicky pain is felt before the menses. There may also be a sensation of the uterus dropping, as if it would fall through the vagina due to congestion in that area.

Folliculinum. This is a new French remedy that can be given on the seventh day of the cycle in a 30 to 200c potency.

PROGESTERONE

Progesterone promotes youthfulness, and is beneficial against cancer and fibrocystic breast disease. Dr. Michael Janson says additional progesterone is especially important for women exposed to exogenous estrogens, found in pesticides, food additives, drugs and other chemicals in the environment. These lead to an overload of estrogen and a deficiency of progesterone. Progesterone is extremely helpful for treating PMS symptoms in such cases. Dr. Bruce Hedendal, a complementary physician in Boca Raton, Florida, recommends a formula derived from Mexican yams. He foresees this treatment as the wave of the future.

REFLEXOLOGY

Reflexology is a science and an art based on the principle that we have reflex areas in our feet that correspond to every part of the body. Massaging specific reflex areas in the feet help to improve the functioning of specific organs and glands.

Laura Norman, a certified reflexologist from New York City, describes three reflexology techniques:

Thumb walking. "This technique can be used on the bottom, tops and sides of the feet, although it is most used on the bottom. The procedure entails bending the thumb at the first joint and inching along the bottom of the foot like a caterpillar, pressing from the heel up to the toe. The right hand is used on the right foot. Taking little tiny bites, press, press, press the whole bottom of the foot."

Finger walking. "This is done in the same way, but bending the finger at the first joint, using the tip of the finger on the outside edge."

Finger rotation. "This is where you rotate the finger into the foot."

Massaging the feet with the above techniques, using a nongreasy, absorbent cream, warms them up and helps promote overall relaxation. For addressing specific problems, reflexology must be applied to specific areas.

Knowing where to massage is fairly simple, as reflex points on the foot correspond to the way the organs and glands are distributed within the body. Laura Norman explains, "If you were to imagine your body reduced, and superimposed onto your feet, the points would be laid out just as they are in your body, from top to bottom. The top of the body is the head, and the toes reflect everything in the head area— the eyes, nose, ears, mouth, teeth, gums, jaw, brain. The ball of the toes represent the chest area, the heart, lungs, bronchial tubes. Then the center of the foot is the internal organs. Working down to the heel and ankle area, you find the pelvic area and reproductive organs. For PMS, these are the points that need to be massaged.

"The pelvic and reproductive organs are located in the heel and ankle area. The uterus point is midway between the ankle bone and the heel, on a diagonal. Thumb walking should be performed around the ankle on the big toe side of the foot. The thumbs should be pressed down, like a caterpillar, all over that inside ankle. Then a circular rotation performed with the thumb can be done on that midpoint. Finger walking can also be used over that area.

"Next, work should be done on the reflex areas that correspond to the ovaries. That is located on the outside of the ankle. With the right foot cradled on the left leg, find the high spot on the ankle bone. Square off the back of the heel and draw an imaginary diagonal line. Divide this line in half and that is where the ovary point is. This outside point of the foot is not visible and must be measured by feel or by using the index or middle finger of the left hand as it wraps around the bottom of the heel. This reflex point is almost always more sensitive than the uterus point, so care should be taken not to use too much pressure. It should help to get the blood circulating.

"Following this, the reflex to the fallopian tubes should be addressed. That goes across the top of the ankle, from ankle bone to ankle bone, on the top of the foot. This connects the ovaries to the uterus. What you need to do is finger-walk from one ankle bone to the other across the top of the foot. Two fingers can be used here, one from each hand.

"Although the focus is on the reproductive organs and glands, all systems should be massaged, as the entire organism is interrelated. It is important, therefore, to massage and press on the entire foot to help all-over relaxation. Sliding the thumbs across the bottom of the feet serves this purpose and feels wonderful."

Reflexology for PMS helps most when performed three or four days before, and during, menstruation. First the right foot is worked on, while resting on the left leg. Then the same actions are repeated on the left side.

Patient Story

LAURA NORMAN

Twenty-five years ago, I had my first reflexology experience. My friend Judy came to visit me from California. At the time, I was suffering from terrible menstrual problems. I was pre-menstrual, bloated, headachy, achy, and feeling awful all over.

She said to me, "Laura, I've been studying something called reflexology, that is such a powerful tool to help you feel better all over, and especially with the menstrual condition." Judy had me take off my shoes and socks, lie down on my bed, and prop my feet up on some pillows. She pulled up a chair to the end of my bed, dimmed the lights, put on some music, and applied some hot, wet washcloths to my feet. She started to rub and press and squeeze my feet with the washcloths. It felt incredible to start with. Then she began massaging my feet with some cream, and this was heavenly. Next, she started to apply pressure to very specific parts of my feet, which she said corresponded to various parts of my body.

I felt fantastic. I was floating. I had never felt so deeply relaxed in my entire life. My symptoms completely disappeared. Afterward I was energized. I was so clear-thinking and productive. At that time I was in college studying for exams, and under a lot of pressure.

Judy continued to work on me, and I continued to find out more about reflexology myself to help myself. I saw a tremendous difference, and it totally changed the course of my life. As a result of pursuing this for my own healing, I ended up doing this professionally, and started a whole career in reflexology.

Now I have been practicing reflexology for twenty-five years and have seen incredible results with all kinds of conditions in all walks of life. I've seen it work on little infants and children and seniors.

Hot News

Studies have shown that PMS patients frequently have insufficient levels of vitamin A, B complex vitamins, copper, zinc, and magnesium, tryptophan, ferritin, and calcium; thus, supplementation of these substances shows promise in easing pre-menstrual symptoms. Dietary strategies that seem to lessen pre-menstrual difficulties include a low-fat regimen, avoidance of sugar and caffeine, and the consumption of a high-carbohydrate, low-protein evening meal in the days before menstruation. Evening primrose oil can reduce both the depression that often accompanies pre-menstrual syndrome and cyclical breast swelling and tenderness. Other treatments that have proven beneficial include exercise regimens, relaxation techniques, and reflexology. *(See below.)*

NUTRITION/DIET

Vitamin A, the B complex, copper, and zinc have been shown to be low in PMS patients.

J. G. Penland and J. Hunt, "Diet Related to Menstrual Symptoms/Nutritional Status and Menstrual-Related Symptomatology," *FASEB Journal* 7 (1993): A379.

Blood levels of copper, zinc, and magnesium are lower in PMS patients than in others, studies show.

C. Posaci et al., "Plasma Copper, Zinc and Magnesium Levels in Patients with Pre-menstrual Tension Syndrome," *Acta Obstet. Gynecol. Scand.* 73 (1994): 452–55.

A study revealed that 45 percent of a PMS patient group had low levels of magnesium.

R. A. Sherwood et al., "Magnesium and Pre-menstrual Syndrome," *Annals of Clinical Biochemistry* 23, no. 6 (1986): 667–70.

Patients with pre-menstrual migraine treated with a magnesium compound had a significantly lower pain index score after 2 months.

F. Faccinetti et al., "Magnesium Prophylaxis of Menstrual Migraine: Effects on Intracellular Magnesium," *Headache* 31 (1991): 298–304.

Magnesium supplementation significantly reduced scores on a menstrual distress questionnaire.

F. Facchinetti et al., "Oral Magnesium Successfully Relieves Pre-menstrual Mood Changes," *Obstet. Gynecol.* 78, no. 2 (1991): 177–81.

Tryptophan depletion increases PMS symptoms, especially irritability, researchers found.

D. B. Menkes et al., "Acute Tryptophan Depletion Aggravates Pre-menstrual Syndrome," *Journal of Affective Disorders* 32 (1994): 37–44.

Increasing calcium reduced pre-menstrual symptoms related to mood, concentration, behavior, and general pain.

J. G. Penland and P. E. Johnson, "The Dietary Calcium and Manganese Effects on Menstrual Cycle Symptoms," *American Journal of Obstetrics and Gynecology* 168, no. 5 (May 1993): 1417–23.

PMS patients received a gram of calcium carbonate daily for 3 months. The result was that 73 percent reported fewer symptoms.

S. Thys-Jacob et al., "Calcium Supplementation in Pre-menstrual Syndrome: A Randomized Crossover Trial," *Journal of Gen. Intern. Med.* 4, no. 3 (1989): 183–89.

Low ferritin levels are linked to increased mood disturbances in pre-menstrual and menstrual phases, and to greater pain during the menstrual phase.

J. G. Penland and J. Hunt, "Diet Related to Menstrual Symptoms/Nutritional Status and Menstrual-Related Symptomatology," *FASEB Journal* 7 (1993): A379.

Caffeine consumption increases PMS symptoms, and its effects are dose-dependent. A survey of 295 students showed that 61 percent of the women who consumed 4.5-15 caffeine-containing drinks daily had moderate to severe PMS. But only 16 percent of those who consumed no caffeine had PMS.

A. M. Rossignol, "Caffeine-Containing Beverages and Pre-menstrual Syndrome in Young Women," *American Journal of Public Health* 75, no. 11 (1985): 1135–37.

Alpha-tocopherol was given to pre-menstrual syndrome sufferers. In three-quarters of the cases, improvement was seen.

R. S. London et al., "The Effect of Alpha-Tocopherol on Pre-menstrual Symptomatology: A Double-Blind Study: II. Endocrine Correlates," *Journal of the American College of Nutrition* 3, no. 4 (1984): 351–56.

Vitamin E has been proven of value to PMS sufferers. In a study of 75 women treated for 2 months with either a placebo or vitamin E, 75 percent of those given the E supplements showed improvement.

R.S. London et al., "The Effect of Alpha-Tocopherol on Pre-menstrual Symptomatology: A Double-Blind Study: II. Endocrine Correlates," *Journal of the American College of Nutrition* 2, no. 2 (1983): 115–22.

Two hundred PMS patients were given the vitamin supplement Optivite. After 3 months, over 96 percent reported significant improvement, and over 30 percent were asymptomatic.

A. Stewart et al., "Effect of a Nutritional Programme on Pre-menstrual Syndrome: A Retrospective Analysis," *Complementary Med. Research*, 5, no. 1 (1991): 8–11.

A low-fat diet was shown to significantly decrease such PMS symptoms as weight gain, bloating, and breast tenderness.

D. V. Jones, "Influence of Dietary Fat on Self-Reported Menstrual Symptoms," *Physiol. Behav.* 40, no. 4 (1987): 483–87.

Reducing dietary fat to 15 percent of caloric consumption, while increasing consumption of complex carbohydrates, reduced PMS breast tenderness and swelling in 6 out of 10 study subjects.

N. F. Boyd et al., "Effect of a Low-Fat High-Carbohydrate Diet on Symptoms of Cyclical Mastopathy," *Lancet* 2 (1988): 128–32.

Consumption of a carbohydrate-rich, protein-poor evening test meal in the late luteal phase improved PMS scores related to depression, tension, anger, confusion, sadness, fatigue, alertness, and calmness.

J. J. Wurtman et al., "Effect of Nutrient Intake on Pre-menstrual Depression," *American Journal of Obstet. Gynecol.*, 161, no. 5 (1989): 1228–34.

PMS has been linked to greater consumption of refined carbohydrates.

G. S. Goei et al., "Dietary Patterns of Patients with Pre-menstrual Tension," *Journal of Applied Nutrition* 34, no. 1 (1982): 4–11.

High sugar intake is associated with PMS.

A. M. Rossignol and H. Bonnlander, "Prevalence and Severity of the Pre-menstrual Syndrome: Effects of Foods and Beverages that are Sweet or High in Sugar Content," *Journal of Reproductive Medicine* 36, no. 2 (1991): 131–36.

In a study on PMS, 100 percent of subjects receiving vitamin A supplementation pre-menstrually showed improvement.

E. Block, "The Use of Vitamin A in Pre-menstrual Tension," *Acta Obstet. Gynecol. Scand.* 39 (1960): 586–92.

HERBS/PLANT EXTRACTS

Evening primrose oil can provide relief of PMS, a study showed.

P. A. Ockerman et al., "Evening Primrose Oil as a Treatment of the Pre-menstrual Syndrome," *Recent Advances in Clinical Nutrition* 2 (1986): 404–5.

A study of 30 patients indicates that evening primrose oil can alleviate the depression associated with PMS.

O. Ylikorkala et al., "Prostaglandins and Pre-menstrual Syndrome," *Prog. Lipd. Research* 25 (1987): 433–35.

Evening primrose oil was shown to be highly effective for depression.

D. F. Horrobin, "The Role of Essential Fatty Acids and Prostaglandins in the Pre-menstrual Syndrome," *Journal of Reproductive Medicine* 28, no. 7 (July 1983): 465–68.

A study of 92 patients with severe cyclical breast pain (and no breast cancer) showed that evening primrose oil either eliminated the pain or reduced it to easily bearable levels.

J. K. Pye et al., "Clinical Experience of Drug Treatments for Mastalgia," *Lancet* 2 (1985): 373–77.

EXERCISE

Regular, moderate exercise reduces PMS symptoms, specifically, impaired concentration, negative affect, behavior change, and pain.

J. A. Aganoff and G. J. Boyle, "Aerobic Exercise, Mood States and Menstrual Cycle Symptoms," *Journal of Psychosometric Research* 38, no. 3 (April 1994): 183–92.

RELAXATION

A 5-month study on 46 women showed that the relaxation response approach produced a 58 percent improvement rate for women with severe PMS.

I. L. Goodale et al., "Alleviation of Pre-menstrual Syndrome Symptoms with the Relaxation Response," *Obstetrics and Gynecology* 75, no. 4 (1990): 649–55.

REFLEXOLOGY

A study of 35 women supports the use of ear, hand, and foot reflexology for PMS treatment.

T. Oleson and W. Flocco, "Randomized Controlled Study of Pre-menstrual Symptoms Treated with Ear, Hand, and Foot Reflexology," *Obstet. Gynecol.* 82, no. 6 (December 1993): 906–11.

CANDIDIASIS

Thirty-two patients with both severe PMS and a history of vaginal candidiasis had failed to respond to various treatments. In a controlled experiment, the treatment group was placed on a sugar-free, yeast-free diet and oral nystatin, and 10 out of the 15 in this group experienced significant relief of PMS. The PMS symptoms of the controls remained unchanged.

J. S. Schinfeld, "PMS and Candidiasis: Study Explores Possible Link," *Female Patient* (July 1987): 66.

SEXUAL ABUSE

A study links sexual abuse to PMS. Of women seeking treatment for PMS, 40 percent have been sexually abused.

"Study Links Abuse, PMS," *Medical Tribune* (April 4, 1991): 3.

23. SEXUAL DYSFUNCTION

Psychologist Dr. Janice Stefanacci says sexual dysfunction stems largely from a society that offers people no models of normal healthy sexuality: "If we look to the media, we see things that are totally aberrant in terms of frequency and potency. We see relationships portrayed between males and females where there is power and domination, or submission and seduction. Role models of healthy sexual communication and actualization are virtually nonexistent. People need a sense of what is normal.

"They also need time to think about sexuality as an integrated part of their personality. Our culture is very fragmented in this regard. Many, many people, men and women, never spend time thinking about their sexuality. In fact, if you were to take an informal survey and ask people, 'What is sexuality?' a good proportion of them would say, 'It's sex. It's something you do, maybe in the bedroom, maybe at night.' Nobody is really sure how often you are supposed to have it or how long it is supposed to last. Most people don't realize that sexuality is a completely integrated part of their personality as much as actualizing in education or interpersonal relationships. Sexuality is very much a part of who we are, how we present ourselves in the world, what we do, and how we think of ourselves. Our adequacy and our self-esteem is tied up in our sexuality."

Our society defines sexuality entirely according to male standards in which sex is a performance, and orgasm is the primary, and perhaps only, yardstick for gauging satisfaction, and hence sexual "function." Some sex researchers are beginning to question the whole concept of sexual dysfunction, promoting broader and less rigid definitions of sexual response and pleasure. "The Masters & Johnson model of sexual response—excitement, plateau, orgasm, and resolution—is very performance-oriented," says Rebecca Chalker, a women's health activist whose upcoming book, *Secrets of Women's Sexuality*, explores ways in which feminists are redefining male standards. "After desire and willingness, the only other compulsory element is pleasure," Chalker points out. "Pleasure and intimacy are the real goals of sexual activity, and if you look at it that way, the concept of sexual dysfunction simply collapses."

Nevertheless, women may worry when they have difficulties achieving orgasms, especially with a partner, and men become concerned if they have difficulties in controlling ejaculations and in getting erections. Both women and men are also distressed when they don't feel sexual attraction. In fact, most people who seek out counseling do so for difficulties with sexual communication and the lack of sexual desire.

Early on, through regular masturbation, boys learn what feels good and how to reliably get orgasms. Girls often wait to begin sexual exploration until they initiate sexual activity and miss out on the benefits of self-exploration. "Learning about sex from boys or men isn't the best thing for women," Chalker says. "Their efficient, orgasm-oriented model doesn't necessarily encompass women's needs and preferences. For example, the repetitive thrusting of intercourse is a pretty efficient way for men to get orgasms, but many women don't easily get orgasms this way. Many need very specific manual stimulation. Another problem is that men get their orgasms relatively quickly, and are then ready for a nap. On average, it takes women much longer to become fully aroused and able to have really strong orgasms." Chalker points out that the biggest difference between women's sexuality and men's is that women have an innate ability to have multiple orgasms. "But under the male standard, many women simply don't have the opportunity to discover this phenomenal facet of their sexuality."

Many sex therapists recommend that women explore their sexual response through masturbation, using a vibrator, sex toys, and sexy videos to stimulate sexual fantasies. You may also want to experiment with things like aromatherapy, oils, and herbs. After sufficient homework, you can try integrating these changes into sex with your partner. Another important change heterosexual couples can make is to try rewriting the "intercourse script." That is, plan to have sexual sessions where intercourse will not take place. Try giving each other maximum pleasure just with your hands. Men can also learn the time-honored technique of postponing intercourse, and hence ejaculation. This ensures that women have time to become fully aroused and can get the maximum pleasure from a sexual session.

As a general rule, young men (we're talking men under forty here) don't have difficulties getting erections. In their forties, however, many men begin to find that erections are less reliable. This problem may in part be caused by lack of desire, but it is also caused by certain diseases, especially diabetes, multiple sclerosis, certain medications, excessive alcohol consumption, prostate surgery, or hardening of the arteries, which is a normal part of aging but is greatly exacerbated by smoking, too much fat in the diet, and not enough aerobic exercise. Other than a healthier, more vigorous lifestyle, there aren't any quick fixes for erectile dysfunction. If, however, men begin to think about sex less as a performance than as an experience in which pleasure and intimacy are the ultimate goal, unreliable erections might become less of an issue. "For some men, taking the focus off erection and expanding it to include full body stimulation may ultimately improve erectile ability," Chalker says.

Early ejaculation can also be a problem for some men, and is often the result of too much direct stimulation of the penis with both hands, or its insertion into the vagina. Men can retrain themselves to delay ejaculation by avoiding immediate penetration and/or direct stimulation of the penis for successively longer periods, or by varying the types of stimulation. Try to encourage your partner to avoid stimulation that brings him quickly to the feeling that orgasm is inevitable. Over time, maybe several months, the time before his ejaculation and orgasm should increase.

Chalker points out that there are two powerful aspects of our sexuality—the physiological and the psychological—and that "neither can live without the other." Unfortunately, psychological problems are the more difficult to deal with and manifest themselves variously. Single people suffer when they cannot find a suitable sexual partner, while people in long-term relationships may find that they are no longer attracted by their partner. In this regard, counseling, as well as exploring a variety of books that are available, can be very helpful. Many people search for aphrodisiacs to stimulate sexual desire, but some research suggests that sexual images—in literature, photographs, or videos—are also quite helpful in stimulating the release of sexual hormones. The booming market in erotica would seem to affirm this idea.

"Today, we have enormous resources available to help with sexual problems that we didn't have a few years ago," Chalker notes. "I've reviewed some of the herbal aids and remedies here, and I encourage the reader to explore the wide range of resources available in book stores or by mail order."

Dr. Vicki Hufnagel reminds us: "Improperly performed episiotomies are another common cause of sexual dysfunction." (*See "Corrective Vaginal Surgery" in* Pregnancy.)

Resources for Sexual Problems

BOOKS

Lonnie Barbach. *For Each Other.* New York: Penguin Signet, 1982.

Rebecca Chalker. *Secrets of Women's Sexuality.* New York: Seven Stories Press, in press.

Mantak Chia. *The Multiorgasmic Man.* New York: HarperCollins, 1996.

Mantak and Maneewan Chia. *Cultivating Female Sexual Energy.* Huntington, N.Y.: Healing Tao Books, 1986.

———. *Cultivating Male Sexual Energy.* Huntington, N.Y.: Healing Tao Books.

Federation of Feminist Women's Health Centers. *A New View of a Woman's Body.* Los Angeles, Calif.: Feminist Health Press, 1995. (Order from Feminist Health Press, 8240 Santa Monica Boulevard, Los Angeles, Calif. 90046.)

Gina Ogden. *Women Who Love Sex.* New York: Simon & Schuster Pocket Books, 1994.

Cathy Winks and Anne Semans. *The Good Vibrations Guide to Sex.* Pittsburgh, Penn.: Cleis Press, 1994.

VIDEO

Betty Dodson. *Sex for One* and *Selfloving: Video Portrait of a Women's Sexuality Seminar.* To order: Box 1933, Murray Hill Station, New York, N.Y. 10156; $45.00.

MAIL ORDER SUPPLIERS

Eve's Garden, 119 West 57th Street, #420, New York, N.Y. 10019-2382.

The Sexuality Library, 938 Howard Street, #101, San Francisco, Calif. 94103: (800) 289-8423.

NUTRIENTS

Studies show that a heightened libido and orgasmic intensity are related to blood levels of histamine. Women who have low histamine levels tend to experience low sexual excitement, while those with a high level are more able to sustain orgasms. Nutrients that increase histamine levels include vitamin B5 and the bioflavonoid rutin. Broccoli, parsley, cherries, grapes, peppers, melons and citrus fruits are good food sources.

AROMATHERAPY

"Aromatherapy is fantastic for helping women regain their sense of sensuality," declares aromatherapist Ann Berwick. These are some of the oils she recommends:

Rose is wonderful for enhancing feminine qualities. It bring out the loving, tender side of us that wants to surrender. Men who have trouble showing their emotions or opening up to their partner can benefit from rose as well.

Clary sage heightens sensation. It takes you out of your body and into a different realm, allowing you to relax and enjoy the romance.

Sandalwood is a wonderful oil for people not in touch with their physical side. It is very earthy and very deep.

Jasmine restores self-confidence in people who have been through traumatic sexual experiences. It can help women who have been abused or who are emotionally closed off from damaging relationships.

"By blending different oils, you can create a formula that enhances the sensual side of your nature," says Berwick. She suggests adding them to the bath or using them while massaging a partner or in self-massage. A personal perfume can be made and used daily. "Surrounding yourself with these glorious scents is a wonderful help."

ORIENTAL PERSPECTIVE

Registered nurse and acupuncturist Abigail Rist-Podrecca explains sexual dysfunction from an Eastern point of view: "Chinese medicine looks to the root of the cause, rather than just the symptoms, and the root seems to be the kidney. The kidneys are called the roots of life. Everything stems from the kidney, they say."

Weak kidney function can be diagnosed in Oriental medicine in multiple ways, including facial diagnosis: "Under the eye is the thinnest tissue in the entire body," explains Rist-Podrecca. "You can see through the skin there. If the blood is not being cleared by the kidneys, and detoxified, then you will see a darkness under the eyes. People will say, 'I haven't had enough sleep,' but it goes beyond that. In Chinese medicine, it says that the kidneys are not functioning optimally, so the blood isn't being cleansed."

She goes on describe various factors that can drain the kidneys. "Cold can deplete the kidneys. Many people can't tolerate cold. This is so because in the winter time, the kidney's function becomes suppressed, much the same way as the sap in a tree runs to the core and into the roots. When people have a compromised kidney situation, where it isn't functioning optimally, they can't stand the cold weather.

"Overwork and tension can also weaken kidney function because the kidneys and the adrenal glands (the adrenal sits on top of the kidney) are considered one and the same in Chinese medicine. So too much stress, and too many chemical toxins, deplete kidney functioning." Hundreds of Chinese herbs nourish kidney function. Here Rist-Podrecca names a few:

Har shar woo. This is an essential herbal formula for nourishing kidney function. It is also said to darken the hair. Hair, bone, teeth, joints, and sexual functions are tied up with the kidney energies. When you energize the kidneys, you affect all these different areas. When combined with *dong quai*, *har shar woo* helps the type of kidney dysfunction that causes low back pain.

Romania is a dark black herb that is high in iron and helps to nourish the blood and improve kidney function.

Dong quai resembles a cross section of the uterus, and has an affinity for this area of the body.

Sexual Abuse

Abuse against women is a problem of staggering magnitude, and it occurs in every socioeconomic and ethnic group. In the United States, it is estimated that 1.8 million women are beaten every year by current or former partners. About 15 percent of women using primary care clinics have been assaulted by partners.

Sexual abuse, even more than physical abuse and battering, is a profoundly invasive violation. It takes what is most pleasurable to us, our sexuality, and turns it into a nightmare of powerlessness and revulsion. Sexual abuse happens to girls and boys, women and men, of all ages. If you have been sexually abused, the most important thing you can do is seek out a counselor, program, or support group that can guide you to recovery and help you become aware of the many resources now available. In addition, there are soothing, empowering products and therapies that may also aid the healing process.

No one deserves to be abused. If you have been abused, you are not the one who has done something wrong. Seek out local support groups, shelter, and legal help. Your state may have a hotline for abused women. Check the Yellow Pages under the following headings: Social Services, Battered Spouses, and Abuse. If danger is imminent, dial 911.

The National Coalition Against Domestic Violence may have a local branch near you. To find the coalition nearest you, call the Washington, D.C., office at (202) 638-6388 (Tuesday, Wednesday, and Thursday from 10 A.M. to 8 P.M. Eastern Time), or call the Denver office at (303) 839-1852 (Monday through Friday).

TRADITIONAL CHINESE PERSPECTIVE

Traditional Chinese medicine sees sexual abuse as an attack on one's energy field. Left uncorrected, this results in physical as well as psychic disturbances. Phyllis Bloom from the Center for Acupuncture and Healing Arts in lower Manhattan describes imbalances which commonly occur, and tells how acupuncture, Chinese herbs, and essential oils can help to restore equilibrium and health: "There are three levels of energy in the body: the protective level, the nutritive level, and the constitutional level. With sexual abuse, any and all of these can be affected. It depends on the situation, for example, whether it is an acute situation or a chronic one that has gone on for a very long time. If the attack is severe, that can cut through all layers.

"The protective level is the surface. It is what we use to defend ourselves. When this level is affected, it can manifest in several ways. A person I treat, who was sexually abused, continually gets flus, sinus problems, and illnesses. This is because her protective layer is overworked and has fallen down. Sometimes people have back pains because they were attacked from the back.

"When the protective layer is overworked, the body delves deeper and undermines the nutritive level. At this level, blood is created and energy flows through all of the organs. People who have problems at this level commonly have problems with various systems. They have digestive or respiratory problems, for example. They often have blood problems too. Women can experience tremendous pain during their periods or stabbing pains in the pelvic area. Other possibilities are masses, fibroids, and cysts. Disturbances in blood also affect a person's ability to express herself in the world. Women suffer from this a great deal."

YUNNAN BAIYAO. "One of the most common formulas for correcting psychic and physical trauma is called *Yunnan baiyao*, meaning the white medicine from Yunnan province. This herbal combination helps the body redirect the blood flow from traumatized areas where the blood becomes stuck. It creates new channels. Once this flow is established, we can work on healing deeper layers of trauma."

ACUPUNCTURE. "Chinese medicine has a five-element system that includes fire, water, metal, earth, and wood. When the nutritive level is affected, the fire element is disturbed. This element is responsible for relationships, intimacy, and boundaries. The organs associated with it are the heart, the heart protector or pericardium, and the small intestine.

"The heart is the center of who we are. Sexual abuse is a shock to the system, and shock is absorbed by the heart. When the heart is affected, we may see memory blocks, insomnia, palpitations and arrhythmia. Acupuncture can help. Sometimes *Yunnan baiyao* can help as well. The acupuncture meridians primarily emanate from the chest out to the inner side of the arm. One in particular that we use is called the Spirit Gate."

AROMATHERAPY. "The essential oil sandalwood can help with palpitations, nervousness, insomnia. Just one drop is needed on the center of the chest."

Herbal Pharmacy

Plants containing phytochemicals with aphrodisiac properties, in order of potency:
> *Vicia faba* (broad bean)
> *Catharanthus lanceus* (lanceleaf periwinkle)
> *Euphorbia lathyris* (caper spurge)
> *Passiflora incarnata* (passionflower)
> *Panax ginseng* (Chinese ginseng)
> *Punica granatum* (pomegranate)
> *Malus domestica* (apple)
> *Zea mays* (corn)

Hot News

Two common causes of sexual dysfunction such as loss of libido, anorgasmia, impotence, and ejaculation difficulties, according to recent studies, are the use of prescription medications—among them guanadrel (Hyorel), Prozac, Marplan, Nardil, Parnate, clomipramine (Anafranil), and amoxapine (Asendin)—and the consumption of alcohol, which can result in a cycle of drinking causing sexual dysfunction, which then leads to more drinking. On the other hand, aerobic exercise has been linked to more sexual activity and greater satisfaction. A natural substance traditionally used to enhance sexuality comes from chaste tree berries, which stimulate and balance the pituitary gland. *(See below.)*

FROM THE MEDICAL LITERATURE ON SEXUAL DYSFUNCTION

MEDICATIONS

There are a number of medications that may lead to sexual dysfunctions such as loss of libido, anorgasmia, impotence, and ejaculation difficulties. Examples include: thiazide diuretics, guanadrel (Hyorel), clonidine (Catapres), methyldopa (Aldomet), propranolol (Inderal), Prozac, Marplan, Nardil, Parnate, clomipramine (Anafranil), trazodone (Desyrel), and amoxapine (Asendin).

"Drugs that Cause Sexual Dysfunction: An Update," *Medical Letter* (August 7, 1992): 34.

ALCOHOL

Although many believe the opposite to be true, consuming alcohol makes women less sexually responsive and aroused. Drinking may also result in the cycle of alcohol leading to sexual dysfunction, which then leads to drinking even more to try to get over the dysfunction. Alcohol use has also been shown to heighten the risk of sexual assault.

J. Norris, "Alcohol and Female Sexuality: A Look at Expectancies and Risks," *Alcohol Health and Research World* 18, no. 3 (Summer 1994): 197.

Despite research evidence to the contrary, a study found that 65 percent of women and 45 percent of men say that alcohol increases sexual pleasure.

M. S. Goldman and L. Roehrich, "Alcohol Expectancies and Sexuality," *Alcohol Health and Research World* 15, no. 2 (Spring 1991): 126.

A study on women and alcohol found that the most powerful predictor of chronic drinking among women and previously nonproblem drinkers was sexual dysfunction.

"Sexual Dysfunction and Drinking," *Women's Letter*, 4, no. 1 (January 1991): 8.

Results of a study on postmenopausal alcoholic women show that those who did not drink for more than one year experienced more sexual satisfaction in their lives compared to those remaining sober over a shorter period of time.

"Abstinence Increases Sexual Satisfaction in Alcoholic Postmenopausal Women," *Brown University Digest of Addiction Theory and Application* 13, no. 8 (August 1994): 11.

EXERCISE

Exercise enhances sexual activity, studies show. Two thousand questionnaires returned by readers of a women's fitness magazine were analyzed, with the results suggesting that aerobic exercise was linked to easier arousal, more sexual activity, and an easier time achieving orgasm. In another study, interviews with male and female swimmers revealed that swimmers in their forties have intercourse rates at levels more in line with the general population of people in their twenties and thirties.

"Can Exercise Help Your Sex Life?" *Consumer Reports on Health* 3, no. 10 (October 1991): 78.

HERBS/PLANT EXTRACTS

Chaste tree berries have traditionally been used by women to increase overall sexual health. Commonly suggested by herbal practitioners as a treatment for hormonal imbalance, they've also been used in some cultures as a means of limiting sexual desire. Research has demonstrated that chaste tree berries act by stimulating and balancing the pituitary gland, thus increasing women's sexual energy when it is too low and lowering it when it is too high. Another herb said to have aphrodisiac effects is damiana, which has a long history of use by Mexican women, primarily as a tea taken approximately an hour before intercourse.

L. Vukovic et al., "Enhancing Female Sexual Response: Exercises and Herbs to Awaken Your Libido," *Natural Health* 23, no. 2 (March–April 1993): 59.

PHYSICAL/SEXUAL ABUSE

Some studies indicate 10 to 20 percent of all women have been sexually abused, while others indicate a rate of 40 to 50 percent.

"Study Links Abuse, PMS," *Medical Tribune* (April 4, 1991): 3.

Women exposed to severe, life-threatening abuse frequently delay seeking the help they need. Of 289 abused women who turned to a battered women's agency, 70 percent waited more than a year to seek help. No association was found between the extent of abuse and the length of delay in seeking help.

R. Reidy and M. Von Korff, "Is Battered Women's Help Seeking Connected to the Level of Their Abuse?" *Public Health Reports* 106, no. 4 (July–August): 360–65.

The national domestic violence hotline was discontinued in June 1992.

T. Randall, "Domestic Violence Hot Line's Demise: What's Next?" *JAMA* 269, no. 10 (March 10): 1223–26.

Results of 150 reports of sexual assault during a one-year period in Omaha, NE, show that women who put up a fight (strong verbal and physical resistance and flight) are more likely to escape rape and no more likely to be injured by the rapist than those who are submissive. These results contradict earlier studies that indicated verbal resistance alone (crying and pleading) could prevent rape.

J. M. Zoucha-Jensen and A. Coyne, "The Effects of Resistance Strategies on Rape," *American Journal of Public Health* 83, no. 11 (November 1993): 1633–35.

Ethanol use is linked to sexual abuse. Alcohol is a factor in 40 percent of beatings.

"Controlling Violence at Home," *University of California, Berkeley Wellness Letter* 10, no. 7 (April 1994): 7.

Women who have been subject to domestic violence are more likely to use alcohol. Statistics also show that abused women are more likely than others to attempt suicide.

J. Abbott et al., "Domestic Violence Against Women: Incidence and Prevalence in an Emergency Department Population," *JAMA* 273, no. 22 (June 14, 1995): 1763–68.

A study of 206 patients with gastrointestinal disorders showed that 44 percent had a history of sexual or physical abuse.

D. A. Drossman et al., "Sexual and Physical Abuse in Women with Functional or Organic Gastrointestinal Disorders," *Annals of Internal Medicine* 113, no. 11 (December 1, 1990): 828–33.

Eating disorders are linked to a history of sexual abuse, studies show.

G. Waller, "Association of Sexual Abuse and Borderline Personality Disorder in Eating Disordered Women," *International Journal of Eating Disorders* 13, no. 3 (1993): 259–63.

A study compared 100 overweight women to 100 slender controls and showed a highly significant correlation between obesity and childhood abuse, both sexual and nonsexual, as well as to early parental loss, parental alcoholism, chronic depression, and dysfunction in the women's own marriages.

V. J. Felitti, "Childhood Sexual Abuse, Depression and Family Dysfunction in Adult Obese Patients: A Case Control Study," *Southern Medical Journal* 86, no. 7 (July 1993): 732–36.

24. TEMPORO-MANDIBULAR JOINT (TMJ) DYSFUNCTION

The temporomandibular joint (TMJ) is a hinged joint that opens and closes the mouth. The jaw is part of a wider system, the craniosacral system, which lies along the center of the body. It begins with the feet, moves up to the knees, the pelvis, the shoulders, and then to the head and jaw. Disruption at any level can result in TMJ pain. The problem may originate with the TMJ itself, or it might start in the feet or with neck tension, for example.

Causes

The two most common causes of TMJ problems are poor bite and stress. Poor bite may be the result of new dental work that affects tooth alignment. Sometimes braces shift the palate, which affects the jaw. In recent years, more adults have been undergoing this procedure, hence, increasing numbers of TMJ disorders. Dentists who specialize in TMJ can diagnose the condition.

Although TMJ dysfunction is not exclusively a woman's problem, it does affect larger numbers of females than males due to stresses brought on by hormonal changes. Dr. Deborah Kleinman, a chiropractor who works with TMJ patients, explains: "There are various stress factors we can talk about that are specific to women. First, we have pre-menstrual tension. This further weakens an already weakened system. I know women who only have a problem with their jaw three days before their period. As soon as their period comes, their pain goes away. This tells me that there is a weakness in the system and that hormones push the body past the point of being able to compensate for it.

"These hormonal changes also occur during pregnancy and menopause. In addition to hormonal changes and added stress, pregnancy creates structural changes through weight gain and the loosening of ligaments. Hormones loosen the pelvis so that the woman is more flexible during delivery. These changes can further aggravate TMJ dysfunction.

"With nursing, postural changes can play a big role. Nursing places stress on the upper back muscles, especially if the woman doesn't use the proper pillows or if she gets lazy and slumps over while feeding her baby. These upper back muscles insert into the occiput, which is part of this craniosacral system. The occiput is the bone at the bottom of the skull. Tightening or pulling on the occiput can affect the head, neck, and TMJ."

Symptoms

Pain can be isolated in the joint itself or it can radiate to the face, neck, ear, and shoulder. Headaches may be a part of the picture. There may be a nagging toothache, even though the tooth is healthy. There can also be difficulty with opening the mouth all the way. If the muscles around the joint become inflamed, they may spasm and lock open. Clicking, grinding or popping noises may accompany chewing or movement of the joint.

Clinical Experience

CRANIOSACRAL THERAPY
Cranio means skull and *sacral* refers to the sacrum, which is a part of the pelvis. This therapy is founded on an understanding of the relationship between these structures and several points in between, including the TMJ. Dr. Deborah Kleinman, who uses a specific form of craniosacral therapy called sacro-occipital technique, explains: "A chiropractor like myself who uses this technique understands that there is a balance between the nervous system and the musculoskeletal system, and a relationship between the pelvis and the sacrum and then the head and the cranium. Between both structures rests the spine, the shoulders, the neck. All of these structures react to shifts in the pelvis and the cranium. The TMJ is part of that." She adds that a stable pelvis balances the body and works in harmony with the cranium. This allows information to flow to the brain smoothly.

A doctor performs a series of tests to determine whether structural stresses exist, and, if so, where. Once this is known, treatment can begin: "We place wedges or blocks under the pelvis. The muscles will relax and contract around these levers in an unforced way, based upon what these levers tell the brain. Then we incorporate breathing techniques to assist the brain in making musculoskeletal changes. This reestablishes the proper craniosacral flow." Sometimes secondary manipulations are necessary to readjust parts of the spine that lie between the pelvis and cranium that get knotted up as a result of compensating for the pelvis and the cranium. Cranial adjustments, made specifically to the temporomandibular joint, also help to reestablish proper balance.

OTHER PHYSICAL THERAPIES

Regularly done isotonic exercise can help some cases of TMJ dysfunction. In addition to jaw exercise, self-treatment for TMJ problems may include jaw awareness, in which the patient tries to notice and avoid clenching and grinding the teeth, as well as biting on gum, ice, or fingernails. Eating soft foods and avoiding resting or sleeping on the stomach can also help, as can learning to rest the jaw and to adopt proper jaw posture. Other potentially helpful techniques include self-massage; relaxed rhythmic opening and closing of the jaw; alternating moist heat (15 minutes) with ice (2–3 minutes) to increase circulation; cool spray/cryotherapy; bite guards; and splints. Surgery should be a last resort when dealing with TMJ problems.

NUTRITION

Nutritional supplements may help in treating TMJ problems. Some of the most useful:

Calcium and magnesium. These minerals are essential for proper muscular function and have a sedative effect.

B-complex vitamins. Take 100 mg, 3 times a day.

Pantothenic acid. 100 mg, twice daily. B-complex vitamins and pantothenic acid are essential for combating stress

Coenzyme Q10. This is another stress fighter;

L-tyrosine and vitamins B6 and C will improve sleep quality and alleviate anxiety and depression.

Multivitamin and mineral complex.

Hot News

Some therapies that have proven helpful in relieving temporomandibular joint dysfunction in studies are acupuncture; biofeedback in combination with intra-oral appliances; progressive relaxation training; and isokinetic exercise. Supplementation of calcium and magnesium citrates serves to relax jaw muscles; another natural remedy is Euphytose, a mixture of plant extracts, including *Passiflora incarnata, Valeriana officials,* and *Cola nitida. (See below.)*

FROM THE MEDICAL LITERATURE ON TEMPOROMANDIBULAR JOINT DYSFUNCTION

ACUPUNCTURE AND OTHER TREATMENTS

Acupuncture can be useful in treating patients with temporomandibular joint dysfunction. In a study, 4 out of 10 patients felt much better, and 6 out of 10 somewhat better, with acupuncture treatment given once a week for 6 to 8 weeks.

A. M. Raustia and R.T. Pohjola, "Acupuncture Compared with Stomatognathic Treatment for TMJ Dysfunction. Part III: Effect of Treatment on Mobility," *Journal of Prosthetic Dentistry* 56, no. 5 (November 1986): 616–23.

In treating TMJ dysfunction, biofeedback in combination with intraoral appliances was more effective than either treatment alone.

D. C. Turk et al., "Effects of Intraoral Appliance and Biofeedback/Stress Managment Alone and in Combination in Treating Pain and Depression in Patients with Temporomandibular Disorders," *Journal of Prosthetic Dentistry* 70, no. 2 (August 1993): 158–64.

Progressive relaxation training was found to help reduce jaw pain and tension; one study found little additional benefit attributable to biofeedback.

R. A. Moss et al., "The Comparative Efficacy of Relaxation Training and Masseter EMG Feedback in the Treatment of TMJ Dysfunction," *Journal of Oral Rehabilitation* 10, no. 1 (1983): 9–17.

Clicking in the jaw is often a sign of craniomandibular disorders. Isokinetic exercise eliminated the clicking in 18 out of 22 subjects (82 percent) participating in a study.

A. R. Au and I. J. Klineberg, "Isokinetic Exercise Managment of Temporomandibular Joint Clicking in Young Adults," *Journal of Prosthetic Dentistry* 70, no. 1 (July 1993): 33–39.

Breathing exercises may help some cases of TMJ pain. Also, craniosacral work by an osteopath can provide relief.

A. Weil, *Natural Health, Natural Medicine* (Boston: Houghton Mifflin, 1990): 322–23.

NUTRITION

Calcium and magnesium (citrates)—1,000 mg of each at bedtime and 200 mg of each 12 hours later—will act as muscle relaxants.

A. Weil, *Natural Health, Natural Medicine* (Boston: Houghton Mifflin, 1990): 322–23.

HERBS/PLANT EXTRACTS

Euphytose is a mixture of plant extracts, including *Passiflora incarnata, Valeriana officinalis*, and *Cola nitida*, among others. Euphytose is used in France to produce anxiety-relieving and/or antidepressant effects. In experimental rats, it acts as an antispasmodic.

M. Valli et al., "Euphytose, an Association of Plant Extracts with Anxiolytic Activity: Investigation of its Mechanism of Action by an In Vitro Binding Study," *Phytotherapy Research* 5 (1991): 241–44.

Passiflora edulis aqueous extract was the subject of a study involving rats, mice, and healthy human volunteers. It was shown to have a nonspecific depressant effect on the central nervous system, and not a hypnotic-sedative effect.

E. Maluf et al., "Assessment of the Hypnotic/Sedative Effects and Toxicity of *Passiflora Edulis* Aqueous Extract in Rodents and Humans," *Phytotherapy Research* 5 (1991): 262–66.

Animal research showed *Harpagophytum procumbens* to have anti-inflammatory and analgesic effects. At 200 mg/kg, its effect was similar to a 68-mg/kg dose of the analgesic acetylsalicylic acid (aspirin).

M. C. Lanhers et al., "Anti-Inflammatory and Analgesic Effects of an Aqueous Extract of *Harpagophytum Procumbens*," *Planta Med.* 58 (1992): 117-123.

25. URINARY INCONTINENCE

Causes

Eighty-five percent of the 13 million people who are incontinent are women. This is because urinary incontinence is commonly set off by childbirth and menopause. Gynecologist Vicki Hufnagel explains: "In many cases, women are given episiotomies after delivery, without proper closure. Since muscles are not put back together correctly, the whole area is unable to provide support." Dr. Hufnagel adds that during menopause, urinary incontinence occurs when a woman is not making enough estrogen. Too little estrogen enters the vaginal tissue, causing the area to become thin, inelastic, and weak.

Urinary incontinence can also be the result of brain and spinal cord lesions, trauma, multiple sclerosis, and allergies.

There are many causes of transient incontinence. Some common ones are infection, strophic urethritis or vaginitis, certain medications (sedatives, hypnotics, diuretics, anticholinergics, alpha-adrenergic agonists or antagonists, and calcium-channel blockers), psychological disorders (especially depression), endocrine disorders, hyperglycemia, restricted mobility, and stool impaction.

Smoking has been found to be the cause of 28 percent of urinary incontinence in women. Smoking increases the odds of both stress and motor urinary incontinence, and with increased daily and lifetime cigarette consumption, the odds for genuine stress incontinence rise. A recent study of 606 women reported in the November 1992 *American Journal of Obstetrics* showed that genuine stress incontinence was twice as common for both former and current smokers as for nonsmokers.

Symptoms

Urinary incontinence is a partial or total loss of control over one's bladder and urinary sphincter muscles. Sometimes, incontinence is accompanied by a feeling of urgency. This is usually the result of a person's inability to sufficiently empty the bladder. Coughing and other stressors are also factors that can set off urinary incontinence. Overflow can occur when the bladder's capacity is small.

Clinical Experience

Women with urinary incontinence are often advised to get bladder surgery, even hysterectomies. But this drastic approach may be completely unnecessary, according to Dr. Hufnagel, who says that women need to be educated about more conservative treatments for this common everyday occurrence.

OUTPATIENT SURGERY AND HORMONE REPLACEMENT
Women need to repair their failed episiotomy, or to receive hormones, Dr. Hufnagel explains. Often, they simply need outpatient surgery to put the muscles and tissues back the way they should have been at the time of delivery.

Regarding menopause, Dr. Hufnagel adds, "We can treat this locally, without surgery, by simply putting hormones into the vagina. One or two months later, we see normal healthy tissue."

ELECTRICAL STIMULATION
This treatment became popular in Europe after it was learned that high voltages of electricity to the vaginal area caused muscles to contract. However, the results were short-lived, and the modality was not problem free. Voltages were applied constantly, which sometimes resulted in tissue burning and nerve damage.

In the United States, electrical stimulation is being performed with lower voltages and a pulsing sequence of one second on and one second off to prevent muscle fatigue. The objective is to strengthen the urethral muscles and the puborectalis sling muscle, which control the opening and closing of the bladder muscles. This form of electrical stimulation, combined with pelvic floor exercises, has produced favorable results in trial studies. It allows for a retraining, toning, and strengthening of muscles so that a patient can regain continence. One electrical product that looks promising is called Cystotron, put out by a company called Biosonics. More information about this system can be obtained on the World Wide Web at www.biosonics.com, or the old-fashioned way, by calling (800) 547-4357.

Hot News

One surprising discovery in recent research is that smoking is the cause of 28 percent of urinary incontinence in women. Studies indicate that surgery and the use of pharmaceuticals are often unnecessary; other methods that have proven effective are behavioral techniques and biofeedback, Kegel exercises, which strengthen pelvic muscles, electrical stimulation of the pelvic floor, and acupuncture. A natural treatment, according to one study, can be extracted from the plant marshmallow; this helps incontinence by treating inflammation of the genito-urinary tract.

SURGICAL TREATMENT

Surgery should be used only as a last resort when dealing with urinary incontinence, and nonpharmacological techniques, such as behavioral methods, should be tried before drugs are used.

M. D. Walters et al., "Nonsurgical Treatment of Urinary Incontinence," *Current Opinions in Obstet. Gynecology* 4, no. 4 (August 1992): 554–58.

EXERCISE

Kegel exercises, to strengthen pelvic muscles, will reduce urinary leakage episodes. A success rate has been reported of from 43 to 95 percent.

B. D. Weiss, "Nonpharmacologic Treatment of Urinary Incontinence," *American Family Practice* (August 1991): 579–86.

Of 36 subjects with stress incontinence, 56 percent substantially improved or were cured after finishing a Kegel exercise program. Proper training in this type of exercise is essential, researchers emphasize.

G. Elia and A. Bergman, "Pelvic Muscle Exercises: When Do They Work?" *Obstetrics and Gynecology* 81 (1993): 283–86.

A pelvic exercise protocol produced results compared to those provided by phenylpropanolamine; this was the finding of a study of 157 women aged 55 to 90.

Thelma Wells et al., "Pelvic Muscle Exercise for Stress Urinary Incontinence in Elderly Women," *Journal of the American Geriatric Society* 39 (1991): 785–91.

BIOFEEDBACK

Biofeedback has been shown to be an effective technique in alleviating urge and stress incontinence.

M. D. Walters et al., "Nonsurgical Treatment of Urinary Incontinence," *Current Opinions in Obstet. Gynecology* 4, no. 4 (August 1992): 554–58.

Four weeks of training with biofeedback improved incontinence in 73 percent of the 22 female patients in a study.

H. Heidler, [Modification of Urge Incontinence by Biofeedback Mechanisms], *Urologe* 25, no. 5 (September 1986): 267–70.

ELECTRICAL STIMULATION

Electrical stimulation was the subject of a study of 38 female patients with frequency, urgency, or urge incontinence. Results: Electrical stimulation of the pelvic floor cured or improved 63 percent. The treatment improved 75 percent of the cases of detrusor instability and hyperreflexia.

M. Zollner-Nielsen and S. M. Samuelsson, "Maximal Electrical Stimulation of Patients with Frequency, Urgency, and Urge Incontinence: Report of 38 Cases," *Acta Obstet. Gynecol. Scand.* 71, no. 8 (December 1992): 629–31.

ACUPUNCTURE

A study of 20 patients showed that 77 percent of those with idiopathic detrusor instability were cured of symptoms with acupuncture treatment.

T. Philip et al., "Acupuncture in the Treatment of Bladder Instability," *British Journal of Urology* 61, no. 6 (June 1988): 490–93.

Frequency, urgency, and painful urination in 22 out of 26 patients improved with acupuncture treatment at the Sp. 6 point.

P.L. Chang, "Urodynamic Studies in Acupuncture for Women with Frequency, Urgency and Dysuria," *Journal of Urology* 40, no. 3 (September 1988): 563–66.

HERBS/PLANT EXTRACTS

Marsh mallow soothes mucous membranes; it's used internally to treat inflammation and mucosal afflictions of the genito-urinary tract, including incontinence.

D. Mowrey, *The Scientific Validation of Herbal Medicine* (New Canaan, Conn.: Keats Publishing, 1986): 33.

26. URINARY TRACT INFECTIONS and INFLAMMATIONS

Urinary tract infections (also known as cystitis and bladder infections) are quite common, accounting for approximately 6 million office visits per year in the United States. *E. coli* and other bacteria that inhabit the large intestine are most often responsible, due to the closeness of the urethra and vagina to the rectum. *(See also chapter 20, Parasites.)*

Dr. Jennifer Brett, a naturopathic physician from Stratford, Connecticut, says only 60 percent of people with symptoms of urinary tract infections (UTI) have true infections; the other 40 percent have inflammations. Three types of infections and inflammations that Dr. Brett commonly sees are true urinary tract infections, urinary tract inflammations, and interstitial cystitis, a more distressing form of inflammation that can last for months or even years.

Causes

The cause of urinary tract inflammations is unknown, but some doctors believe it may be due to viruses, food allergies, candida in the colon, hormonal changes, new sexual partners, or vigorous sexual activity. Similarly, some believe that interstitial cystitis may be from candida or allergic reactions to foods and additives. "These irritants inflame the pelvis and bladder, and the body responds by increasing blood flow to the area," Dr. Brett explains. "Pelvic congestion causes further irritation and pressure on the bladder. Again, the body responds by sending more blood. This becomes a vicious cycle."

HIGH-RISK GROUPS. David Kauffman, M.D., a specialist in women's urological problems at St. Luke's Roosevelt Hospital in New York City, says that there are basically four types of women at high risk: "The most common patients are young, sexually active females. Another large group at risk are postmenopausal women. In fact, 8 to 10 percent of all women over 60 will get a bladder infection at some point. We also see a lot of patients who are hospitalized. The risk of bladder infection increases about 5 percent per day for every day that a catheter is in place. For this reason, medical doctors try to get catheters out as quickly as possible. The last high-risk group are patients with neurological problems. An example would be multiple sclerosis, where patients do not completely empty their bladder.

"Many sexually active women get cystitis as a result of intercourse because the bacteria that normally live in the vaginal vault area get pushed up into the urethra. A woman's urethra is only about an inch and a half long, while in men it is much longer. In females, it doesn't take too much for bacteria to migrate from the outside of the urethra to the inside of the bladder. That's why we see so many more young women with bladder infections.

"It is very important for women to know that their partners are not giving them infections. The bacteria starts in their vaginal area and simply gets pushed into the bladder during intercourse."

HORMONAL IMBALANCE. "You might be asking yourself, why don't all sexually active women get bladder infections? There are many reasons for this. One of the more interesting ones has to do with the woman's hormonal environment. We know that there are estrogen and progesterone receptors on the lining cells of the urethra. In some women bacteria sticks to these receptors due to hormone levels. Imagine bacteria as little organisms with Velcro hooks. Picture the lining cells of the urethra with the opposite kind of hooks. Bacteria just hooks on to the Velcro on the receptor sites. In most women, the urinary stream washes away most bacteria. But in these women, the hormonal environment will not allow for it to be expelled that easily. These are the women we see in our office with recurrent bladder infections."

Dr. Kauffman adds that postmenopausal women tend to get urinary tract infections for this reason as well. Their low estrogen levels cause their urethral linings to be "stickier" for bacteria. "One way to treat that is simply to administer low-dosage estrogen cream into the vaginal vault, about once a week," he advises. "Many women are on estrogen pills, but that does not have the same protective influence on the urinary tract as does estrogen cream."

WEAKENED IMMUNITY. Linda Wharton, a naturopathic physician and acupuncturist from New Zealand and author of *Natural Woman Health: A Guide to Healthy Living for Women of All Ages,* says recurrent bladder infections reflect a state of lowered immunity and weakened vitality: "Remember that cystitis is an infection, and as in the case with all infections, individuals with lowered nutritional status, poor cellular health, and lowered immunity are much more susceptible to its threat. Women don't always develop acute cystitis each time a stray bacteria finds its way into the bladder. As is often the case with many other genitourinary infections, it is common to play host to these potentially problem-causing bacteria for weeks or months or even a lifetime without them actually resulting in acute symptoms. It is only when the health of the whole body is reduced that an explosion of this bacterial population takes place. This may occur, for example, when a woman goes through a period of great stress, such as a divorce or the death of a loved one."

STRUCTURAL PROBLEMS. Wharton adds that other causes of cystitis are often overlooked: "Pelvic floor muscles can weaken as a result of pregnancy and childbirth. When these muscles are weakened, the bladder may prolapse and bulge forward into the wall of the vagina. If the back part of the bladder droops below the neck of the bladder, it becomes virtually impossible to empty the bladder properly. This leaves an almost permanent reservoir of urine in the bladder. In time, the stagnant urine becomes a haven for bacteria to multiply, should they be present." Wharton further states that a prolapsed transverse colon, brought on by childbirth, age, abdominal fat, poor posture, and spinal problems, can result in bladder compression. In time this can cause the transverse colon, which lies across the abdomen, to sag, compressing the organs beneath it, including the bladder. Blood flow is impeded, and the oxygen-starved bladder becomes ripe for infection. She adds, "This same downgrading of tissue health can occur as a direct result of a chronic back problem. All the pelvic organs receive nervous impulses from the spine, and a chronic lower back problem can interfere with these nervous impulses from the spinal cord." Wharton advises women with these concerns to see an osteopath or chiropractor.

CONSTIPATION. "Waste materials are excreted from our bodies through several different channels. The bowels excrete in the form of feces; the lungs gets rid of toxins in the form of carbon dioxide; the skin eliminates toxins as perspiration; and the kidney and bladder pass toxins out in the form of urine. If any one of these waste disposal systems is functioning inadequately, it places an excessive load on the others. If you only manage a half-hearted bowel movement every two or three days, you are placing undue stress on your kidneys and bladder, as accumulated toxins are passed out this way instead. In a sense, then, there is actually a direct link between chronic constipation and repeated urinary tract infections."

Symptoms

Typical symptoms of urinary tract infections and inflammations are frequent urination, a sensation that the bladder is never quite empty, and a burning sensation upon urination. Often women get up at night to urinate. There may be cramps, and the urine may be dark and foul-smelling. In severe cases, there may be blood in the urine as well.

Clinical Experience

DIAGNOSIS
A diagnosis of cystitis is usually made by collecting a midstream urine sample, and testing for the presence of bacteria. If the problem stems from an inflammation, no pathogenic bacteria will be found in the urine. Further, a vaginal culture will not reveal vaginal secretions.

CONVENTIONAL TREATMENTS
The usual treatment for cystitis is a course of antibiotics, and standard therapy for chronic cystitis generally consists of repeated rounds of the same therapy.

In the long term, this practice may actually exacerbate the condition rather than cure it. It is well known that broad-spectrum antibiotics are indiscriminate killers that destroy colonies of friendly gut bacteria along with problem-causing organisms. Once the delicate gastrointestinal microflora is upset, less desirable strains of bacteria proliferate, virtually unchecked. This includes *E. coli*, the prime cause of cystitis, and candida overgrowth, a suspected cause of inflammations.

Dr. Kauffman says that antibiotics should be a last-ditch effort, used only when various holistic protocols fail to achieve results. Even then, mild medicines should be used: "What of women who do all the right things, and still come back with bladder infections? In these cases, we need to turn to more traditional medical approaches. The gold standard for treating patients who do everything right and still get infections is a very gentle, bacteriostatic antibiotic. A bacteriostatic antibiotic does not kill the bacteria, but limits bacterial growth. It is gentler on the system, and generally does not cause yeast infections or GI disturbances. I am not big on taking antibiotics, but this is a better alternative than constant infections."

Dr. Brett reports that radical therapies are sometimes used for persistent cases: "Treatments I have read about in recent medical journals include surgery to cut nerves to reduce irritation to the bladder, hormonal therapy, and even antidepressive medications to help women sleep better, even though this doesn't get at the root cause of the problem."

NATUROPATHIC TREATMENTS

Most cystitis sufferers do well with these naturopathic therapies:

WATER. It is important to drink plenty of pure water, about one 8-ounce glass each hour. "If you are in agony and you don't know what to do, start drinking water, and don't stop," advises Dr. Wharton. "Stay away from tea, coffee, soft drinks, and alcohol, but drink plenty of water."

UNSWEETENED CRANBERRY JUICE OR CRANBERRY CAPSULES. Cranberries change the pH of the urine, making it more acidic and less hospitable to bacteria. It also contains powerful antibacterial substances. In fact, studies reveal that as little as 15 ounces of cranberry juice cause an 80 percent inhibition of bacterial growth. Bacteria loses its ability to cling to the bladder wall, and must exit the system along with urine. Other research indicates that cranberry juice combined with vitamin C acidifies the urine further. The effect is therefore much greater when both are taken together.

OTHER DRINKS. Other drinks useful for temporarily acidifying the urine include lemon juice and water, buttermilk, or simply mixing two teaspoons of apple cider vinegar into a glass of water. Drink any of these substances three or four times a day.

ACIDIC DIET. During an acute attack of cystitis, the diet can be temporarily changed to further acidify the urine. Dr. Wharton warns that this is recommended only for short periods of time, during an acute infection: "Eat plenty of acidic foods, such as grains, nuts, seeds, fish, dairy products, meat and bread, and cut back on fruit and vegetables."

VITAMINS

VITAMIN C. An ascorbic acid form of vitamin C acidifies the urine, and should be taken to bowel tolerance with cystitis or any infection. Bowel tolerance is where the stool becomes quite loose, almost to the point of diarrhea. Any time the body is fighting an infection, it tolerates large amounts of C, sometimes as much as 10,000 to 15,000 mg orally each day (and even more intravenously). Ascorbic acid should be taken every two to three hours since it is water-soluble, which means that it is rapidly excreted from the body.

Dr. Wharton says that ascorbic acid fights infections in several ways: "Vitamin C concentrates in very high levels in the urine and exerts a direct bactericidal effect. It also supports systemic immune system function by helping to activate neutrophils, the white blood cells most involved in the front line defense against infection. It also works to stimulate the production of lymphocytes, which are important for coordinating immune function at the cellular level."

VITAMIN A. In addition to vitamin C, think about vitamin A. An easy way of supplementing with this vitamin is to use halibut or cod liver oil capsules, up to 25,000 IU a day, during acute phases of infection. Vitamin A helps protect the mucous membrane lining of the bladder and urethra from irritation during infection. It also improves antibody response and white blood cell function. Just a word of warning here: if you are pregnant, do not supplement with these high doses of vitamin A, as it has been associated with birth defects. Beta carotene, with which the body can make vitamin A as it is needed, is a safer alternative.

ZINC. This nutrient is essential for increasing white blood activity in response to infection. When cystitis is acute, approximately 50 mg elemental zinc is needed daily.

BOTANICALS
The classes of herbs used to treat cystitis include antiseptic herbs, demulcents, and diuretics. Antiseptic herbs for bladder infections include uva-ursi, buchu, goldenseal, juniper berries, and garlic. "Think garlic whenever you have any type of infection, including cystitis," says Dr. Wharton. Demulcents soothe inflamed mucous membranes inside the bladder and urethra, and include marsh mallow root, juniper berry, and corn silk. Diuretic herbs stimulate the production and excretion of urine, which helps to wash out bacteria. Common diuretics are parsley and goldenrod.

Dr. Wharton recommends these old naturopathic herbal remedies for treating burning urine: "Mix together equal parts of fennel, burdock, and slippery elm. Steep a teaspoon of this mixture in a cup of boiled water for about 20 minutes. Have one cup before each meal, and one before bed."

She also recommends flaxseed tea or a combination of uva-ursi and buchu: "For either tea, use one teaspoon of the dried herb(s) to a cup of boiling water. Again, let it steep for 15 to 20 minutes. Then drink one cup, three or four times a day. The results more than compensate for the awful taste."

Dr. Joseph Pizzorno adds this bit of advice: "After sexual intercourse, women should wipe the opening to the urethra with a dilute solution of Betadine or a strong solution of goldenseal tea to wash away any bacteria that may have been forced up into the urethra."

HYDROTHERAPY. This is another traditional naturopathic method for helping people overcome the discomforts of cystitis. Sitz baths or hot compresses stimulate blood circulation and remove toxins from the pelvic area. Dr. Wharton explains how this is done: "You can use a hot compress by dipping a small hand towel into a basin of water, as hot as you can possibly tolerate it. Ring out the water and quickly apply the cloth to the area just above the pubic bone. As the cloth cools, repeat the process. In total, apply the compress eight or nine times. Repeat this process two to three times throughout the day. It actually feels wonderful and gives quite a bit of local relief to the symptoms.

"Alternatively, you can try making a sitz bath. Fill a small tub with water, once again, as hot as you can bear it. Add six drops of bergamot oil, and sit in the bath so that water actually covers your pelvis and lower abdomen. Stay there for around half an hour. As the water cools, keep replenishing with fresh, hot water to keep the water up to a hot, even temperature. Just a word of warning: If you have a problem with a weak heart or high blood pressure, hot sitz baths aren't really for you. You are better off just using a local compress."

ACUPUNCTURE. Dr. Wharton reports impressive results in the treatment of chronic cystitis with acupuncture, when it is accompanied by lifestyle and dietary changes: "Usually an acute attack of cystitis responds to two to four acupuncture sessions, spaced two or three days apart. Chronic cystitis sufferers often benefit from an extended course of acupuncture treatment to prevent the reoccurrence of their problem."

AROMATHERAPY. Essential oils can enhance any treatment program, according to aromatherapist Ann Berwick. To help clear up a urinary tract infection, eighteen to twenty drops of juniper and cedarwood can be added to one ounce of lotion and massaged into the lower abdomen. Also, six to eight drops of juniper, bergamot, or sandlewood can be added to a sitz bath or full bath.

For urinary inflammation not caused by bacteria, Dr. Brett suggests the following:

DIET. Avoidance of foods that encourage candida growth, such as wheat, simple sugars, white flour, pastries, candies, alcohol, aged cheeses, vinegar, and even fruit. Avoid known food allergens. It is a good idea to get a test to determine if there are any other foods in the diet that are acting as irritants.

WATER. Again, one 8-ounce glass of water every hour is needed. It is also a good idea to drink a glass of water and to urinate immediately after sexual intercourse. This tends to reduce bladder irritation that sexual intercourse may cause.

CLOTHING. Avoid tight-fitting pants, nylon underwear, and pantyhose. They encourage candida growth in the vaginal tract, which irritates the bladder and urethra.

VITAMINS. 2,000–6,000 mg buffered vitamin C, 100–200 mg vitamin B6, 4–6 capsules evening primrose oil.

HERBS. Herbs that soothe the bladder include althea or marsh mallow, corn silk, slippery elm, and goldenrod.

HOMEOPATHY. The remedy cantharis is often effective in reducing bladder and urethra irritations.

When the diagnosis is interstitial cystitis, Dr. Brett says, "the basic way to treat this condition is to remove congestion from the pelvis." These are the therapies she suggests:

TESTS. To remove the source of irritation, it is a good idea to be tested for food allergies to see if a food is causing an antibody-antigen reaction and irritating the bladder. It is also important to test for candida in the colon because candida can cause irritations and antibody reactions that irritate the bladder. Next, check to see that the hormones are in balance. If they are not, they can be treated with vitamin B6, evening primrose oil, and herbs.

AEROBIC EXERCISE. Doing aerobic exercise every day helps to remove blood congestion from the pelvis. This means walking, jogging, swimming, bicycling, anything that moves the blood.

INVERSION EXERCISE. Specific exercises to remove the blood involve turning upside down. In yoga, this is accomplished with the headstand or shoulderstand. It can also be achieved by raising the legs up and bicycling. But if there is a back or neck problem, a simple solution is the slant board. This can be made simply by taking an old door or a couple of one-by-four boards. One end can be placed on the couch, and the other end on the floor. Once it is stable, the person lies upside down, that is, with the head near the floor and the feet near the couch. The blood is automatically pulled out of the pelvis by gravity, and moved into the chest and head. Remaining too long can cause dizziness; five or ten minutes works for most people.

HERBS. The soothing herbs previously mentioned are useful here as well: marsh mallow, corn silk, slippery elm, and goldenrod.

DIET. A low-acid diet decreases irritations. High-acid foods to omit are red meat, dairy, shellfish, and citrus fruits. The diet should include whole grains, beans and vegetables. Essential fatty acids, such as those found in flaxseed oil, evening primrose oil, and fish oils, can help reduce inflammation. In interstitial cystitis, they are key for reversing the cycle of irritation and blood congestion.

"If you follow these basic points," says Dr. Brett, "within three to four weeks, you are likely to notice that your ability to sleep through the night is improved, and that your cramping and pain during the day is significantly lessened."

PREVENTION. Long-term preventive changes obviously make a lot more sense than simply dealing with each acute infection as it arises. Here are some simple personal hygiene measures to reduce the likelihood of reinfection:

After a bowel movement, wipe from front to back, away from the vagina.

Encourage your partner to wash thoroughly before any sexual contact.

Avoid the transfer of bacteria from the anus to the vagina during lovemaking.

During a period, change pads and tampons frequently.

Do not wear tight-fitting jeans or nylon pantyhose or pants. Cotton pants and stockings with garters allow more air flow and ventilation.

Make a habit of drinking lots of water. Aim for seven to eight glasses each day. This keeps the urine dilute so that bacterial proliferation is less likely. It also prompts frequent urination, which washes out problematic bacteria. Reduce intake of coffee and tea.

Make a habit of emptying your bladder frequently. Research shows that women who ignore their urge to urinate for long periods of time are much more likely to develop cystitis. The motto here is when you need to go, go right away. Urinate after sexual intercourse. This will help to wash out any of the bacteria that may have been pushed up into the urethra.

Try not to urinate before sex so that more bacteria is pushed out after sex. A glass of water right before intercourse will further increase the volume of liquid in the bladder for the washout of bacteria later on.

If infections are an ongoing problem, try this. Take a detachable shower and direct a stream of water into the vaginal area before sex. This will dilute the bacteria and decrease their numbers so that less bacteria gets pushed up into the bladder during intercourse.

Avoid chemical irritation to the urethra by staying away from perfumed or colored personal hygiene products. Diaphragms and birth control pills, as a means of contraception, often promote urinary tract infections and should not be used by women who tend to get the condition. Condoms or a properly fitted cervical cap are better.

See a registered osteopath or chiropractor if you think you may have a spinal problem that can be contributing to your recurring cystitis.

"Remember that your bladder health reflects your overall health," says Dr. Wharton, "so take a good look at your lifestyle. Ask yourself, "Do I eat a nutritious, balanced diet? Do I get enough relaxation and sleep? Am I under stress?" Maybe you drink too much coffee or alcohol or smoke or use recreational drugs. If your lifestyle is unhealthy, your body will be too."

ORIENTAL PERSPECTIVE

Dr. Brett explains that traditional Chinese medicine views cystitis as the end result of an accumulation of damp and heat in the bladder: "Often there is a weak flow of *chi* (energy) in the kidney and the spleen meridians. Weakness of spleen energy leads to the formation of damp in the body, which, in turn causes a stagnation of energy. As in nature, whenever anything builds up, there is friction. A stagnation of *chi* eventually leads to the development of heat, what we in the West interpret as cystitis.

"Spleen *chi* is easily injured through dietary indiscretion. Overeating can damage the spleen *chi*, as well as drinking with meals, or an overconsumption of damp-forming foods, such as dairy products, chilled foods or drinks, and raw fruits and vegetables. Greasy foods, such as take-out foods, also damage spleen *chi*.

"What you do with your mind actually affects spleen energy as well. An overuse of the mind, particularly through chronic anxiety and worry, or through many years of overstudying, also tends to deplete spleen energy.

"When the cooling yin energy of the kidneys is weakened, cystitis becomes much more likely as well. Kidney yin is consumed with age, but it can also prematurely diminish through lifestyle. The long-term overwork, stress, and exhaustion that form a part of many American lives these days, along with an overconsumption of alcohol and too much sex, all deplete the vital kidney energy." Acupuncture, combined with lifestyle changes, can help to balance energy and eliminate cystitis.

Herbal Pharmacy

Plants containing phytochemicals with antibacterial properties, in order of potency:

> *Coptis chinensis* (Chinese goldthread)
> *Coptis* sp. (generic goldthread)
> *Mangifera indica* (mango)
> *Coptis japonica* (huang lia)
> *Hydrastis canadensis* (goldenseal)
> *Hamamelis virginiana* (witch hazel)
> *Phyllanthus emblica* (emblic)
> *Punica granatum* (pomegranate)
> *Quercus infectoria* (aleppo oak)
> *Berberis vulgaris* (barberry)
> *Phellodendron amurense* (huang po)

Argemone mexicana (prickly poppy)
Fragaria sp. (strawberry)
Rheum rhaponticum (rhubarb)
Glycine max (soybean)

Hot News

An important factor in the development of urinary tract infections, studies indicate, is the overuse of antibiotics. Natural preventatives include cranberry juice, lactobacilli, progesterone extracted from the wild yam, buchu leaf, the plant marsh mallow, cornstalk, and uva-ursi. A technique useful in reducing infection recurrence is hydration monitoring with a hand-held probe.

FROM THE MEDICAL LITERATURE ON URINARY TRACT INFECTIONS

NUTRITION/DIET

Drinking 4 to 6 ounces of cranberry juice almost daily for 7 weeks was shown to prevent urinary tract infections in 19 of 28 nursing home patients. Researchers suggest that cranberry juice is preventive, rather than curative, of urinary tract infections.

L. Gibson et al., "Effectiveness of Cranberry Juice in Preventing Urinary Tract Infections in Long-Term Care Facility Patients," *Journal of Naturopathic Medicine* 2, no. 1 (1991): 45–47.

A placebo-controlled study led researchers to conclude that cranberry juice may be effective in the treatment of urinary tract infections.

J. Avorn et al., "Reduction of Bacteriuria and Pyuria after Ingestion of Cranberry Juice," *JAMA* 271, no. 10 (March 9, 1994): 751–54.

A study found that 73 percent of subjects suffering from urinary tract infections who consumed 16 ounces of cranberry juice per day experience relief. The recurrence rate was 61 percent when the treatment was withdrawn.

P. N. Prodromos et al., "Cranberry Juice in the Treatment of Urinary Tract Infections," *Southwest Med.* 47 (1968): 17.

A study of seven juices—cranberry, blueberry, grapefruit, guava, mango, orange, and pineapple—found that only two—cranberry and blueberry—are helpful as treatments for bladder infection.

Ofek et al., "Anti-escherichia Adhesin Activity of Cranberry and Blueberry Juices," *New England Journal of Medicine* 324 (1991).

Five female subjects were treated twice a week with intravaginal and perineal implantation of *Lactobacillus casei* GR-1 and experienced relief from recurrent urinary tract infections. The treatment resulted in infection-free periods ranging from 4 weeks to 6 months, and all of the patients preferred it to antibiotics.

A. W. Bruce and G. Reid, "Intravaginal Instillation of Lactobacilli for Prevention of Recurrent Urinary Tract Infections," *Canadian Journal of Microbiology* 34, no. 3 (March 1988): 339–43.

Studies support the use of lactobacillus an effective means of treating and preventing urinary tract infections and cystitis.

G. Reid et al., "Is There a Role for Lactobacilli in Prevention of Urogenital and Intestinal Infections?" *Clinical Microbiology Review* 3, no. 4 (October 1990): 335–44.

HERBS/PLANT EXTRACTS

Progesterone extracted from the wild yam has been used in a number of conditions common to women, including urinary tract infections.

N. Barnard, "Natural Progesterone: Is Estrogen the Wrong Hormone?" *Good Medicine* (Spring 1994): 11–13.

A known urinary antiseptic, buchu leaf, is used to treat inflammation and infection and has been used in patients suffering from cystitis and urinary tract infections. Other herbs used to heal the urinary tract have been marsh mallow, cornstalk, and uva-ursi.

D. Mowrey, *The Scientific Validation of Herbal Medicine* (New Canaan, Conn.: Keats Publishing, 1986): 273.

TRADITIONAL CHINESE MEDICINE

Female urinary tract infection patients given *yishenkang* granules experienced enhanced immune function, with a cure rate reaching over 68 percent.

J. S. Sun, [Prevention and Treatment of Recurrent Urinary Tract Infection with a *Yishenkang* Granule], *Chung Hsi I Chieh Ho Tsa Chih* 9, no. 8 (August 1989): 452, 469–71.

HYDRATION MONITORING

A study of premenopausal women who had had at least two urinary tract infections in the previous 6 months found that the use of simple hydration monitoring with a hand-held probe led to a reduction in infection recurrence.

S. D. Eckford et al., "Hydration Monitoring in the Prevention of Recurrent Idiopathic Urinary Tract Infections in Pre-Menopausal Women," *British Journal of Urology* 76, no. 1 (July 1995): 90–93.

ANTIBIOTICS

The overuse of antibiotics should be considered one important factor involved in the development of urinary tract infections. Amoxicillin was found to reduce the normal periurethral anaerobic flora, and promoted colonization of gram-negative enterobacteria.

K. J. Lidefelt et al., "Changes in Periurethral Microflora After Antimicrobial Drugs," *Archives of Disease in Children* 66 (1991): 683–85.

INTERSTITIAL CYSTITIS

The medical profession has failed to reach agreement on what interstitial cystitis actually is, as well as on what causes it and how best to treat it. One study found that IC causes such misery that it makes sufferers contemplate suicide four times more often than the general population does. Thirty percent of those with the condition can't work full time. Stress levels or dietary changes have been seen to trigger symptoms, and some people have benefited from transcutaneous electrical nerve stimulation.

E. Zamula, "Interstitial Cystitis: Progress Against Disabling Bladder Condition," *FDA Consumer* 29, no. 9 (November 1995): 28.

While men do suffer from interstitial cystitis, it is 50 times more common in women. Adherence to a low-acid diet has been found to be an effective means of managing the condition in some patients; this involves the elimination of spicy foods, coffee, tomatoes, citrus fruit, tea, alcohol, and chocolate. Acupuncture and biofeedback have also shown some promise. Researchers have suggested such potential causes of the condition as allergic reactions, hormone disturbances, autoimmune disease, abnormalities of the spine, and scarring from hysterectomy or endometriosis.

R. Hughes, "Two Types of Misery," *Harvard Health Letter* 20, no. 3 (January 1995): 3.

A review article argues that silk may be a cause of interstitial cystitis, due to its allergenic properties.

D.H. Hollander, "Interstitial Cystitis and Silk Allergy," *Medical Hypotheses* 43 (1994): 155–56.

An article recommends the following supplements for incorporation into the interstitial cystitis treatment protocol: vitamins C, D, B12, and B6, as well as bioflavonoids, zinc, vitamin K, calcium, magnesium, quercetin, EFA's Calc Sulph and Kali Sulph cell salts, *Zea mays* (sweet corn), cranberry, and *kava kava*. Diathermy, sitz baths, and Kegel exercises may also help.

T. Hudson, "Interstitial Cystitis," *Townsend Letter for Doctors and Patients* (December 1995): 128–29.

27. VAGINAL YEAST SYNDROME (CANDIDIASIS)

Dr. William Crook, author of *The Yeast Connection and Women,* says that yeast overgrowth is the result of antibiotics, and that women are especially susceptible: "The yeast we're talking about normally live in the body of every man, woman, and child. It's called *Candida albicans.* When you are healthy, there are no problems, but when you take a lot of antibiotic drugs you begin to get complications. Antibiotics knock out the normal, friendly bacteria while they are fighting off enemies. As a result the yeast overgrows, and a woman may get a vaginal yeast infection, a child may develop thrush or diaper rash, and a man or woman may get bloating, constipation, and digestive symptoms.

"But that's not the major problem. This yeast puts out toxins that weaken the immune system. It so disturbs the interior membrane of the intestinal tract that you absorb food allergens that would normally be excreted. People truly become sick all over."

Causes

"There are several reasons why a woman is more susceptible to yeast infections than a man," says Dr. Crook. "Since her genitalia is internal, yeast is able to grow on the warm anterior membranes of the body. The little tube going from the urinary bladder to the outside is only a fraction of an inch in a woman, whereas in a man it is many inches long. This allows the bacteria to get up into the woman's bladder much more easily. Women have fifty times more urinary tract infections than men, and they are given antibiotic drugs as treatment. Birth control pills further promote yeast growth. So does pregnancy. And teenage girls with a few pimples on their face are much more likely to run to the dermatologist and get tetracycline, an antibiotic that makes yeast grow."

Nutritionist Gracia Perlstein adds these causes to the list: "Some women are susceptible at the end of each month's menstrual flow. Low estrogen levels present at menopause, and also pregnancy, where the rate of infection can be as high as 20 percent toward the end. Also women who have diabetes have an increased risk.

"Stress is another factor. Many people have two or three jobs. They are running around, eating on the run, not really paying attention to their diet. When people do that, they tend also to overdo sweets and processed foods that weaken the immunity and set up a perfect environment for the candida overgrowth."

Complementary physician Dr. Robert Sorge says candida is the result of drug pollution. In addition to antibiotic overuse mentioned earlier, he adds the following: "The most likely candidate for candida overgrowth is a person who has been on steroids, hormone medication, cortisone, the entire gamut of prescriptions and over-the-counter drugs, especially ulcer medications like Tagamet and Zantac, and oral contraceptives. As far as I'm concerned, the sugar and junk food diet that most people have is also a drug."

Symptoms

Classical symptoms of a yeast infection are itching, redness, irritation, and a cottage-cheese-like curdly white discharge. Symptoms are not always obvious, but a gynecologist can often confirm whether or not a yeast infection exists by looking at a smear under the microscope or creating a culture to see if yeast colonies form.

Clearing up immediate symptoms is relatively simple. Many over-the-counter preparations, including homeopathic remedies, exist for that purpose. The trick, according to Dr. Marjorie Ordene, a holistic gynecologist from Brooklyn, New York, is to treat the overall yeast syndrome, not just the local infection. "Often the vaginal itching will be the impetus for the person to come to the doctor, but it is not the only problem they have. Unless the whole person is treated, the yeast is bound to recur." Dr. Ordene breaks down symptoms of a yeast syndrome into five categories:

General symptoms: low energy and fatigue, brain fog, depression, headaches, muscle and joint paints, memory loss, extreme sensitivity to chemicals, recurrent urinary infections, light-headedness.

Digestive symptoms: gas, bloating, intermittent constipation and diarrhea, indigestion, intestinal cramps.

Respiratory symptoms: chronic post nasal drip, frequent coughs, sore throats, colds, asthma, allergies.

Skin problems: eczema, itching, rashes, fungal infections.

Hormonal problems: menstrual irregularities, menstrual cramps, pre-menstrual syndrome, mood swings, problems with the endocrine glands, hypothyroidism, hypoglycemia or diabetes.

Clinical Experience

TESTING. Since the intestines serve as a reservoir for much of the yeast, a stool study may reveal an overgrowth. Excess yeast here indicates that yeast is present in other parts of the body, including the vagina, and causing recurrent yeast infections.

A simple skin test may reveal a yeast allergy as well. Red or itchy skin indicates a problem. Often the results are seen quickly, within ten to fifteen minutes, although sometimes there is a delayed reaction or none at all.

These tests are not always reliable, according to Dr. Crook: "Although we physicians generally like to have a test that can say you do or do not have a particular condition, such as a chest x-ray to see whether your heart is enlarged, there is not presently a single, simple laboratory test that can say whether you do or do not have a yeast-related problem. If a woman has a vaginal infection, a lab study of the secretion may help identify the yeast. Sometimes a culture may. But they are not 100 percent accurate. They may not be more than 50 percent accurate. There are studies done on stools because yeast grows there, but those are not reliable either. The best we can do is to suspect it, and then to note the response of a person to a sugar-free special diet, and oral anti-yeast medication, both prescription and non-prescription."

YEAST-FREE DIET. A yeast-free diet is both diagnostic and therapeutic. If a woman feels better when following the diet, this indicates a yeast sensitivity. The diet should be observed for several weeks at a minimum, and may be followed indefinitely. Some people feel much better and choose to eat this way permanently. Foods can be added back gradually, however, to see their effect. If symptoms recur, the reintroduced food should be avoided.

The yeast-free diet attacks on two fronts:

Avoid sweets. The relationship between sugar and yeast was seen in a study performed at St. Jude Hospital in Memphis, Tennessee, where mice who were fed sugar had 200 times greater yeast concentration than mice who were not. Yeast feeds on sugar, causing many symptoms, especially digestive problems such as gas and bloating. Avoiding sugar entails more than just not adding granulated sugar to cereal or tea; it means checking labels and staying away from corn syrup, maltose, artificial sweeteners, fructose, corn starch, sodas, and lactose, a milk sugar found in dairy products.

Avoid foods containing yeasts and molds. These include baked foods such as breads, muffins, cakes, cookies, and other refined carbohydrates, commercial fruit juices, tomato sauce (unless homemade with fresh tomatoes), foods containing vinegar, pickled foods, smoked foods, alcohol, fermented foods, smoked meats, dried fruits, mushrooms (except for shiitake), pistachio nuts, and peanuts. Leftovers may be moldy as well.

What you can eat are healthful foods that do not contain yeasts and molds. Included are whole grains, such as brown rice, millet, amaranth, quinoa, and barley, as well as fresh vegetables. Lots of steamed green vegetables are particularly beneficial because they are abundant in purifying chlorophyl. Also allowed are sea vegetables, whole wheat matzo, sourdough rye bread, popcorn, tortillas, tofu, miso, plain yogurt, lean meats, fresh fish, organically fed, free-range poultry and eggs from free-range chickens. Organic extra virgin olive oil, when used sparingly, can inhibit yeast overgrowth, according to recent studies. Raw garlic or lightly cooked garlic helps get rid of candida in the intestines.

SUPPLEMENTS. Sometimes diet alone is not enough. After all, yeast has been in the body for years. These supplements provide additional needed help:

Flora. The flora found in lactobacillus acidophilus and bifida bacteria can be taken in powder form or as sugar-free yogurt. The effectiveness of flora was noted in a New York Medical School study of women with recurrent vaginal yeast infections. Those eating sugar-free yogurt had fewer infections than those who did not. Flora repopulate the intestinal tract with good bacteria, which in turn crowd out the yeast. The effects of flora are temporary, so the powder or yogurt should be consumed on a daily basis.

Antifungal, antiyeast agents. Over-the-counter preparations, such as citrus seed extract, kyolic garlic, caprylic acid, pau d'arco, and berberine, may be helpful. Sometimes prescription agents such as nystatin are needed. These remedies get rid of excess yeast only. Since they are not absorbed into the blood, they are safe to take, even during pregnancy and while nursing.

Homeopathic candida. Helps desensitize the body to yeast.

Garlic suppositories. Simple insertion of a clove of garlic into the vagina has a powerful healing effect. *The New Our Bodies, Ourselves* suggests that the clove should be peeled but not nicked, and then wrapped in gauze before inserting.

A strong body is better able to rebalance its health. In addition to supplements that target yeast infections specifically, these nutrients provide overall nutritional support:

Multivitamin/mineral supplement. Formulas containing zinc, magnesium, yeast-free vitamins, trace minerals, and essential fatty acids boost immune function and help prevent recurrent yeast infections.

Chlorophyl cleanses the intestines and purifies the blood.

Essential fatty acids. 3,000 mg of evening primrose, borage, or black currant seed oil daily in three divided doses, or one tablespoon of organic flaxseed oil. (Never cook flaxseed oil, and keep refrigerated.)

Vitamin C. 3,000–5,000 mg daily in three divided doses helps fight infections.

B complex. 50–100 mg with each meal combats stress.

HERBS. The following Oriental and Western formulas can help alleviate yeast problems:

Oriental formulas:

Digestive Harmony and Herbastatin. Digestive Harmony is a combination of bitter herbs that work together to cleanse the digestive tract and other internal organs of yeast infections. Herbastatin gets rid of yeast caused by phlegm. These products can be ordered from Health Concerns in Oakland, California (1-800-233-9355).

Yudaiwan. This Chinese remedy helps to eliminate creamy discharges.

Ku shen. Used as a wash to clean the vagina.

Western herbs:

Garlic. Excellent for fighting infections. Can be eaten raw, lightly cooked, or taken in capsule form. Odorless brands are sold in health food stores.

Black walnut tincture. Thirty drops three times daily, added to water before meals.

Pau d'arco has wonderful immune-enhancing and antifungal properties. As a tea, three to four cups can be taken daily.

Summa. This is another good herbal tea for helping the immune system.

Also helpful are goldenseal, bearberry, Oregon grape, German chamomile, aloe vera, rosemary, ginger, alfalfa, red clover, and fennel.

COLON THERAPY. "My battle with candida lasted a long time," says colon therapist Tovah Finman-Nahman. "I tried everything, including a strict diet, antifungals, and vitamin C drips. But I never got it under control until I started doing colonics. Then I saw quick results. The gas and the bloating went away, and my chronic fatigue amazingly disappeared. I have seen similar results with a lot of people who come to see me. I can't stress how good colonics are."

What makes colon therapy such an effective treatment? First, it creates a clean internal environment. "We want a good environment so that flora can grow and flourish. That is paramount when we have candida overgrowth," says Finman-Nahman. Second, colonics calm an irritated colon: "Herbs can be added to the water, such as pau d'arco, which has antifungal properties. Yellow dock can also be added to soothe any inflammation. Fennel can be used to dissipate gas and eliminate the bloating that a lot of people with candida tend to get. Aloe vera gel is absolutely wonderful. It is very soothing to an inflamed colon. And of course, it can be taken orally in the form of aloe vera juice.

"In conjunction with colonics, psyllium can be taken orally. This moisturizes impacted fecal material in the congested colon, which further aids cleaning.

"People ask, 'How many colonics should I get?' That depends on the individual. The more the merrier. For a healthy person I recommend at least ten in a series, and then a maintenance program. Sometimes, it can take as long as six months to get candida under control because it is a very hearty bacteria. When yeast is at the point of being candidiasis, it can grow through the colon walls and run rampant. The more we cleanse, the better our chance of getting it under control and regaining health."

AROMATHERAPY. Tea tree oil is scientifically shown to be anti-fungal, anti-yeast, and anti-viral. One tablespoon of the oil added to a pint of water, and used in a douche, helps to eliminate yeast infections. This can be followed with the placement of acidophilus tablets or capsules into the vagina to reestablish proper vaginal bacteria.

LIFESTYLE FACTORS. Perlstein notes these important habits for minimizing the incidence of vaginal infections:

Wear underpants with a cotton crotch so that air can circulate. Avoid pantyhose or any tight-fitting clothing for the same reason.

Develop good toilet habits of always wiping from front to back. This keeps anal bacteria from entering the vagina. Avoid feminine hygiene sprays and powders, which can cause irritation. Douching is not necessary; a healthy vagina is naturally clean.

Keep stress under control. Take a few deep breaths. Go for a brisk walk in the open air. Do something to alleviate the stress that builds up.

HOMEOPATHY. Since homeopathy treatments are chosen according to symptoms, deciding on a remedy depends on the quality of the discharge and the sensations, according to Dr. Ken Korins. Here he offers some of the major remedies for vaginal yeast infections:

Pulsatilla. This remedy is often indicated in vaginitis. The woman has a thick, yellowish-to-green discharge. Sometimes the consistency is milky or creamy. Mentally, she is often moody, gentle, and weepy, and craves sympathy.

Silica. The main symptom is an itching of the vulva and vagina. It is sensitive to touch. The discharge tends to be thin, and sometimes curdly.

Kreosotum. The person has violent symptoms. Discharges are excoriating, burning is profuse, and there is a foul odor, as well as violent itching and a burning and swelling of the labia. Discharge tends to be yellow and may actually be a watery, bloody type of consistency.

Hephera sulph. Symptoms are similar to silica, but more chronic. There is itching of the vagina, particularly after sexual intercourse, and it often has an odor similar to that of old cheese. Both hephera sulph and silica can be used to treat sores or cysts, particularly Bartholin cysts.

Kali bichromium. Here discharges tend to be thick, green, and sometimes jelly-like.

Alumina. Discharge is thick and transparent.

Nitric acid. Helps when there are sores or ulcers on the vaginal mucosa. The sensation tends to be a sharp, sticking pain. Discharges are brown. Often, there is a stain on underwear that leaves a yellow perimeter.

Mercurius. The discharges are excoriating but greenish and bloody. There is a sensation of rawness.

Medorrhinum. Discharge is thick and acrid, with a sensation way up in the uterus.

Herbal Pharmacy

Plants containing phytochemicals with antibacterial/antifungal activity, in order of potency:

Coptis chinensis (Chinese goldthread)
Coptis sp. (generic goldthread)
Mangifera indica (mango)
Coptis japonica (huang lia)
Hydrastis canadensis (goldenseal)
Hamamelis virginiana (witch hazel)
Phyllanthus emblica (emblic)
Punica granatum (pomegranate)
Quercus infectoria (aleppo oak)
Berberis vulgaris (barberry)
Phellodendron amurense (huang po)
Argemone mexicana (prickly poppy)
Fragaria sp. (strawberry)
Rheum rhaponticum (rhubarb)
Glycine max (soybean)

Hot News

Vaginal candidiasis is associated with a mild zinc deficiency, with low vaginal cell concentrations of beta carotene, and with iron deficiency, according to recent research; these studies suggest that supplementation of zinc, beta carotene, and iron may help combat candida. Another significant relationship is between *Candida albicans* and baker's yeast; a study recommends eliminating yeast foods from the diet of candidiasis patients. On the other hand, yogurt containing *lactobacillus acidophilus* is helpful in the diet, as are evening primrose oil, fish oil, and linseed oil, which contain essential fatty acids that appear to have antifungal actions, grapefruit seed extract, water extracts of the herb *Cassia alata,* and kyolic garlic extract.

Natural substances that can be used as external treatments for candida, according to studies, are honey, used in an undiluted and unprocessed form as a dressing, boric acid suppositories, lactate-gel, an acid cream, and a solution of tea tree oil used as a douche.

FROM THE MEDICAL LITERATURE ON VAGINAL YEAST SYNDROME

NUTRITION AND DIET

A study suggests that mild zinc deficiency is associated with recurrent vaginal candidiasis, and may play a role in women's susceptibility to candidiasis.

J. Edman et al., "Zinc Status in Women with Recurrent Vulvovaginal Candidiasis," *American Journal of Obstet Gynecol* 155, no. 5 (November 1986): 1082–85.

Vaginal cell concentrations of beta carotene are significantly reduced in women with vaginal candidiasis, a study found. Reduced beta carotene may affect the local immune response, resulting in altered vaginal flora and the subsequent development of vaginal candidiasis. If this hypothesis proves correct, then increased intake of carrots, green leafy vegetables, and other beta carotene-rich foods might help to prevent vaginal candidiasis.

M. S. Mikhail et al., "Decreased Beta-Carotene Levels in Exfoliated Vaginal Epithelial Cells in Women with Vaginal Candidiasis," *American Journal of Reproductive Immunology* 32 (1994): 221–25.

A study showed a significant relationship between *Candida albicans* and baker's yeast in humans; the author recommends eliminating yeast foods from the diet of candidiasis patients for at least 3 to 4 months, with reintroduction of those foods done gradually and carefully monitored.

B. B. Jorgensen, "Baker's Yeast Allergy in Candidiasis Patients," *Journal of the Advancement of Medicine* 7, no. 1 (Spring 1994): 43–49.

In a study of 92 women with chronic fungal vaginal infection, boric acid suppositories achieved a 98 percent cure rate.

R. Jovanovic et al., "Antifungal Agents Versus Boric Acid for Treating Chronic Mycotic Vulvovaginitis," *Journal of Reproductive Medicine* 36 (1991): 593–97.

Honey, in an undiluted and unprocessed form, inhibits the growth of the fungi *Aspergillus fumigatus, Pencisillium citrium, Trichophyton rubrum, Trichophyton tonsurans,* and *Candida albicans.*

S. E. E. Efem et al., "Honey Dressing Effective Treatment for Wound Infections/The Antimicrobial Spectrum of Honey and its Clinical Significance," *Infection* 20 (1992): 227–29.

Researchers found a threefold decrease in candida infections when patients consumed yogurt containing *lactobacillus acidophilus* for a period of 6 months. The authors conclude that daily ingestion of 8 ounces of yogurt containing lactobacillus decreases both candida colonization and infection.

Eileen Hilton et al., "Ingestion of Yogurt Containing *Lactobacillus Acidophilus* as Prophylaxis for Candidal Vaginitis," *Annals of Internal Medicine* 116, no. 5 (March 1, 1992): 353–57.

Evening primrose oil, fish oil, and linseed oil are rich in linoleic, linolenic, and eicosapentaenoic acid, essential fatty acids that appear to have anti-bacterial, anti-fungal, and anti-viral actions.

U. N. Das, "Antibiotic-Like Action of Essential Fatty Acids," *Canadian Medical Association Journal* 132, no. 12 (1985): 1350.

Lactate-gel, an acid cream, used in the vagina daily for 7 days, proved in one study to be as effective as oral metronidazole as a treatment of bacterial vaginosis.

B. Andersch et al., "Treatment of Bacterial Vaginosis with an Acid Cream: A Comparison Between the Effect of Lactate-Gel and Metronidazole," *Gynecological Obstetric Investigations* 21, no. 1 (1986): 19–25.

C. albicans was isolated more often and in greater number from the saliva of malnourished patients with mouth lesions, who had anemia and a deficiency of iron. Therapy with oral ferrous sulfate was associated with a rapid clearing of the mouth lesions and a fall in salivary candida count.

J. Fletcher et al., "Mouth Lesions in Iron-Deficient Anemia: Relationship to *Candida Albicans*, Saliva and to Impairment of Lymphocyte Transformation," *Journal of Infectious Disease* 131 (1975): 44–50.

Several patients with chronic mucocutanous candidiasis associated with reduced cellular immunity and iron deficiency demonstrated rapid improvement in clinical manifestations following iron administration.

J. M. Higgs and R. S. Wells, "Mucocutaneous Candidiasis," *British Journal or Dermatology* 86, suppl. (1972): 88–102.

A commercial caprylic acid preparation has proven highly effective in eliminating candidiasis.

W. J. Crinnion, "Clinical Trial Results on Nessbry's Capricin," unpublished paper, September 10, 1985.

HERBS/PLANT EXTRACTS

The essential oil of the plant *Leonotis nepetaefolia* found to have antibacterial activity; it also was found to inhibit dermatophytic fungi and suppress other aerial fungi. Hence the oil may be quite useful in skin infections due to dermatophytes even with secondary bacterial infections.

R. H. Gopal et al., "Antimicrobial Activity of Essential Oil of *Leonotis Nepetaefolia*," *Ancient-Sci-Life* 14, no. 1–2 (July–October 1994): 68–70.

Berberine sulfate blocks the adherence of streptococci to host cells, making it an effective treatment for streptococci infections.

D. Sun et al,. "Berberine Sulfate Blocks Adherence of Streptococcus Pyogenes to Epithelial Cells, Fibronectin, and Hexadecane," *Antimicrobrial Agents in Chemotherapy* 32 (1988): 1370–74.

Berberine sulfate, an alkaloid extracted from an Indian medicinal herb, inhibits the growth of *Candida albicans*, as well as 10 other fungi.

V. M. Mahagan et al., "Antimyotic Activity of Berberine Sulphate: An Alkaloid from an Indian Medicinal Herb," *Sabouraudia* 20 (1982): 79–81.

Water extracts of *Cassia alata* (ringworm senna) showed strong antibacterial (against *E. coli*) and antifungal (against *C. albicans*) activities when evaluated relative to those of the standard antibacterial agent choloraphenicol and antifungal agent amphotericin B.

C. O. Crockett et al., "*Cassia Alata* and the Preclinical Search for Therapeutic Agents for the Treatment of Opportunistic Infections in AIDS Patients," *Cellular Molecular Biology* 38, no. 5 (1992): 505–11.

A study showed that bromelain appeared as effective as antibiotics in treating a variety of infectious processes, including pneumonia, skin, staph infections, kidney infections, and bronchitis, and that bromelain is particularly useful as a supplement to antibiotics.

R. A. Neubauer, " A Plant Protease for the Potentiation of and Possible Replacement of Antibiotics," *Experimental Med Surgery* 19 (1961): 143–60.

Echinacin greatly accentuates the efficacy of a topical antimycotic agent (econazol nitrate) in preventing recurrence of vaginal candidiasis. Standardized skin tests were used to show that echinacea's effects were due to boosting of cell-mediated immunity.

E. G. Coeugniet and R. Kuhnast, "Recurrent Candidiasis: Adjuvant Immunotherapy with Different Formulations or Echinacin," *Therapiewoche*, 36, 1986, p. 3352-3358.

Oral grapefruit seed extract has proven be effective against candida, *Geotricum* sp., and hemolytic coliforms.

G. Ionescu et al., "Oral Citrus Seed Extract in Atopic Eczema: In Vitro Studies on Intestinal Microflora," *Journal of Orthomolecular Medicine* 5 (1990): 155-157.

Tea tree oil possesses significant antiseptic properties and is regarded by many as the ideal skin disinfectant—active against a wide range of organisms, having good penetration, and nonirritating to the skin. Tea tree oil has been used in the following conditions: acne, aphthous stomatics (canker sores), athlete's foot, boils, burns, carbuncles, corns, emphysema, gingivitis, herpes, impetigo, infections of the nail bed, insect bites, lice, mouth ulcers, psoriasis, root canal treatment, ringworm, sinus infections, sore throat, skin and vaginal infections, tinea, thrush, and tonsilitis.

P. M. Altman, "Australian Tea Tree Oil," *Australian Journal of Pharmacy* 69 (1988): p. 276-278.

A 40 percent solution of tea tree oil emulsified with isopropyl alcohol and water was shown to be highly effective for the treatment of vaginal candidiasis as well as cervitis, chronic endovervicitis, and trichomonal vaginitis.

E. O. Pena, "Melaleuca Alternifolia Oil: Uses for Trichomonal Vaginitis and Other Vaginal Infections," *Obstet Gynecol* 19 (1962): 793–95.

A review article states that kyolic garlic extract enhances the elimination of *Candida albicans* in infected animals.

P. P. Tadi et al., "Anticandidal and Anticarcinogenic Potentials for Garlic," *International Clinical Nutrition Review* 10, no. 4 (October 1990): 423–29.

TRADITIONAL CHINESE MEDICINE

A study suggests that a combination of *Shouhu-san* and mequitazine is a useful treatment for recurrent vaginal candidiasis.

T. Chimura and T. Funayama, [Clinical Effect of Combined Use of *Shouhu-san* and Mequitazine in Recurrent Vaginal Candidiasis Received Protracted Antibiotic Therapy], *Japanese Journal of Antibiotics* 47, no. 5 (May 1994): 553–60.

HOMEOPATHY

Homeopathic remedies for vaginitis include pulsatilla (windflower), kreosotum (beechwood creosote), borax, hydrastis (goldenseal), sepia (cuttlefish), graphites (plumbago), and calcarea carbonica (carbonate of lime).

Frans Vermeulen, *Concordant Materia Medica* (Haarlem, The Netherlands: Merlijn Publishers, 1994).

28. VARICOSE VEINS

This common condition, which usually affects women's lower extremities, is the result of damaged valves in the veins. Normally, these tiny valves ensure that the blood will fully return to the heart. But when they become injured, some blood in the veins runs backwards, pools, and finally engorges the vessels. Valve damage may be congenital, or it may be the result of thrombophlebitis, pregnancy, or obesity. Varicose veins are large, contorted, unsightly, and sometimes even painful.

Clinical Experience

Standard procedures for treating varicose veins range from elevating the legs, wearing elastic stockings, and even surgery in more severe instances. With early intervention, the following natural remedies have a high rate of effectiveness:

NUTRIENTS AND HERBS

Certain foods and supplements may strengthen the integrity of the vein wall. These include dark-skinned fruits and berries, such as blueberries, cherries, and purple grapes. Vitamin C with bioflavonoids, especially quercetin or bilberry, improves elasticity, so that blood can return more effectively to the heart.

Astringent herbs, such as horse chestnut, witch hazel, gota kola, and butcher's broom are good to take, although the first two should not be used when pregnant or lactating. Naturopathic physicians often recommend 1,000 mg of butcher's broom, two to three times daily, for pregnant women in their third trimester, who are troubled by varicose veins as well as hemorrhoids.

Another factor to consider is dietary support for the liver. This is because a congested liver backs up venous circulation, and places additional pressure on the veins, which can then damage valves. Foods, such as beets and artichokes, and herbs, such as milk thistle and dandelion, can improve liver circulation. At the same time, it is important to refrain from substances known to cause liver damage, such as drugs, alcohol, and other harsh chemicals.

EXERCISE

Exercise is important for keeping weight optimal. This lessens stress to the body, which, in turn, decreases one's chance of damaging the valves in the veins. In addition, exercise improves overall circulation in the arteries and veins.

Of particular benefit are postures that take pressure off the legs, such as inverted postures in yoga or even just lying on a slant board with the legs elevated for a few minutes a day. *(See "Inversion Exercise" in Urinary Tract Infections.)* Medical magnets can be placed over the feet for added healing power. These exercises are particularly useful for people who work in occupations in which they are constantly on their feet.

Another form of exercise to consider is *qi gong*, which strengthens the vein's ability to pump blood back to the heart.

CHELATION THERAPY

Many people know that chelation therapy improves arterial integrity, but few realize that it can aid venous circulation as well, thereby helping varicose veins. Chelation therapy also helps to overcome liver congestion and thrombophlebitis, two conditions that put women at risk for varicose veins. *(See sections on chelation therapy in chapter 1, Aging, and chapter 12, Heart Disease.)*

Hot News

Researchers have found promise in a number of plant extracts for treating varicose veins: an extract from the plant *Centella asiatica,* which has a regulatory effect on connective tissue of the vascular wall; witch hazel; bilberry (*Vaccinium myrtillus*), which lessens swelling, numbness, and cramps in the legs; bromelain (from the stem of the pineapple plant); a component from the horse chestnut (used topically; horse chestnut is toxic used internally); the rhizome of butcher's broom (*Ruscus aculeatus*), an active ingredient of which, ruscogenins, produce anti-inflammatory and vasoconstrictor effects. Another promising substance is pycnogenol, effective in treating nightly leg cramps. Interestingly, one study has demonstrated that varicose veins show unusually strong response to placebo ointments. *(See below.)*

NUTRITION/DIET

Pycnogenol produced improvement in 93 percent of those treated for nightly leg cramps. Ninety milligrams daily produced clear improvement in 77 percent of those with varicose veins, a German study showed.

W. V. Bowles, "A New Super Antioxidant: Pycnogenol," *Total Health* 16, no. 2 (April 1994): 36–39.

The recommended diet for avoidance of varicose veins is high in fiber and low in fat and refined carbohydrates. Substances to be avoided include animal protein, refined foods, sugar, salt, fried food, junk food, alcohol, and cheese. Recommended supplements: DMG (gluconic), vitamin C plus bioflavonoids, brewer's yeast, lecithin, potassium, B complex (with extra B12 and B6), D, E, and zinc.

J. F. Balch and P. A. Balch, *Prescription for Nutritional Healing* (Garden City Park, New York, 1990): 307–8.

HERBS/PLANT EXTRACTS

A study assessing the use of *Centella asiatica* extract on patients with varicose veins confirmed the treatment's regulatory effect on connective tissue of the vascular wall.

M. R. Arpaia et al., "Effects of *Centella Asiatica* Extract on Mucopolysaccharide Metabolism in Subjects with Varicose Veins," *International Journal of Clinical Pharmacol. Research* 10, no. 4 (1990): 229–33.

Witch hazel leaf can help in treating hemorrhoids and varicose veins.

D. B. Mowrey, *The Scientific Validation of Herbal Medicine* (New Canaan, Conn.: Keats Publishing, 1986): 272.

Bilberry (*Vaccinium myrtillus*) is beneficial in the treatment of symptoms of varicose veins in the legs, i.e., swelling, numbness, and cramps.

R. McCaleb, "Bilberry for Circulatory Health," *Better Nutrition for Today's Living* 55, no. 6 (June 1993): 54–57.

The effectiveness of bilberry extract in prevention of platelet aggregation and reduction of tension of blood vessel walls is proven in ex vivo and animal studies. The extract contains flavonoids called anthocyanosides that are potent antioxidants, improving microcirculation and protecting blood vessels.

M. R. Werbach and M. T. Murray, *Botanical Influences on Illness* (Tarzana, Calif.: Third Line Press, 1994).

Bromelain (from the stem of the pineapple plant) has fibrinolytic activity, and is useful in the treatment of thrombophlebitis, deep vein thrombosis, and varicose veins. In a study, bromelain lowered the number of hematomas in varicose vein patients. Sixty-five out of 90 of those treated for 2 weeks had no hematomas, versus 32 out of 90 untreated patients.

Werbach and Murray, *Botanical Influences on Illness*.

Horse chestnut (*Aesculus hippocastanum*) is used to treat varicose veins and hemorrhoids; the active component is escrin, which can be used orally (some say) or topically. A study of 22 patients with chronic venous insufficiency showed that after 3 hours of treatment with horse chestnut seed extract (50 mg escin), treated subjects showed a decrease of 22 percent in capillary filtration coefficient (there was an increase in the placebo group).

Werbach and Murray, *Botanical Influences on Illness*.

Horse chestnut should be considered toxic, and is not recommended for internal use. Components of horse chestnut may help those with chronic venous insufficiency by reducing edema and improving venous compliance.

Lawrence Review of Natural Products (February 1995): 1–2.

Procyanidolic oligomers, or PCOs (complexes of flavonoids) stabilize collagen, including collagen structures supporting arteries, capillaries, and veins. PCOs also increase intracellular levels of vitamin C and scavenge oxidants and free radicals. They may be useful in the treatment of varicose veins.

Werbach and Murray, *Botanical Influences on Illness*.

The rhizome of butcher's broom (*Ruscus aculeatus*) has been used to treat venous disorders, including hemorrhoids and varicose veins. Its active ingredients, ruscogenins, produce anti-inflammatory and vaso-constrictor effects. Standardized ruscus extract has been used together with trimethyl hesperidine chalcone and ascorbic acid in studies on patients that demonstrated its effectiveness for venous insufficiency.

Werbach and Murray, *Botanical Influences on Illness*.

Padma 28 is a Tibetan formula containing 28 herbs; a study of 36 patients indicates its effectiveness in reducing intermittent claudication. Other research shows that treatment with Padma 28 increases the distance that patients can walk pain-free.

Werbach and Murray, *Botanical Influences on Illness*.

Herbs recommended to minimize varicose veins include buckthorn bark, collinsonia root, red grapevine leaves, stone root, and uva-ursi.

Balch and Balch, *Prescription for Natural Healing*.

PLACEBO EFFECT

A placebo ointment applied daily for 24 days produced a reduction in night cramps (by 66 percent), leg heaviness (by 69 percent), tiredness from standing (by 62 percent), and itching (by 45 percent). Conclusion: Varicose vein symptoms show a strong response to placebo ointments.

E. Ernst et al., "The Powerful Placebo," *Lancet* 337 (March 9, 1991): 611.

contributors

ACUPUNCTURE

DR. PAT GORMAN
5 East 17th Street
New York, NY 10003
(212) 620-0506

Dr. Gorman, a licensed acupuncturist, has been in practice for many years and writes and lectures on acupuncture, Chinese philosophy, and *tai chi*. She is on the
faculties of the Traditional Acupuncture Institute in Mary-
land and the Worsley Institute of Classical Acupuncture
in Florida. Her private practice specializes in Five Element diagnosis.

PHYLLIS BLOOM
150 Fifth Avenue
New York, NY 10011
(212) 675-1164

Dr. Bloom has studied acupuncture and traditional Chinese medicine in China and the United States, and has a
background in massage and social work. The focus of her
practice is acupuncture, massage, and healing arts by
women for anyone.

GINA MICHAELS
Mille Fleurs Day Spa
130 Franklin Street
New York, NY 10013
(212) 966-3656

Ms. Michaels, director of the Mille Fleurs Day Spa in Soho,
New York City, has been practicing as a licensed acupuncturist for twelve years and as a massage therapist for twenty
years. Mille Fleurs offers treatments including herbal body
wraps, facials, and body work.

ABIGAIL RIST-PODRECCA, R.N., O.M.D.
Herbs and Acupuncture Center
431 5th Avenue, 4th floor
New York, NY 10016
(212) 679-1554

Abigail Rist-Podrecca is a licensed acupuncturist and
holds a Chinese Medical Doctorate in Women's Health. She
has practiced preventive medicine for fifteen years using
traditional Chinese medicine, acupuncture, and herbal
therapy.

AROMATHERAPY

SHARON OLSON, PH.D.
20-61 32nd Street
Astoria, NY 11105
(718) 726-3817
(718) 545-1408 (fax)

Dr. Olson is a professor in the psychology department of
Montclair State University, and a certified psychologist in
New York State. Her clinical practice includes aromatherapy and Bach Flower Remedies. She is also a certified hypnotherapist and a certified Reiki practitioner.

AYURVEDA

NANCY LONSDORF, M.D.
Maharishi Ayurveda Center
4910 Massachusetts Avenue, Suite 315
Washington, DC 20016
(202) 244-2700
(800) THE-VEDA (general information)

Dr. Lonsdorf, author of *A Woman's Best Medicine*, received
her M.D. from Johns Hopkins University and completed postgraduate studies in psychiatry at Stanford. Trained in Maharishi Ayurveda in India and the United States, she has been
director of the Maharishi Ayurveda Center in Washington,
DC for nine years.

BIRTH CONTROL

REBECCA CHALKER, M.A.
c/o WomanCap
25 Fifth Avenue, Suite 1A
New York, NY 10003
(212) 529-8489

Rebecca Chalker is a women's health activist and director of WomanCap, New York's leading cervival cap provider. She is the author of several acclaimed books on subjects of importance to women. They include *A Woman's Book of Choices* (with Carol Downer), *Overcoming Bladder Disorders* (with Kristine Whitmore, M.D.), and *The Complete Cervical Cap Guide*.

BARBARA SEAMAN
110 West End Avenue, #5D
New York, NY 10023
(212) 580-1838

Well-known columnist and author, Barbara Seaman's works include the now-classic trilogy *The Doctors' Case Against the Pill, Free, Female and Women*, and *The Crisis in Sex Hormones*. She is a cofounder of the National Woman's Health Network and a trustee of the National Council on Women's Health.

CHIROPRACTIC

DR. DEBORAH KLEINMAN
33 Sandy Hollow Road
Port Washington, NY 11050
(516) 883-4252

Dr. Deborah Kleinman is a chiropractor and also does cranial-sacral work on Long Island.

DR. MITCH PROFFMAN
The Healing Center
175 West 72nd Street
New York, NY 10023
(212) 501-7110, and
144-02 69th Avenue
Flushing, NY 11367
(718) 268-9080

Dr. Proffman, a graduate of New York Chiropractic College, has done advanced studies in nutrition, stress management, and exercise physiology and practices in Queens and Manhattan. He is a vegetarian and runs marathons.

STEFANIE ODINOV PUKIT, D.C., C.C.H.
(*See* Homeopathy)

DR. RICHARD STATLER
577 W. Jericho Turnpike
Huntington, NY 11743
(516) 424-BACK

Dr. Statler, a certified chiropractic sports practitioner, an emergency medical technician, and a certified personal fitness trainer, has ten years of chiropractic experience. He teaches postgraduate sports programs, served on the Chiropractic Advisory Committee for the 1996 Atlanta Paralymbic Games, and consults with various teams and other groups.

DR. MARY E. OLSEN
42 High Street
Huntington, NY 11743
(516) 427-3724

In practice for seven years as a chiropractor in Huntington, New York, Dr. Olsen specializes in diversified adjustments, craniosacral therapy, and applied kinesiology. She lectures on natural approaches to menopause and other health issues.

COLON THERAPY

ANITA LOTSON
The Healing Center
175 West 72nd Street
New York, NY 10023
(212)496-6529

Ms. Lotson is a certified colonic therapist at The Healing Center in New York City, where reflexology and massage are used in conjunction with colonic treatments.

TOVAH FINMAN-NAHMAN
Lifeline Hygienics
150 Theodore Fremd, Suite B15
Rye, NY 10580
(914) 921-5433

Ms. Finman-Nahman is a colonic therapist and director of Lifeline Hygienics in Rye, New York, using colonic irrigation and nutritional counseling.

COMPLEMENTARY MEDICINE

DAHLIA ABRAHAM, N.D.
252 W. 79th Street
New York, NY 10024
(212) 799-7378

Dr. Abraham is a naturopath in practice in New York City. She focuses on prevention and providing individualized nutritional programs and conducting health seminars.

DR. RICHARD ASH
800A 5th Avenue
New York, NY 10021
(800) 628-3009

As director of the Fifth Avenue Medical Clinic in New York City, Dr. Ash's practice of environment medicine incorporates a variety of nutritional therapies and cutting-edge techniques, including reconstructive therapy.

ROBERT C. ATKINS, M.D.
152 E. 55th Street
New York, NY 10022
(212) 758-2110

Dr. Atkins graduated from Cornell University Medical College and has hospital affiliations with both Columbia and Rochester Universities. He is the founder and executive medical director of the Atkins Centers for Complementary Medicine, established in 1970, and president of the Foundation for the Advancement of Innovative Medicine. Among his many best-selling books is the classic *Dr. Atkins' Diet Revolution*. He specializes in treating a wide variety of disorders, including asthma, cancer, chronic fatigue, hypoglycemia and immune system disorders.

DR. ERIC BRAVERMAN
PATH Medical
212 Commons Way, Building 2
Princeton, NJ 08540
(609) 921-1842
(800) 224-7105

Dr. Braverman is the founder and director of Princeton Associates for Total Health, a clinical practice devoted to mind and body wellness. He conducts research on diagnosing and treating brain illness, epilepsy, head trauma, substance abuse, reversing heart disease, preventing stroke, and general medical wellness and prevention of aging. PATH Medical produces a 500-page Wellness Manual that describes everything they do in both conventional and nontraditional medicine, as well as a 20-minute video describing the center's activities.

DR. CHRISTOPHER CALAPAI
18 E. 53rd Street, 3rd floor
New York, NY 10022
(212) 838-9100
1900 Hempstead Turnpike
East Meadow, NY 11554
(516) 794-0404

An osteopathic physician, Dr. Calapai is board-certified in family practice. He specializes in a variety of treatment modalities, including intravenous vitamin therapy, chelation, and reconstructive nerve therapy.

DR. PAUL CUTLER
652 Elmwood Avenue
Niagara Falls, NY 14301
(716) 284-5140

Dr. Cutler specializes in heart patients and chelation and practices in Niagara Falls, New York, and St. Catherine's, Ontario. He has been a fellow on the American Board of Chelation since 1993.

DR. MARTIN DAYTON
18600 Collins
N. Miami Beach, FL 33160
(305) 931-8484
(305) 936-1849 (fax)

Board certified in chelation therapy and in family medicine, Dr. Dayton is an internationally known lecturer on chelation therapy and teacher of family medicine for physicians, medical students, and the public. He maintains a private practice as a licensed osteopathic physician and surgeon in southeast Florida.

DR. MARTIN FELDMAN
132 East 76th Street
New York, NY 10021
(212) 744-4413

For twenty years Dr. Feldman was assistant professor of neurology at Mount Sinai Medical School. For the past fifteen years he has been a licensed complementary, nutritional M.D. His practice employs a variety of nutritional therapies to treat such conditions as allergies, digestive problems, and hormonal imbalances.

DR. HERBERT GOLDFARB
29 The Crescent
Montclair, NJ 07042
(201) 744-7470

Dr. Goldfarb is the author of *The No Hysterectomy Option* and *Overcoming Infertility*. He attended medical school at New York University School of Medicine, where he is now an assistant clinical professor.

WILLIAM J. GOLDWAG, M.D.
7499 Cerritos Avenue
Stanton, CA 90680
(714) 827-5180

Dr. Goldwag is the medical director of the Center for Preventive/Holistic Medicine located in Southern California, and is on the board of directors of the American Holistic Medical Association. He has been one of the pioneers in the use of chelation therapy and other nutritional and complementary medical therapies for the treatment of chronic health disorders.

DR. BRUCE HEDENDAL
301 Crawford Boulevard, Suite 206
Boca Raton, FL 33432
(407) 391-4600
(800) 726-8404 (to order *For Women Only* series on tape and other material)

Dr. Hedendal holds a Ph.D. in nutrition and has practiced holistic chiropractic for twenty years. He directs the Hedendal Chiropractic and Nutrition Center, specializing in chiropractic, acupuncture, clinical nutrition, detoxification, craniopathy, and biofeedback. An expert on herbs and homeopathy, Dr. Hedendal is internationally recognized as a health researcher, author, and clinician.

DR. MICHAEL JANSON
Center for Preventive Medicine
275 Millway
P.O. Box 732
Barnstable, MA 02630
(508) 362-4343

Dr. Janson, the author of *The Vitamin Revolution in Health Care*—a practical guide detailing the most recent developments in medical approaches to health care and preventive medicine—has been in practice for twenty years, using nutrition and dietary supplements with his patients.

DR. DAVID KAUFMAN
425 West 59th Street, Suite 3A
New York, NY 10019
(212)523-7754

Dr. Kaufman has been in practice for over seven years. His focus is on infertility, sexual dysfunction, and urinary problems.

DR. STEVEN RACHLIN
1510 Old Northern Boulevard
Roslyn, NY 11576
(516) 625-6884

Dr. Rachlin received his medical degree from the University of Bologna in Italy and did his internship and residency in internal medicine. He has been practicing complementary medicine since 1981.

DR. MICHAEL SCHACHTER
2 Executive Boulevard, Suite 202
Suffern, NY 10901
(914) 368-4700

Dr. Schachter, coauthor of *Food, Mind, and Mood* and author of *A Natural Way to a Healthy Prostate*, has been using alternative cancer therapies for most of that time. His practice in Suffern, New York employs physicians and health care practitioners who serve patients with a variety of medical and emotional problems.

DR. STEVEN SILVERMAN
8 Haven Avenue
Port Washington, NY 11050
(516) 944-9633

Dr. Silverman graduated from the New York Chiropractic College in 1980, and taught anatomy and holistic health at New Rochelle College. He is now in private practice in Port Washington and Hauppauge, New York.

DR. CHARLES SIMONE
123 Franklin Corner Road, Suite 108
Lawrenceville, NJ 08648
(609) 896-2646

Dr. Simone is a medical oncologist and tumor immunologist practicing in Lawrenceville, New Jersey.

DR. ROBERT H. SORGE
208 3rd Avenue
Asbury Park, NJ 07712
(908) 775-7575

Dr. Sorge, a graduate of the United States School of Naturopathy and Applied Sciences and the Anglo American Institute of Drugless Therapy, has been in private practice since 1964. He is director of Abunda Life Holistic Clinic and editor of *Abunda Life Times*.

DR. DAVID STEENBLOCK
Health Restoration Center
26381 Crown Valley Parkway, Suite 130
Mission Viejo, CA 92691
(714) 367-8870

Dr. Steenblock is director of the Health Restoration Center in Mission Viejo, California, the first comprehensive stroke and brain injury center to use hyperbaric oxygen as a method of treatment.

DR. ELIZABETH VLIET
P.O. Box 64507
Tucson, AZ 85728
(520) 797-9131
(800) 509-1688

Dr. Vliet is the founder and medical director of the Women's Center for Health Enhancement and Renewal at All Saints Hospital, Fort Worth, Texas, and at an evaluation-retreat center in Tucson, Arizona. She is currently on the faculty of the Department of Family Medicine at the University of Arizona College of Medicine and the University of North Texas Health Science Center.

DR. PAVEL YUTSIS
1309 W. 7th Street
Brooklyn, NY 11204
(718) 259-2122
(212) 399-0222

Dr. Yutsis is director of the Department of Allergy and Environmental Medicine at the Atkins Center for Complementary Medicine in New York City and medical director of the Advanced Preventative Medical Group. His expertise includes clinical ecology, nutritional therapy, and chelation therapy.

DETOXIFICATION THERAPIES

SUSAN LOMBARDI
We Care Health Center
18000 Long Canyon Road
Desert Hot Springs, CA 92241
(800) 888-2523

Founder and president of the We Care Health Center in Palm Springs, California, Susan Lombardi is a yoga instructor, massage therapist, colon therapist, and lymphologist. She is the author of *Ten Easy Steps for Complete Wellness* and the producer of *Three Minute Vegetarian Cooking*.

ENVIRONMENTAL ILLNESS

HEATHER MILLAR, B.S.N., R.N.
1515 W. 2nd Avenue, #543
Vancouver, BC
Canada V6J 5C5
(604) 733-6530

Ms. Millar, along with Myrna Millar, B.Ed., M.B.A., is coauthor of *The Toxic Labyrinth*, the story of a family's successful battle against environmental illness, as well as *Overcoming Environmental Illness*.

GYNECOLOGY/FEMALE RECONSTRUCTIVE SURGERY

VICKI HUFNAGEL, M.D.
Center for Female Reconstructive Surgery
Herbody Clinics
433 S. Beverly Drive
Beverly Hills, CA 90212
(310) 553-5821
(310) 553-7525 (fax)
New York Office
(212) 639-9868
WWW.//HerBody.com

Dr. Hufnagel's sensational bestseller *No More Hysterectomies* has radically changed traditional perceptions about the role and function of the female reproductive system. In an ongoing effort to educate, inform, and empower women about their health care rights and surgical options, Dr. Hufnagel has appeared on numerous television and radio programs, and has been featured in print media around the world. She received her education at the University of California at Berkeley, where she was a founding member of the Berkeley Women's Health Collective, founded the nation's first free clinic for women, and contributed to the first edition of *Our Bodies Ourselves*. Trained as an Ob-Gyn surgeon, Dr. Hufnagel is currently the medical director and founder of the Center for Female Reconstructive Surgery in Beverly Hills and New York.

DR. MARJORIE ORDENE
2515 Avenue M
Brooklyn, NY 11210
(718) 258-7882

Dr. Ordene, a holistic family physician, graduated from Cornell University Medical College, where she was trained in obstetrics, gynecology, and pediatrics. Her practice in Brooklyn, New York, specializes in nutrition, herbal medicine, and classic homeopathy.

HELLERWORK

SARAH SUATONI
The White Street Center for Movement and Bodywork
43 White Street
New York, NY 10013
(212) 966-9005
(212) 219-3053 (fax)

A certified Hellerwork practitioner, Ms. Suatoni works with Dr. David Kaufman at the Pelvic Floor Rehabilitation Laboratory at Saint Luke's Hospital, New York City. She is also cofounder and codirector of the White Street Center for Movement and Bodywork in New York.

HERBOLOGY

LETHA HADADY
Karma Unlimited Inc.
245 Eighth Avenue, Suite 364
New York, NY 10011

Ms. Hadady, an acupuncturist, herbalist, and author trained in New York and China, teaches classes in traditional Chinese herbology. Her latest book is *Asian Health Secrets: the Complete Guide to Asian Herbal Medicine*.

LIN SISTER
18A Elizabeth Street
New York, NY 10013
(212) 962-5417

Lin Sister is an herbal shop in Chinatown that is an excellent source for a variety of herbs, and also sells herbs by mail order.

HEALTH CONCERNS
8001 Capwell Drive
Oakland, CA 94621
(800) 233-9355

A mail-order source for herbs.

HOMEOPATHY

DR. JANE CICCHETTI
Five Element Center
115 Route 46W
Mountain Lake, NJ 07046
(201) 402-8510

Ms. Cicchetti, a registered member of the North American Society of Homeopaths and director of the Five Elements School of Classical Homeopathy, is the author of *Homeopathy for Injury* and *Trauma and the Five Elements Handbook* and creator of the Homeopathy Workshop audiocassette program.

DR. KEN KORINS
200 W. 57th Street, Suite 1205
New York, NY 10019
(212) 246-5122

Dr. Korins, a M.D. and homeopath, was trained in traditional medicine at Syracuse Medical School and has studied homeopathy for ten years. Having given up his allopathic practice in favor of alternative methods, he is now a doctor of traditional homeopathy at The Healing Center in New York City.

DR. GENNARO LOCURCIOAS
(212) 696-2680

Dr. Locurcioas is a medical doctor and a doctor of homeopathy. He is a member of the faculty at the Royal London Homeopathy Hospital, and also practices in Manhattan and New Jersey.

ERIKA PRICE, D.I. HOM., D.H.M.
130 W. 16th Street, Suite 66
New York, NY 10011
(212) 645-7544

Erika Price is a doctor of homeopathic medicine and practices classical homeopathy and holistic healing. She earned her doctorate of homeopathic medicine from the British Institute of Homeopathy and was awarded Fellow of the British Institute of Homeopathy.

STEPHANIE ODINOV PUKIT, D.C., C.C.H.
20 W. 20th Street, Suite 1002
New York, NY 10011
(212) 206-8100

Dr. Odinov Pukit, founder and director of the Soho Chiropractic Clinic, is certified by the National Council for Homeopathic Certification, and has practiced and taught homeopathy for seventeen years. Her chiropractic work includes Cranial SOT, Applied Kinesiology, Nutrition, and Body Integration ™; currently she also uses Network Spinal Analysis to allow patients to experience the true healing art of chiropractic. She has been a Buddhist practitioner since 1970 and is a senior meditation instructor and teacher.

IMMUNO-AUGMENTIVE THERAPY (IAT) FOR CANCER

DR. JOHN CLEMENT
P.O. Box 22579
Ft. Lauderdale, FL 33335
(809) 352-7455

Having studied with Dr. Lawrence Burton for many years, Dr. Clement now directs Dr. Burton's clinic in the Bahamas.

MAGNETIC HEALING

SUSAN BUCCI
86 Coppersmith Road
Levittown, NY 11756
(516) 731-4648
(800) 285-3430 (for catalogue)

As a holistic nurse, Ms. Bucci has used magnet therapy as part of her practice for four years. She also lectures and trains other professionals in magnet use.

MASSAGE THERAPY

SUSAN LACINA, R.N., M.S., N.P.
The Healing Center
175 West 72nd Street
New York, NY 10023
(212) 439-4781

Ms. Lacina, who has completed studies to be a nurse practitioner, has been a practicing registered nurse since 1982 and a massage therapist since 1986. Her specialties include Swedish, pregnancy, and sport massage, reflexology, and aromatherapy.

JAMES F. KRESSE
43 Sheep Lane
Levittown, NY 11756
(516) 731-1973

Schooled and certified in Austria at the Dr. Vodder Clinic, James Kresse is a licensed and registered massage therapist in New York State. He practices in Levittown, Long Island, specializing in the Dr. Vodder Method of manual lymph drainage; he is also an aromatherapist and a metaphysical practitioner.

MIDWIFERY

JEANETTE BREEN
Baldwin Midwifery Service
660 Merrick Road
Baldwin, NY 11510
(516) 223-1251

Ms. Breen is a nurse-midwife, specializing in home births, birth center births, and water births. She maintains a well woman's gynecological practice using herbs, homeopathy, and other natural remedies.

NATURAL HYGIENE

ANTHONY PENEPENT, M.D., M.P.H.
P.O. Box 220289
Great Neck, NY 11022
(212) 239-9582

Dr. Penepent was raised according to natural hygienic precepts. He practices nutritional medicine with homeopathy in Manhattan, Great Neck, and Huntington, New York.

NATUROPATHY

DR. JENNIFER BRETT
998 Nichols Avenue
Stratford, CT 06497
(203) 377-1525

Dr. Brett has been practicing homeopathy in Connecticut since 1988, emphasizing natural, preventive women's health care. She writes two newsletters, *Nutrition and Health* and *Naturopathic Center Newsletter*.

DR. LANCE MORRIS
1601 North Tucson Boulevard, Suite 37
Tucson, AZ 85716
(520) 322-8122

Dr. Morris, who received his naturopathic medical degree from Bastyr University in Seattle, Washington, is the cofounder of Solsstice Clinica. He uses nutrition, Oriental medicine and acupuncture, homeopathy, and alternative treatments, specializing in chronic and degenerative disease.

LINDA RECTOR-PAGE, N.D., PH.D.
167050 Via Esta
Sonora, CA 95370
(800) 736-6015

Dr. Rector-Page has been working in the fields of nutrition and herbal medicine, both professionally and as a personal lifestyle choice, since the early '70s. She is a certified Doctor of Naturopathy and a Ph.D., with extensive experience in formulating and testing herbal combinations. She is the author of several successful books, including *Healthy Healing*, *Cooking for Healthy Healing*, *How to be Your Own Herbal Pharmacist*, and *Party Lights*, as well as a Library Series of specialty booklets on nutritional healing. Dr. Rector-Page speaks nationwide regarding Lifestyle therapy on radio and TV talk shows and at conventions.

DR. JANE GUILTINAN
Natural Health Clinic
Bastyr University
Seattle, WA
(206) 632-0354

Dr. Guiltinan, chief medical officer at Bastyr University, Seattle, Washington, has been a naturopathic physician for ten years, specializing in women's health care and immune system disorders. She was named physician of the year by the American Association of Naturopathic Physicians.

DR. TORI HUDSON
2067 Northwest Lovejoy
Portland, OR 97209
(503) 222-2322

Dr. Hudson graduated from the National College of Naturopathic Medicine in 1984 and is currently a professor of gynecology and a supervising physician, maintains a private practice, and is a lecturer and author. She has consulted with the newly formed office of the Study of Alternative Medicine and served as advisor to the Department of Health and Human Services on health reform issues.

ROGER HIRSCH, O.M.D.
9730 Wilshire Boulevard, Suite 105
Beverly Hills, CA 90212
(800) 967-3898

Dr. Hirsch, who has twenty years' experience in acupuncture, is in private practice in California, where he has been an author and medical examiner. He has served as an adjunct faculty member of several colleges and is a member of the board of directors of the China Medical University.

DR. JOSEPH PIZZORNO
Bastyr University
14500 Juanita Drive N.E.
Bothell, WA 98011
(206) 823-1300

Cofounder and founding president of Bastyr University, Dr. Pizzorno has led Bastyr to become the first accredited, multidisciplinary university of natural medicine in the United States. Senior editor and coauthor of the internationally acclaimed *Textbook of Natural Medicine* and member of several editorial boards, he has helped define the standard of care for naturopathic medicine, documented the scientific validity of natural medicine, and pushed forward the frontiers of our understanding of healing. As lecturer, bestselling author of the *Encyclopedia of Natural Medicine*, researcher, and expert spokesman, he has introduced and taught credible natural medicine to medical and lay audiences throughout the United States and Europe.

NUTRITION

NINA ANDERSON
P.O. Box 36
E. Canaan, CT 06024
(860) 824-5301

Nina Anderson is an author and a nutritional researcher in Connecticut. She is researching the anti-aging effects of foods, enzymes, minerals, and the power of the mind. She is the coauthor with Howard Peiper of the book, *Over 50, Looking 30: The Secrets of Staying Young*.

GAR HILDEBRAND
(619) 759-2967

Gar Hildebrand is the author of "Five-year Survival Rates of Melanoma Patients Treated by Diet Therapy After the Manner of Gerson: A Retrospective Review." Currently he is president of the Gerson Research Organization in San Diego, California.

LINDA OJEDA, PH.D.
c/o Hunter House
P.O. Box 2914
Alameda, CA 94501
(800) 266-5592
(510) 865-5282

Dr. Ojeda has a doctorate in nutrition and began studying non-medical approaches to menopause more than ten years ago. A frequent media guest, she is a health consultant to business and a lecturer on fitness and nutrition.

RAY PEAT, PH.D.
P.O. Box 5764
Eugene, OR 97405
(541) 345-9855

Ray Peat has his Ph.D. in biology from the University of Oregon and wrote his dissertation on age and hormone-related oxidative changes. He has taught biochemistry, endocrinology, and nutrition at several colleges and universities. He has authored several books, including *Nutrition for Women*, *Progesterone in Orthomolecular Medicine*, *Generative Energy*, and *Mind and Tissue*.

ROSS PELTON, R.PH., PH.D.
P.O. Box 81365
San Diego, CA 92138-1365
(619) 275-2456

Dr. Pelton is a pharmacist, nutritionist, author, and health educator. He is the coauthor of *How To Prevent Breast Cancer*, and the author of *Alternatives is Cancer Therapy* and *Mind, Food, and Smart Pills*. Dr. Pelton graduated from the University of Wisconsin with a degree in Pharmacy and received his Ph.D. in Psychology and Holistic Health from the University of Humanistic Studies in San Diego, California.

GRACIA PERLSTEIN
20 Lower Devon Road
Belle Terre, NY 11777
(516) 331-9210
Wild By Nature
198 Route 25A
E. Setauket, NY 11833
(516) 246-5500

Ms. Perlstein, who maintains a private practice in Belle Terre, New York, has been involved in alternative health care for twenty-eight years and has worked as a nutritionist with holistically oriented M.D.s for twenty years. She is also part of the management/development team for Wild By Nature, a natural foods supermarket.

DOLORES PERRI, M.S., R.D., C.N.S.
The Healing Center
175 West 72nd Street
New York, NY 10023
(212) 787-2404

Dolores Perri, a nutritionist in private practice in New York, offers caring, individualized counseling to enhance wellness and heal conditions such as allergies, hormonal imbalance, cancer, and Alzheimer's disease. Her research is on the cutting edge of traditional and nontraditional therapies.

GARY S. ROSS, M.D.
500 Sutter Street, Suite 300
San Francisco, CA 94102
(415) 398-0555

Dr. Ross is a graduate of George Washington University School of Medicine. He has been practicing nutritional, preventive medicine for 20 years, specializing in the treatment of chronic fatigue syndrome and hormonal imbalance. He is the coauthor of the "Natural Treatment Series" audio tapes and is working on an upcoming anti-aging book.

PODIATRY

HOWARD ROBINS, D.P.M.
175 West 72nd Street
New York, NY 10023
(212) 721-9202
20 Park Place
Great Neck, NY 11021
(516) 482-1224

Dr. Robins is a podiatrist in practice in New York City. Once a foot surgeon, he has been active since 1979 as an outspoken advocate of holistic methods of foot care and the prevention of foot surgery.

PSYCHOLOGY

JANICE STEFANACCI, PSY.D.
Center for Wholistic Health, Education and Research
6801 Jericho Turnpike
Syosset, NY 11791
(516) 365-7924
5 Travers Street
Manhasset, NY 11030

Dr. Stefanacci, a clinical psychologist, is director of psychological services at the New Center for Wholistic Health, Education and Research in Syosset, New York. She is an author, columnist, and lecturer to lay and professional groups, with a private practice in Manhasset, New York.

ALEXANDER SCHAUSS, PH.D.
P.O. Box 1174
Tacoma, WA 98401
(206) 922-0448

Dr. Schauss, author of *Diet, Crime and Delinquency*, directs the Institute for Biosocial Research in Tacoma, Washington. As an eating disorders specialist, he emphasizes the connection between diet and behavior.

PSYCHONEUROIMMUNOLOGY

DR. CARL SIMONTON
Simonton Cancer Center
P.O. Box 890
Pacific Palisades, CA 90272
(310) 459-4994

Dr. Simonton, head of the Simonton Cancer Center, is a psychotherapist who has pioneered the use of guided imagery for people recovering from cancer.

READINGS

CARLA HARKNESS
(510) 526-8568

Ms. Harkness is the author of *The Fertility Book*.

SUSAN MOSS
4767 York Boulevard
Los Angeles, CA 90042
(213) 255-3382
(800) 231-1776 (to order book)

Susan Moss was a high-risk candidate for breast cancer, but decided against surgery when she found that she had a lump in her breast and a tumor in her uterus. Instead, she devised a health program covering every aspect of her life and was rid of the tumor and lump in two months. This experience inspired her to write *Keep Your Breasts: Preventing Breast Cancer the Natural Way*. Ms. Moss has a B.A. in art and psychology from the University of Nevada.

DR. RON SCOLASTICO
P.O. Box 6556
Woodland Hills, CA 91365
(800) 359-3771 (to order book)

Dr. Scolastico, an academic psychologist and spiritual counselor, has studied human consciousness for twenty-five years. He is the author of four books, including *Doorway to the Soul* and *Healing the Heart, Healing the Body*.

REFLEXOLOGY

GERRI BRILL
14 E. Broadway
Port Jefferson, NY 11777
(516) 474-3137

Ms. Brill has had twenty years' experience in hospital nursing. She has received certification in reflexology at New York University from Laura Norman and training in therapeutic touch with Doris Krieger, and has a private practice in Port Jefferson, New York.

LAURA NORMAN
Laura Norman and Associates
41 Park Avenue, Suite 8A
New York, NY 10016
(212) 532-4404

Laura Norman, a registered, certified reflexologist and New York State-licensed massage practitioner, has been in private practice for twenty-five years, and has established the Laura Norman Reflexology Training Center in New York City. She is currently revising her book, *Feet First: A Guide to Foot Reflexology*.

REIKI

NILSA VERGARA
76-09 34th Avenue
Jackson Heights, NY 11372
(718) 651-2260

Ms. Vergara, a traditional *reiki* master offering classes in first and second master levels of *reiki*, has been a psychotherapist for twenty years and is a Minister of Spiritual Healing. She uses these modalities to facilitate change and empower the individual.

YOGA

BONNIE MILLEN
P.O. Box 100
Huntington, NY 11743
(516) 271-5601

A registered physical therapy assistant, with a master's degree in dance education, Bonnie Millen specializes in movement analysis and injury prevention. She is a certified practitioner of the American Oriental Body Work Therapy Association, has designed corporate fitness programs, and teaches yoga and movement arts in New York City.

JOHN GOFMAN, M.D., PH.D.
P.O. Box 421993
San Francisco, CA 94142
(415) 664-1933

Dr. Gofman is a professor of molecular and cell biology at the University of California at Berkeley, and the author of the book, *Preventing Breast Cancer: The Story of a Major, Proven, Preventable Cause of this Disease*.

WILLIAM G. CROOK, M.D.
(901) 423-5400

Dr. Crook is a fellow of the American Academy of Pediatrics and the American College of Allergy and Immunology. He is also a member of the American Academy of Allergy and Immunology, Alpha Omega Alpha, and many other medical organizations. Dr. Crook is the author of eleven books, including *The Yeast Connection* and *The Women*.

index